Handbook of Pediatric Infectious Disease and Antimicrobial Therapy

Handbook of Pediatric Infectious Disease and Antimicrobial Therapy

STANFORD T. SHULMAN, M.D.
Head, Division of Infectious Diseases
Associate Dean for Academic Affairs and
Professor of Pediatrics
Northwestern University Medical School
The Children's Memorial Hospital
Chicago, Illinois

WILLIAM P. MacKENDRICK, M.D.
Clinical Instructor of Pediatrics
Northwestern University Medical School
Fellow, Division of Neonatology
The Children's Memorial Hospital
Chicago, Illinois

JULIE KIM STAMOS, M.D.
Clinical Instructor of Pediatrics
Northwestern University Medical School
Fellow, Division of Infectious Diseases
The Children's Memorial Hospital
Chicago, Illinois

Mosby
Year Book

St. Louis Baltimore Boston Chicago London Philadelphia Sydney Toronto

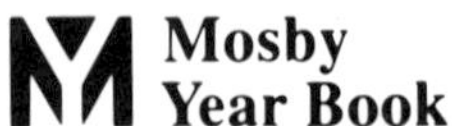

Dedicated to Publishing Excellence

Sponsoring Editor: Laurel Craven
Assistant Editor: Lauranne Billus
Assistant Managing Editor, Text and Reference: George Mary Gardner
Production Manager: Nancy C. Baker
Proofroom Manager: Barbara M. Kelly

Mosby, 11830 Westline Industrial Drive, St. Louis, MO 63416

1 2 3 4 5 6 7 8 9 0 CL/ML 97 96 95 94 93

Library of Congress Cataloging-in-Publication Data

Shulman, Stanford T.
Handbook of pediatric infectious disease and antimicrobial therapy
Stanford T. Shulman, William P. MacKendrick, Julie Kim Stamos.
p. cm.
Includes bibliographical references and index.
ISBN 0-8151-7805-0
1. Communicable diseases in children—Pathogenesis.
2. Communicable diseases in children—Treatment. 3. Infection in
children—Pathogenesis. 4. Infection in children—Treatment.
I. MacKendrick, William P. II. Stamos, Julie Kim. III. Title.
[DNLM: 1. Anti-Infective Agents—therapeutic use.
2. Communicable Diseases—drug therapy. 3. Communicable
Diseases—in infancy & childhood. WC 195 S562h]
RJ401.S58 1992 92-49179
618.92'9—dc20 CIP
DNLM/DLC
for Library of Congress

We dedicate this work to our wonderfully understanding spouses: Claire Shulman, Jim Stamos, and Anne Minciotti.

PREFACE

This handbook has been developed to serve as a practical resource for the physician actively involved with providing medical care to children. We have attempted to fill this volume with useful information and tables that will be of assistance to medical students and house officers who treat sick children, as well as practitioners who have completed their training but need a convenient quick reference for specific information.

Throughout this work we have tried to emphasize principles of pathogenesis of specific infections as well as therapeutic issues, and have focused to some degree on the interface between the infectious agent and the defenses of the host.

The field of infectious diseases is increasingly focused on the patient who is immunocompromised by a serious medical condition and/or by therapies that cause immune impairment as a side effect. Both the spectrum and the frequency of infections that occur with oncology, organ transplantation, HIV infection or immunosuppression continue to expand. In addition, with the increasing internationality and worldwide travel of our patient populations, tropical and "exotic" illnesses are encountered with surprising frequency. Thus we have provided much information about these infections and their therapy in this handbook. At the same time, we have addressed the diagnosis and treatment of more routine pediatric infections.

Recently the United Nations estimated that 250,000 children die each week, the vast majority as a result of infectious diseases. Most of these deaths are preventable. We hope that this handbook will assist those whose efforts are devoted to providing improved pediatric care throughout the world.

Stanford T. Shulman, M.D.
William P. MacKendrick, M.D.
Julie Kim Stamos, M.D.

CONTENTS

IMMUNIZATIONS 1

I. GOAL:

The goal of immunization is prevention of disease. The ultimate goal of immunization is eradication of disease, as exemplified by smallpox, the last case occurring in October 1977. Vaccines available in the United States are listed in Table 1–1.

II. ACTIVE IMMUNIZATION:

A. Definition:

1. Active immunization induces the recipient to respond immunologically (usually by antibody production) to a vaccine.
2. The vaccine may consist of either live (usually attenuated) or killed agents or components or products produced by an infective agent.
3. The vaccine does not result in immediate protection, but protection is usually of long duration.
4. Some vaccines induce protection for life; others must be readministered periodically. Some induce complete protection, whereas others induce only partial protection.

B. Vaccine constituents:

1. Immunizing antigen: e.g., pneumococcal polysaccharide, tetanus toxoid, or attenuated measles virus.
2. Adjuvant: A compound (frequently aluminum salt) used to increase antigenicity, especially for vaccines that incorporate inactivated microorganisms.
3. Suspending fluid: Sterile water or saline solution. However, this may also contain proteins derived from the medium in which the vaccine was produced (e.g., egg antigens).
4. Stabilizers: Low concentrations of chemicals (e.g., neomycin, mercurials) used to prevent bacterial growth or to stabilize the antigen.

TABLE 1–1.
Vaccines Available in the United States

Vaccine	Type	Age at Vaccination
Anthrax*	Cell-free protein antigen	>6 mo
Cholera*	Inactivated *Vibrio cholerae*	>6 mo
Diphtheria, tetanus, pertussis (DTP)	Toxoids and inactivated bacteria	2,4,6,15–18 mo; 4–6 yr; then DT q10yr
Diphtheria, tetanus, acellular pertussis (DTaP)	Toxoids and purified pertussis components	Use as doses 4 and 5 of DTP series
Hepatitis B	Purified hepatitis B surface antigen	Birth; 1, 6 mo
Hemophilus B (Hib)	Polysaccharide-protein conjugate	2,4,6,15 mo: HbOC; 2,4,12 mo: PRP-OMP
Influenza*	Inactivated virus	>6 mo
Measles, mumps, rubella	Live attenuated viruses	15 mo; repeat at 5 or 12 yr
Meningococcus*	Polysaccharide	>2 yr
Plague*	Inactivated bacteria	>6 mo
Pneumococcus*	Polysaccharide	>2 yr
Poliomyelitis		
Oral	Live attenuated virus (trivalent)	2,4,15–18 mo; 4–6 yr
Inactivated	Inactivated virus (trivalent)	2,4,15–18 mo; 4–6 yr, then q5yr
Rabies*	Inactivated virus	Any
Smallpox*	Live attenuated virus	>6 mo
Tuberculosis* (BCG)	Live attenuated organisms	Any
Tularemia*	Live attenuated bacteria	>6 yr
Typhoid*	Inactivated *Salmonella typhi*	>6 mo
Yellow fever*	Live attenuated virus	>9 mo

BCG = bacille Calmette-Guérin, HbOC = diphtheria CRM_{197} protein, PRP-OMP = meningococcal cell membrane protein.
*Use selectively.

C. Routine immunizations

1. DTP:
   a. Type: Diphtheria toxoid, tetanus toxoid, and inactivated whole *Bordetella pertussis* organism.
   b. Route: Intramuscular.

c. Schedule: 2, 4, 6, and 18 months; 4 to 6 years; then dT (full dose of tetanus toxoid with reduced dose of diphtheria toxoid) q10yr.
d. Adverse reactions (primarily due to pertussis component):
   1) *Common:* Slight fever and irritability, local irritation.
   2) *Rare:* Extreme irritability, temperature >40.5°C, seizures, hyporesponsive state.
      NOTE: Family history of seizure disorder is not a contraindication to pertussis immunization
e. Contraindications to reimmunization:
   1) Encephalopathy within 7 days of immunization.
   2) Seizure within 72 hours.
   3) Persistent screaming within 48 hours.
   4) Hyporesponsive episode within 48 hours.
   5) Temperature ≥40.5°C. within 48 hours without other cause.
   6) Anaphylactic reaction to vaccine.
f. Comments: Diphtheria and tetanus toxoids and acellular pertussis vaccine (DTaP; ACEL-IMUNE) recently was licensed for use as the fourth and fifth doses of DTP series in children aged 15 months through 6 years. Its efficacy is comparable to whole-cell DTP. Local and systemic reactions occur less frequently with DTaP.

2. MMR:
   a. Type: Live attenuated viruses of measles, mumps, and rubella.
   b. Route: Subcutaneous injection.
   c. Schedule: 15 months; immunization before 15 months is indicated in epidemic or highly endemic circumstances. These children should be reimmunized at 15 months of age. In addition, reimmunization on entrance to grade school or to junior high school is recommended for all children immunized at 15 months.
   d. Adverse reactions: Five percent to 15% of children develop fever (temperature up to 39.5°C) 5 to 12 days after immunization, lasting 1 to 2 days. Mild rash, arthralgia, and lymphadenopathy may occur after primary rubella immunization.

e. Comments: Two million children still die of measles each year worldwide.

3. OPV:
   a. Type: Live attenuated poliovirus, serotypes I, II, and III.
   b. Route: Oral.
   c. Schedule: 2, 4, and 18 months; 4 to 6 years.
   d. Indications:
      1) Normal infants and children receiving routine immunizations.
      2) Unimmunized or partially immunized children at imminent risk of poliovirus exposure.
      3) Adults who have received ≥ 1 doses of IPV or OPV and are at future risk of polio exposure.
      4) Adults who are unimmunized or who had partial or complete IPV series and are at imminent risk of polio exposure.
   e. Adverse reactions: Approximately one in 7.8 million doses results in paralysis in an immunologically normal vaccine recipient. Approximately one in 5.5 million doses results in paralysis in a household contact. Immunocompromised individuals who receive OPV vaccine are at increased risk for paralytic disease and therefore should receive IPV.
   f. Comments: Five million cases of paralytic polio are estimated to have been prevented through the use of OPV.
4. IPV:
   a. Type: Inactivated poliovirus vaccine (trivalent).
   b. Route: Subcutaneous.
   c. Schedule: 2, 4, and 10 to 16 months of age; then q5yr thereafter.
   d. Indications:
      1) Unimmunized or partially immunized persons with compromised immunity.
      2) HIV-infected persons (symptomatic or asymptomatic).
      3) Household contacts of an immune-deficient (including HIV) person.

4) Partially immunized or unimmunized adults in households of children to receive OPV.
5) Unimmunized or partially immunized adults at future risk of polio exposure.
6) Adults who had primary IPV series and who are at future risk of polio exposure.
7) Individuals who refuse OPV.

e. Adverse reactions: IPV has no serious side effects.

5. Hib:
   a. Type: *Hemophilus influenzae* type b polysaccharide linked to a protein carrier: diphtheria CRM_{197} protein (HbOC) or meningococcal cell membrane protein (PRP-OMP).
   b. Route: Subcutaneous or intramuscular.
   c. Schedule: HbOC: 2,4,6,15 months; PRP-OMP: 2,4,12 months
   d. Adverse reactions: One in 67 patients develops local irritation; one in 100 develops fever (temperature ≥38.5°C).
6. Pneumococcal vaccine:
   a. Type: Capsular polysaccharides of common serotypes.
   b. Route: Subcutaneous, intramuscular.
   c. Schedule: Children ≥24 months with functional or anatomic asplenia, nephrotic syndrome, HIV infection, sickle cell disease, immunosuppression, CSF leaks, cystic fibrosis, or those about to undergo cytoreduction therapy for Hodgkin's disease. Adults ≥65 years, or with chronic cardiac or pulmonary disease, lymphatic malignancy, or chronic liver disease.
   d. Indications:
      1) Primary targets:
         a) Children with chronic pulmonary disease.
         b) Children with significant cardiac disease.
         c) Children receiving immunosuppression therapy.
         d) Children with sickle cell disease and other hemoglobinopathies.
         e) Children in nursing homes or other chronic care facilities.

   2) Others at high risk:
      a) Children with diabetes, chronic renal and metabolic diseases.
      b) Children with symptomatic HIV infection.
      c) Children receiving long-term high-dose aspirin (e.g., for juvenile rheumatoid arthritis).
   3) Contacts:
      a) Close contacts of high-risk patients.
      b) Hospital personnel, teachers.
e. Adverse reactions: No serious side effects known.
f. Comments: Pneumococcal vaccine contains capsular polysaccharide antigens of 23 serotypes that cause 88% of pneumococcal bacteremia and meningitis in adults and nearly 100% of bacteremia and meningitis in children. Efficacy is estimated to be about 60% in high-risk populations.

7. Hepatitis B vaccine (HBV): Purified HBsAg.
   a. Route: Intramuscular.
   b. Schedule: 0,1,6 months.
      1) Alternative schedule for infants born to HBsAg-negative women: 1 to 2, 4, and 6 to 18 months.
      2) Infants born to HBsAg-positive women also should receive hepatitis B immune globulin at birth.
      3) Adolescents should be immunized with HBV (3 doses: 0,1,6 months) if resources permit.
   c. Indications:
      1) Preexposure vaccination with HBV vaccine:
         a) Staff and residents of institutions for the mentally disabled.
         b) Recipients of certain blood products (e.g., hemophiliacs).
         c) Hemodialysis patients.
         d) Household and sexual contacts of HBV chronic carriers, including adoptees from HBV-endemic areas.
         e) All neonates.
         f) Heterosexually active persons with multiple partners or with recent sexually transmitted disease.
         g) Homosexually active males.

- h) Intravenous drug users.
- i) International travelers (>6 mo in an HBV-endemic area).
- j) Health care workers.
- k) Inmates of long-term correctional facilities.

2) Postexposure vaccination with HBV vaccine:
- a) Infants born to HBV carrier mothers or to mothers with acute hepatitis B in third trimester.
- b) Accidental percutaneous or permucosal exposure to HBsAg-positive blood.
- c) Sexual partners of persons with acute HBV infection.
- d) Household contacts of persons with acute HBV infection.

d. Adverse effects: No serious side effects.
e. Comments: 80% to 95% effective.

8. Influenza vaccine.

a. Type: Inactivated whole virus or split virus vaccines. Only the split vaccine is used for children <13 years.
b. Route: Intramuscular.
c. Schedule: This vaccine is reformulated each year because of yearly variation in circulating influenza strains. Dosage is 0.25 mL of the split vaccine for children 6–35 months, and 0.5 mL for those 3–8 years. Two doses are given, 1 month apart, if child is receiving influenza vaccine for the first time. Children 9–12 years receive one 0.5-mL dose of split vaccine, and those >12 years one 0.5-mL dose of whole or split vaccine.
d. Indications

1) Primary targets.
- a) Children with chronic pulmonary disease.
- b) Children with significant cardiac disease.
- c) Children receiving immunosuppression.
- d) Children with sickle cell disease and other hemoglobinopathies.
- e) Children in nursing home or other chronic care facilities.

2) Others at high risk.
   a) Children with diabetes, chronic renal and metabolic diseases.
   b) Children with symptomatic HIV infection.
   c) Children receiving long-term high-dose aspirin therapy (e.g., for juvenile rheumatoid arthritis).
3) Contacts.
   a) Close contacts of high-risk patients.
   b) Hospital personnel, teachers.

e. Adverse reactions: Generally well-tolerated. Contraindicated in children with anaphylactic egg hypersensitivity.

III. PASSIVE IMMUNIZATION: ADMINISTRATION OF PREFORMED ANTIBODY.

A. Indications:

1. Individuals incapable of an active antibody response to immunization.
2. When no vaccine is available (e.g., hepatitis A).
3. When time does not allow for adequate protection by active immunization after exposure has occurred (e.g., rabies, measles, tetanus).
4. When antibody may ameliorate a disease already present (e.g., diphtheria, tetanus, botulism).
5. As an immunomodulator (e.g., anti-D [RhoD]).

B. Types:

1. Standard human immune serum globulin (ISG):
   a. Consists of at least 95% IgG, pooled from large groups (>1,000) of adult donors.
   b. Not known to transmit hepatitis or other infectious agents, including HIV.
   c. Available for intramuscular use.
   d. Indications for ISG:
      1) Replacement therapy in antibody-deficient disorders.
      2) Hepatitis A prophylaxis; give within 14 days of exposure.
      3) Measles prophylaxis; prevents or modifies infection if given within 6 days of exposure. Exposed

infants <1 year of age should receive immune globulin (ISG).

4) Unproved uses of ISG include hepatitis B prophylaxis, non-A, non-B hepatitis, rubella in pregnancy.

e. Adverse reactions:

1) Discomfort and pain at intramuscular injection site.
2) Less commonly, flushing, headache, chills, and nausea.
3) Serious reactions uncommon.
4) Contraindicated in persons with selective IgA deficiency.

2. Intravenous gammaglobulin: Almost pure IgG from more than 1,000 adult donors, chemically treated to contain mostly monomeric IgG.

a. Indications:

1) Treatment of humoral immune deficiency states.
2) Idiopathic thrombocytopenic purpura.
3) Kawasaki disease.
4) Of possible value in pediatric HIV infection, when CD4 count >200/mm^3.
5) May be somewhat effective in decreasing the incidence of infection in low birth weight infants.

b. Adverse reactions: Few.

3. Specific Human IGs: Prepared from donors known to have high titers of the desired antibody, either naturally acquired or induced by immunization. Preparations and indications for use include:

a. Hepatitis B immune globulin (HBIG): Ideally given within 24 hours of exposure to needlestick from persons known to be HBsAg positive or to be at high risk of having HBsAg-positive blood but whose status is unknown and cannot be tested. Also indicated for neonates born to HBV-positive women.

b. Varicella zoster immune globulin (VZIG). To prevent or ameliorate varicella in immunocompromised hosts with recent exposure (within 96 hours).

1) Indications:

a) Individuals at risk (if exposed):

i) Susceptible, immunocompromised children or adults.

ii) Normal susceptible persons ≥15 years old, particularly if pregnant. Determine serologic status.
iii) Neonate whose mother had onset of varicella 5 days before delivery to 48 hours after delivery.
iv) Hospitalized premature infant (≥28 weeks gestation) with negative maternal history of varicella.
v) Hospitalized premature infant (<28 weeks or ≤1,000 gm), regardless of maternal history.

b) Significant exposure history:
i) Household contact with varicella or zoster.
ii) Playmate contact (>1 hour of indoor play) with varicella or zoster.
iii) Hospital contact in same two to four-bed room, adjacent beds in large ward, or prolonged face-to-face contact with patient or staff member with varicella or zoster.
iv) Neonate whose mother had onset of varicella 5 days before delivery to 48 hours after delivery.

c) VZIG should be given when a person at risk (a) has had significant exposure (b), and when VZIG can be given within 96 hours.

c. Rabies immune globulin (RIG): Should be given together with active rabies immunization within 24 hours of exposure.
d. Tetanus immune globulin (TIG): Highly effective in preventing tetanus if administered soon after injury.
e. RhoD immune globulin (Rho-Gam): Highly effective in preventing Rh hemolytic disease of the neonate. Indicated after inadvertent transfusion of Rh-positive blood to an Rh-negative recipient and in Rh-negative women who have delivered an Rh-positive infant or have aborted.

C. Antibodies of nonhuman origin:

1. The following preparations are available:
   a. Botulism antitoxin: Effective in neutralizing unbound toxin even after clinical disease is present.
   b. Diphtheria antitoxin: Effective in neutralizing non-tissue-bound toxin.
   c. Antirabies serum: Use only when human preparations (RIG) are unavailable. See Table 1–2.
   d. Tetanus antitoxin: Use only when human preparations (TIG) are unavailable. See Table 1–3.
   e. Antivenoms for use in snake bites and spider bites.
   f. Antithymocyte globulin (ATG) or antilymphocyte globulin (ALG): Use for prevention and/or treatment of organ transplant rejection.
   g. Murine monoclonal antibodies directed against T lymphocytes (OKT3): Use for prevention of organ transplant rejection.
2. Adverse reactions:
   a. Acute febrile reactions: Common, mild; may be treated with antipyretics.

TABLE 1–2.
Rabies Prophylaxis: General Guide*

Animal Species	Condition of Animal at Attack	Treatment of Exposed Human
Wild animal: skunk, bat, fox, raccoon, coyote, other carnivore	Consider rabid until laboratory tests prove otherwise	RIG and HDCV
Domestic animal: dog, cat	Healthy, under surveillance	None, but start RIG and HDCV at first sign of animal rabies during 10-day holding period
	Unknown or escaped	Call public health officer for advice
	Rabid or suspected rabid	RIG and HDCV
Livestock, rodents, rabbits, hares		Individualize; these animals are very rarely infected

*Adapted from *Redbook.* Elk Grove Village, Ill, 1991, American Academy of Pediatrics.
RIG = rabies immune globulin, HDCV = human diploid cell vaccine.

TABLE 1–3.
Tetanus Prophylaxis for Wounds

Doses of Tetanus Immunization	Clean, Minor Wounds		All Other Wounds	
	Td	TIG	Td	TIG
Unknown or <3	Yes	No	Yes	Yes
≥3	No*	No	No†	No

Td = adult tetanus and diphtheria toxoids, TIG = tetanus immune globulin.
*Yes if >10 years since last dose.
†Yes if >5 years since last dose.

b. Serum sickness:
   1) Manifestations consist of maculopapular rash, fever, arthralgia, lymphadenopathy, and urticaria.
   2) Symptoms usually begin 7 to 10 days after exposure.
   3) Edema, glomerulonephritis, Guillain-Barré syndrome, peripheral neuritis, and myocarditis may occur.
   4) May resolve spontaneously within a few days to 2 weeks.
   5) Management may include antihistamines, anti-inflammatory agents, or corticosteroids.

c. Anaphylaxis: Usually begins within minutes of exposure to the provoking agent.
   1) Management includes epinephrine, antihistamines, intravenous fluids to maintain blood pressure, and corticosteroids; occasionally emergency establishment of an airway.
   2) All personnel administering these products should be prepared to treat anaphylaxis.

d. Individuals to receive an animal serum should be tested prior to its administration by a scratch test, followed by intradermal skin test. Desensitization may be necessary.

IV. Immunizations in special circumstances:

A. Pregnancy:

1. Pregnant women should receive vaccines only when urgently needed.

2. In the U.S., tetanus and diphtheria are the only vaccines recommended during pregnancy.
3. Pregnancy is a contraindication to administration of live virus vaccines except when the disease to be prevented poses a greater threat to the woman or fetus than vaccination, *and* exposure is highly probable.

B. Pre-term infants:

1. Prematurely born infants should be immunized at the usual chronological age.
2. Vaccine doses are the same as for term infants.

C. Immunodeficient children:

1. Live virus vaccines and BCG are contraindicated in patients with congenital immune disorders.
2. Immunologically normal siblings and other household contacts of individuals with immune deficiency should not receive OPV because live attenuated poliovirus is shed in stool, and may be transmitted to the immunocompromised individual by the fecal-oral route.
3. Live virus vaccines should be given no less than three months after immunosuppressive therapy is discontinued.
4. Normal children receiving short-term (less than 2 weeks) low to moderate doses of systemic corticosteroids, maintenance physiologic doses, or topical steroids may receive live virus vaccines.
5. Recommendations for children with HIV infection are included in Table 1–4 and in Chapter 5.

TABLE 1–4.
Immunization of HIV-Infected U.S. Children*

Vaccine	Asymptomatic HIV Infection	Symptomatic HIV Infection
DTP	Yes	Yes
OPV	No	No
IPV	Yes	Yes
MMR	Yes	Yes
Hib conjugate	Yes	Yes
Pneumococcus	Yes	Yes
Influenza	Yes	Yes

*Modified from *Redbook.* Elk Grove Village, Ill, 1991, American Academy of Pediatrics.

D. Asplenic children:

1. All asplenic persons, regardless of the reason they are asplenic, are at increased risk for fulminant sepsis. This includes patients with sickle-cell disease, who are functionally but not anatomically asplenic.
2. *Streptococcus pneumoniae* is the most important cause of septicemia in this population, followed by *H. influenzae*, *Neisseria meningitidis*, and *Escherichia coli*.
3. Polyvalent pneumococcal vaccine and quadrivalent meningococcal polysaccharide vaccine are recommended for all asplenic individuals ≥2 years.
4. Conjugated Hib vaccine should be given at the appropriate ages.

E. Children with chronic disease:

1. In general, immunizations recommended for normal children should be given, unless the child has an immunologic disorder.
2. Children with certain chronic diseases (involving the heart, lungs, kidneys; diabetes and metabolic diseases; hematologic diseases and malignancies; and immunocompromised states) may be at increased risk for complications of influenza and pneumococcal infection and should receive pneumococcal and yearly influenza vaccines.

F. Children with neurologic disorders:

1. Children with certain neurologic disorders are at increased risk for complications after pertussis and measles vaccines.
2. However, because of current risks of natural measles, vaccination for measles is recommended even in children with a history of seizures.
3. Pertussis vaccine should be deferred if the neurologic status is not stable.
4. Family history of seizures is not a contraindication for measles or DPT vaccine.

APPROACH TO INFECTIONS BY SYMPTOMS AND SIGNS 2

I. FEVER OF UNKNOWN ORIGIN (FUO):

A. Definition:

1. There is no consistent definition of FUO in the pediatric literature.
2. Useful working definition: Fever for at least 7 days in a child in whom the initial history and physical examination and preliminary laboratory data have not indicated the source of the fever.

B. Etiology:

1. Pediatric FUOs usually represent uncommon manifestations of common disorders.
2. Approximate breakdown by etiologic category:
   a. Infectious: 40% to 50%.
   b. Collagen-vascular: 10% to 20%.
   c. Neoplasms: 5% to 10%.
   d. Miscellaneous: 10% to 15%.
   e. Undiagnosed: 20% to 30%.

C. Evaluation:

1. A thorough history is essential and should include:
   a. Careful description of the fever pattern: Is it continuous (e.g., in typhoid fever), remittent, relapsing (e.g., in malaria and borreliosis)?
   b. Attention to associated findings at the time of fever, including tachycardia, skin warmth, and diaphoresis. Absence of these findings may suggest factitious fever.

   c. Exposure to ill contacts.
   d. Animal exposures.
   e. Travel history (recent and remote).
   f. Dietary history (raw meat/fish ingestion, unpasteurized milk, pica).
   g. Family history (ethnic background may support diagnoses such as familial Mediterranean fever, familial dysautonomia).
2. Careful physical examination, searching for:
   a. A focus of infection or findings to suggest an occult infectious process.
   b. Findings suggesting a noninfectious disease that could explain the FUO (e.g., rashes, vasculitic lesions or arthritis suggesting a collagen-vascular disease; smooth tongue and lack of tears suggesting familial dysautonomia; conjunctival injection, swollen hands and feet or other features to suggest Kawasaki disease [KD]).
3. Laboratory data and ancillary tests:
   a. Preliminary:
      1) Complete blood cell (CBC) count with differential, platelet count.
      2) Erythrocyte sedimentation rate (ESR; may help to direct further evaluation).
      3) Aerobic and anaerobic blood cultures.
      4) Urinalysis and urine culture.
      5) Chest x-ray film.
      6) Tuberculin skin test with control.
      7) Serologic testing (especially "febrile agglutinins," useful in diagnosing salmonellosis, brucellosis, tularemia, or rickettsial infection).
      8) Any other tests or studies indicated by the history or physical findings (e.g., antinuclear antibody [ANA], anti-DNA antibodies if systemic lupus erythematosus [SLE] is suspected).
   b. Secondary or advanced studies (if needed):
      1) Sinus x-ray or CT studies.
      2) Bone scan.
      3) Bone marrow examination and culture (helpful in diagnosing neoplastic or hematologic disorders;

culture may aid in diagnosing a variety of infections, including typhoid fever, brucellosis, disseminated tuberculosis [TB]).

4) Radiographic evaluation of the gastrointestinal tract (to search for inflammatory bowel disease or other intra-abdominal pathologic conditions).
5) Abdominal ultrasound or CT scan (helpful in detecting occult tumor or abscess).
6) Gallium scan.
7) Echocardiogram (to help rule out subacute bacterial endocarditis).
8) Computed tomography (CT) scan of the head and lumbar puncture merit consideration if complaints of headache or vague neurologic symptoms are present.

4. Therapy:
   a. Empiric antibiotic trials are rarely helpful and may serve to obscure and delay diagnosis.
   b. Treatment with a nonsteroidal anti-inflammatory drug may be appropriate when juvenile rheumatoid arthritis (JRA) remains as a diagnosis of exclusion after an exhaustive evaluation.

II. FEVER AND SEIZURE:

A. Etiology:

1. Seizures with fever may be seen in central nervous system (CNS) infections because of direct cortical inflammation and/or lowering of the seizure threshold by fever.
2. Febrile seizures are seizures that are associated with fever (temperature usually >38.5°C) in the absence of CNS infection or underlying seizure disorder. The infection causing the fever is most commonly a viral upper respiratory tract infection, viral gastroenteritis, or roseola. By definition, febrile seizures occur in children 3 months to 5 years of age (usually 6 months–3 years). They are typically nonfocal and of short duration. The exact mechanism by which fever triggers a febrile seizure is unknown.

3. Fever caused by any non-CNS infection may lower the seizure threshold in a child with a known seizure disorder or CNS abnormality that predisposes to seizures.

B. Clinical findings:

1. Seizures caused by meningitis or other CNS infections are typically associated with persistently altered mental status or other signs of raised intracranial pressure, such as altered reflexes, Babinski's sign, pupillary changes, and/or altered respiratory pattern. Nuchal rigidity is a reliable indicator of meningitis in older children but is difficult to elicit in children <18 to 24 months of age.
2. Simple febrile seizures are single, generalized tonic-clonic convulsions lasting <15 minutes and are followed by fairly prompt return to the patient's baseline neurologic and mental status. Complex febrile seizures, by definition, are focal, last more than 15 minutes, or recur within 24 hours. Symptoms of the precipitating infection are usually present.

C. Diagnostic approach:

1. The most critical aspect of evaluating the child with fever and seizure is assessing presence or absence of CNS infection. Lumbar puncture is indicated in the following circumstances:
   a. Any child with signs and symptoms of meningitis or sepsis.
   b. Any patient with a first seizure associated with fever, particularly those <12 to 24 months of age, because signs of meningitis are unreliable in this age group.
2. If CNS infection has been ruled out, evidence supporting the diagnosis of febrile seizure should be sought.
   a. Seizure description, as noted earlier, should be obtained, and the height of the associated fever documented.
   b. Signs and symptoms of an associated febrile infection should be sought but are not always present, because febrile seizures often occur early in febrile illnesses.
   c. Immunizations, particularly against pertussis and measles, may cause postvaccination fevers of sufficient magnitude to result in a febrile seizure.

d. A history of previous febrile seizures is important, as is a family history of febrile seizures.

3. Evidence of a neurocutaneous disorder, cerebral palsy, or other static CNS abnormality should be sought on physical examination.
4. Cranial CT scan is indicated if an anatomic CNS abnormality is suspected.
5. Electroencephalograms are of limited value in the acute setting, because they remain abnormal in many patients with febrile seizures for 7 to 10 days after the seizure.

III. FEVER AND LYMPHADENOPATHY:

A. Fever with generalized lymphadenopathy:

1. Most children have palpable lymph nodes, especially in the cervical and inguinal regions. Nodes <10 mm in diameter are usually normal. Generalized lymphadenopathy can be defined as node enlargement in more than two noncontiguous areas.
2. Etiologic categories:
   a. **Infectious:** Viral (human immunodeficiency virus [HIV], Epstein-Barr virus [EBV], cytomegalovirus [CMV], measles), fungal (disseminated histoplasmosis or coccidiodomycosis), toxoplasmosis, secondary syphilis, bacterial infection with hematogenous spread.
   b. **Collagen-vascular:** JRA, SLE, serum sickness.
   c. **Neoplastic:** Lymphoma, leukemia, neuroblastoma.
   d. **Miscellaneous:** Histiocytosis, sarcoidosis.
   e. **Drug reaction:** Phenytoin, allopurinol, antileprosy medications.
3. Approach to evaluation:
   a. **History:** Duration of lymphadenopathy, associated symptoms, current and recent medications, travel history, ill contacts, risk factors for HIV infection.
   b. **Physical examination:** Lymph node size and character, hepatosplenomegaly, tonsillar hypertrophy, rash or skin lesions, arthritis.
   c. If patient is taking a medication known to cause generalized lymphadenopathy (see section A.2.e. above), discontinue that medication.

d. If history and physical do not suggest a diagnosis, proceed with screening tests: CBC with differential; EBV, CMV, HIV, toxoplasma titers; ANA; blood cultures; TB skin test; chest x-ray film; fungal titers.
e. If history, physical examination, and screening tests do not suggest a diagnosis, excisional node biopsy is generally indicated. Bone marrow examination may be the diagostic procedure of choice if hematologic abnormalities are present.

B. Fever with cervical lymphadenopathy:

1. Etiologic categories:
   a. **Infectious:** Viral upper respiratory tract infection, group A β-hemolytic streptococcus (with pharyngitis), anaerobic bacteria (with dental infections), *Staphylococcus aureus,* EBV, CMV, toxoplasmosis, mycobacteria (especially atypical mycobacteria), cat-scratch disease, leptospirosis, tularemia, and brucellosis.
   b. **Neoplastic:** Neuroblastoma, leukemia, lymphoma, rhabdomyosarcoma, and sinus histiocytosis.
   c. **Miscellaneous:** KD, sarcoidosis.
   d. Other neck masses such as infected branchial cleft cysts and cystic hygromas may be confused with cervical lymphadenopathy but can usually be distinguished by careful physical examination, ultrasound, or CT scan.
2. Approach to evaluation:
   a. **History:** Associated symptoms, weight loss, ill contacts, TB exposures, animal exposures, ingestion of undercooked meat, and duration of associated fever.
   b. **Physical examination:** Thorough head and neck examination, including precise documentation of lymph node size and character, rash or skin lesions, hepatosplenomegaly, and other lymph node sites.
   c. If history and physical examination do not suggest a diagnosis, initial screening tests can be done: CBC count, ESR, chest x-ray film, throat culture for group A streptococcus, EBV serology (heterophile antibody test is unreliable in young children), TB skin test, *Toxoplasma* and CMV serologies, and needle aspira-

tion of the node if fluctuant. Optional studies include skin test with cat-scratch antigen (if available), serologies for leptospirosis, brucellosis, and tularemia.

d. If the previous evaluation is not diagnostic, observation for 4 to 6 weeks is appropriate. If node size is decreasing, further observation is acceptable; otherwise, excisional node biopsy is indicated.

IV. FEVER AND ABDOMINAL PAIN:

A. General considerations:

1. Possible diagnoses can be grouped broadly by patient age and findings on abdominal examination (Table 2–1).
2. Accurate diagnosis by noninvasive means may be difficult, especially in young children and infants who cannot describe their pain.

B. Diagnostic considerations by category (Table 2–1):

1. Infants with abdominal tenderness or distention:
   a. Presence of copious diarrhea suggests gastroenteritis; fecal leukocytes, stool cultures and assay for rotavirus may be helpful tests.
   b. Necrotizing enterocolitis (NEC) is seen in neonates, especially prematures; abdominal radiographs demonstrating pneumatosis intestinalis or portal venous gas are diagnostic.
   c. Hirschsprung's enterocolitis must be considered in an infant with a history of constipation.
   d. Sepsis may induce ileus with abdominal distention.
   e. Appendicitis is uncommon in this age group and very difficult to diagnose before perforation.
2. Children and adolescents with epigastric or right upper quadrant (RUQ) pain:
   a. Right middle lobe or right lower lobe pneumonia may produce pleural irritation resulting in pain referred to the RUQ; chest x-ray film is diagnostic.
   b. RUQ tenderness is common in the preicteric phase of viral hepatitis; liver enzyme levels and appropriate serologic tests are diagnostic.
   c. Pancreatitis caused by viral infections, especially mumps, or after use of certain medications is usually

TABLE 2–1.
Major Differential Diagnoses of Abdominal Pain by Age, Symptoms, and Examination Findings*

Infants with abdominal tenderness or distention
Gastroenteritis (viral/bacterial)
NEC
Hirschsprung's enterocolitis
Sepsis
Appendicitis (uncommon)
Children/adolescents with epigastric or RUQ pain
Pneumonia
Hepatitis
Pancreatitis
Gastritis/gastroenteritis
Children/adolescents with umbilical/lower quadrant pain
Gastroenteritis
Appendicitis
UTI
Inflammatory bowel disease
Mesenteric lymphadenitis
PID in female adolescents
Children/adolescents with diffuse pain and tenderness
Ruptured appendix
Spontaneous bacterial peritonitis
Familial Mediterranean fever
HSP or other vasculitides
Children/adolescents with diffuse pain but minimal tenderness
UTI
Streptococcal pharyngitis

*NEC = necrotizing enterocolitis; UTI = urinary tract infection; PID = pelvic inflammatory disease; HSP = Henoch-Schönlein purpura.

accompanied by low-grade fever and epigastric pain. Serum amylase and lipase levels will aid in diagnosis.

d. Appendicitis involving a retrocecal appendix may manifest with epigastric or RUQ pain.

3. Children and adolescents with umbilical or lower quadrant pain:
   a. Appendicitis classically manifests with periumbilical pain later localizing to the right lower quadrant

(RLQ); onset of emesis follows the onset of pain. Diarrhea, if present, is mild. In contrast, gastroenteritis begins with emesis, followed by or coincident with abdominal pain, and copious diarrhea is usually present. Barium enema and/or ultrasound of the RLQ may be helpful in diagnosing appendicitis but should not be the sole basis for establishing a diagnosis.

   b. Inflammatory bowel disease may manifest insidiously with an elevated ESR, low serum albumin level, weight loss, abdominal pain, and fever. Barium enema, small bowel series, or colonoscopy are usually diagnostic.
   c. Mesenteric lymphadenitis may be caused by adenovirus (look for an associated pharyngitis), *Yersinia enterocolitica, Yersinia pseudotuberculosis,* or rarely by *Mycobacterium tuberculosis*. It may closely mimic appendicitis and may be distinguishable from appendicitis only at laparotomy.
   d. Pelvic inflammatory disease classically manifests in female adolescents with cervical motion tenderness, adnexal tenderness, fever, leukocytosis, and elevated ESR. Careful pelvic examination is essential. However, presenting signs and symptoms frequently vary, and direct laparoscopy is the most accurate diagnostic method. Adnexal ultrasound may be helpful in demonstrating an inflammatory adnexal mass.
   e. Urinary tract infections may manifest with diffuse lower quadrant or periumbilical pain.
4. Children and adolescents with diffuse abdominal pain and tenderness:
   a. Perforated appendix must be considered in a patient with an antecedent history of appendicitis followed by a period of improvement and subsequent deterioration.
   b. Spontaneous peritonitis occurs mainly in children who have ascites secondary to nephrotic syndrome or other causes.
   c. Familial Mediterranean fever occurs in certain Middle Eastern ethnic groups and is characterized by recurrent episodes of fever and polyserositis (peritonitis, pleuritis, and synovitis).

   d. HSP is accompanied by low-grade fever in 50% of cases and frequently manifests with crampy abdominal pain. Other features of HSP (nephritis, arthritis, and characteristic rash) are usually also present.
5. Children and adolescents with diffuse abdominal pain but minimal tenderness:
   a. Urinary tract infections frequently manifest with emesis and abdominal pain; urinalysis and urine culture are diagnostic.
   b. Streptococcal pharyngitis may be accompanied by abdominal pain; rapid streptococcal antigen testing and/or throat culture is diagnostic.

V. FEVER AND DIARRHEA:

A. Etiology:

1. Infectious gastroenteritis is the chief cause of fever and diarrhea and may be divided into three classes according to pathogenic mechanism (see also Chapter 6, section I):
   a. Rotavirus, Norwalk virus, *Giardia lamblia, Vibrio cholerae,* and enterotoxigenic *Escherichia coli* cause noninflammatory diarrhea through enterotoxin production or reduction of absorptive surface.
   b. *Shigella, Salmonella, Campylobacter,* enteroinvasive *E. coli,* and *Entamoeba histolytica* cause inflammatory diarrhea through mucosal invasion.
   c. *Salmonella typhi* and *Yersinia* multiply intracellularly and produce enteric fever syndromes in which systemic illness is more apparent.
2. Appendicitis may manifest with fever and some degree of diarrhea, among other symptoms.
3. Fever and diarrhea may be presenting symptoms of either ulcerative colitis or Crohn's disease.

B. Epidemiology:

1. Rotavirus and Norwalk virus are prevalent causes of gastroenteritis in the winter, whereas bacterial gastroenteritis is generally seen in the summer and fall.
2. Place of acquisition is also an important epidemiologic consideration:
   a. "Traveler's diarrhea," which may affect 20% to 60%

of North American travelers to developing countries, is usually caused by enterotoxigenic *E. coli*.

b. Enteric infections are a common problem in day-care centers and are most commonly caused by *Giardia,* rotavirus, *Shigella,* and *Campylobacter*.

3. Gastroenteritis in the immunocompromised host may be caused by unusual organisms such as CMV, *Candida,* and mycobacteria, whereas common causes of gastroenteritis in normal children, such as *Cryptosporidium,* may cause a life-threatening infection in these patients.
4. Causative organisms also vary with patient age, as summarized in Table 2–2.

C. **Diagnosis:**

1. Fever and diarrhea caused by inflammatory bowel disease may be differentiated from acute infectious gastroenteritis by the chronicity of symptoms and presence of signs of systemic illness, but the distinction is not always readily apparent by history. Associated physical findings, such as oral ulcers or perianal fissures in the case of Crohn's disease, may be helpful. The diagnosis of inflammatory bowel disease usually requires barium enema and/or colonoscopy.
2. Appendicitis is usually distinguishable from other causes of fever and diarrhea on the basis of history and physical examination.
3. Consideration of the epidemiologic factors outlined earlier, together with the type of diarrhea, usually allows approximate determination of the most likely causative agent in cases of gastroenteritis. Frankly bloody diarrhea is usually bacterial in origin, whereas watery diarrhea can be caused by nearly any organism.
4. Laboratory tests to further define the cause of a given case of gastroenteritis are warranted if epidemiologic information is needed or if a treatable cause is suspected.
   a. Rotavirus in the stool can be reliably detected by enzyme-linked immunosorbent assay (ELISA).
   b. Bloody diarrhea, unusually severe or persistent symptoms, or history of exposure to a known bacterial enteritis warrant stool culture. Organisms that

TABLE 2–2.
Organisms Causing Infectious Diarrhea

Organism	Age Groups	Comments
Rotavirus	Infants and children	Occurs in day-care epidemics and in winter; often accompanied by vomiting
Norwalk virus	Older children, adult	Prevalent in winter; accompanied by vomiting ("winter vomiting disease")
Enterotoxigenic *E. coli*	All ages	Usual cause of "traveler's diarrhea"; important cause of childhood diarrhea in tropics but less so in United States
Enteropathogenic *E. coli*	Neonates	May cause nursery outbreaks of diarrhea
Campylobacter	All ages	Causes bloody diarrhea
Yersinia	All ages	Causes acute watery diarrhea in children <5 yr; may manifest as pseudoappendicitis or mesenteric adenitis in older children and adolescents
Salmonella	All ages, particularly young children	Bloody diarrhea; concomitant bacteremia frequent in infants
Shigella	All ages, especially day care	Bloody, mucoid diarrhea; Shiga's toxin may produce neurologic symptoms
Giardia	All ages	Prevalent in day-care settings

can be readily identified in culture include *Salmonella, Shigella, Yersinia,* and *Campylobacter*. Systemic illnesses such as hemolytic-uremic syndrome also must be considered.

c. Presence of fecal leukocytes in stool specimens suggests but does not confirm a diagnosis of bacterial enteritis.

d. Stool examination for ova and parasites is warranted if there is a history of travel to a developing country, if the illness was acquired in a day-care setting, if symptoms are persistent, or if other evidence of intestinal parasitic disease is present.

VI. FEVER AND HEPATOSPLENOMEGALY:

A. General considerations: A variety of illnesses may manifest with fever associated with hepatosplenomegaly. Generalized lymphadenopathy is also often present as another manifestation of reticuloendothelial hypertrophy. EBV-related infectious mononucleosis (IM) is the most common illness that manifests in this manner. (See Chapter 8, section III, C.)

B. Etiologic possibilities:

1. Infectious:
   a. **EBV** IM: Usually associated with acute pharyngitis and hepatic enzyme elevation.
   b. **CMV** mononucleosis is less often characterized by pharyngitis and cervical adenopathy, and splenomegaly is usually less prominent than in EBV IM.
   c. **Toxoplasmosis** may produce a syndrome resembling classical EBV IM, although pharyngitis and anterior cervical adenitis are less common than in EBV IM.
   d. Acute **HIV** infection may manifest with an IM-like illness that lasts several weeks.
   e. Acute hepatitis often manifests with fever and hepatomegaly, with splenomegaly sometimes present, particularly with acute hepatitis B.
   f. Other less common etiologies:
      1) **Cat-scratch disease** occasionally causes hepatosplenomegaly in addition to its more common manifestations of fever and lymphadenitis.
      2) Disseminated **tuberculosis** may manifest with fever and hepatosplenomegaly, usually with pulmonary manifestations.
      3) Acute disseminated **histoplasmosis** in young children generally manifests as fever, hepatosplenomegaly and general lymphadenopathy.
      4) *Hepatosplenic candidiasis* or *mycosis* is an increasingly diagnosed entity in immunocompromised hosts (most typically patients with neoplasms) with fever and hepatosplenomegaly.
2. Noninfectious
   a. Hematologic *malignancy,* particularly acute childhood leukemia, frequently presents with fever, hepa-

tosplenomegaly, and usually other associated symptoms. Neuroblastoma and hepatoblastoma can also mimic this presentation.

b. *Still's disease,* systemic-onset juvenile rheumatoid arthritis, often is manifested by fever and hepatosplenomegaly, together with rash and sometimes arthritis.

C. **Approach to evaluation**

1. Careful history that focuses upon potential exposures (contact with IM, ingestion of raw meat, exposure to cat litter, recent blood transfusion, unprotected sexual contact, IV drug abuse, cat exposure, contact with TB, travel or residence in area of histoplasmosis endemicity, exposure to hepatitis) and associated signs and symptoms (arthritis, rash, lymphadenopathy, pharyngitis) is the first step.
2. Physical examination may yield clues to the diagnosis, including evidence of cat scratches, presence or absence of associated findings like generalized or localized lymphadenopathy, pharyngitis, rash, evidence of toxicity, icterus, arthritis, and pallor.
3. Laboratory investigations:
   a. Routine screening tests such as CBC and ESR may reveal anemia, and very elevated ESR (seen particularly with noninfectious disorders or disseminated infections, e.g., TB or histoplasmosis).
   b. Monospot test is reliable in children with IM ≥ 4 years old but may need to be repeated after 1 week if results initially are negative. EBV serologic tests (e.g., IgM-VCA antibody) can detect recent or current infection.
   c. Serologic tests for antibodies to CMV, toxoplasmosis, and HIV (if indicated) and urine culture for CMV are useful but may require convalescent sera for interpretation.
   d. Chest radiograph abnormalities may assist in diagnosing TB or histoplasmosis.
   e. Serum transaminase levels indicate whether an active hepatitic process is present. If levels are elevated, IgM-anti-HAV, HBsAg, and anti-HBc are indicated to establish the presence of acute hepatitis A or B.

f. In compromised hosts, abdominal CT scan is essential to diagnose hepatosplenic candidiasis or mycosis.

VII. FEVER AND LIMP:

A. Etiology:

1. Limp with fever is a common problem in childhood, and the differential diagnosis is extensive, including both infectious and noninfectious causes. The area of involvement is often difficult to localize, especially in younger children, and may include the joints (hip, knee, or ankle), bones, or soft tissues.
2. Infectious:
   a. **Septic arthritis** (see Chapter 6, section K, 1): Septic arthritis (SA) is a medical emergency, particularly when it involves the hip, and a delay in diagnosis and therapy may lead to loss of joint function. Fever and joint effusion are the usual findings; however, effusion of the hip joint may be difficult to detect. Synovial fluid analysis is critical for establishing the diagnosis.
   b. **Osteomyelitis** (see Chapter 6, section K, 2): Osteomyelitis typically manifests with fever and localized bone pain. Osteomyelitis may be complicated by SA, especially in infants and when it involves the proximal femur.
   c. **Rheumatic fever** (see Chapter 12, section A): The clinical manifestations of acute rheumatic fever include fever, polyarthritis, and carditis and usually occur at least 7 days after the onset of a group A streptococcal pharyngeal infection. Diagnosis is established based on the Jones criteria.
   d. Other infectious causes of limp and fever include Lyme disease, KD, and reactive arthritis, which may be seen with some diarrheal illnesses (e.g., *Yersinia enterocolitica, Shigella*).
3. Noninfectious:
   a. **JRA:** Systemic-onset JRA often manifests with high fevers and joint effusion. Other findings may include rash, hepatosplenomegaly, anemia, and rheumatoid factor. This disorder is usually a diagnosis of exclusion.

b. **Leukemia:** Leukemia in children often manifests with fever and bone pain, which is caused by periosteal invasion and subperiosteal hemorrhage. Other findings may include lymphadenopathy, splenomegaly, anemia, thrombocytopenia, and blasts in the blood smear.

c. Noninfectious etiologies of limp and fever in children also include vaso-occlusive crisis in sickle cell disease (SCD), HSP, serum sickness, toxic synovitis, and arthritis associated with inflammatory bowel disease.

B. **Approach to evaluation:**

1. **History:** Duration of illness, height of fever, associated symptoms (e.g., sore throat, diarrhea, weight loss, upper respiratory tract infection, easy bruisability), past history (e.g., similar episodes previously, presence of SCD, history of tick bite), travel history, or trauma history.
2. **Physical examination:** General appearance of the child, vital signs, growth parameters, localization of pain, presence of joint effusion, rash, hepatosplenomegaly, lymphadenopathy, and mucous membrane changes.
3. **Laboratory data:**
   a. Blood culture may be positive with SA or osteomyelitis.
   b. CBC count with differential, platelet count, and ESR: ESR is usually markedly elevated with acute osteomyelitis, acute rheumatic fever, KD, and JRA. Anemia is usually found in chronic osteomyelitis, KD, JRA, and leukemia. Thrombocytosis is found in KD (usually a later finding), and thrombocytopenia is often seen with leukemia. Sickle cell prep should be done if the status is unknown.
   c. Aspiration of synovial fluid for analysis is indicated in patients with fever and joint effusion. See Table 2–3 for interpretation of joint fluid.
   d. Roentgenogram of the involved extremity and radionuclide bone scan should be performed when the diagnosis of osteomyelitis is being entertained. X-ray studies of the affected areas are generally normal during the acute stage.

TABLE 2–3.
Synovial Fluid

	Normal	Septic Arthritis	Non-septic Inflammatory	Reactive Arthritis
Color	Pale-yellow	Yellow-green	Yellow	Clear—slightly turbid
Clarity	Clear	Cloudy	Cloudy	Variable
Viscosity	High	Low	Low	Variable
WBC/mm^3	< 200	≥ 70,000	3000–50,000	5000–30,000
%Neutrophils	< 25%	> 90%	70%	Variable
Mucin clot	Good	Poor	Poor	Fair—Good
Gluose (% blood)	80–100	< 60	< 80	< 80

e. Tests for streptococcal antibodies (anti-streptolysin O, anti-DNase B), C-reactive protein and electrocardiogram (P-R interval prolongation) should be performed in patients suspected to have rheumatic fever.
f. If the diagnosis of Lyme disease is entertained based on epidemiologic and clinical evidence, serologic tests (ELISA or Western blot assays) should be obtained.
g. Echocardiograms should be performed on patients suspected of having KD.
h. Immunologic work-up should be pursued if the history and examination do not reveal an etiology and the bone scan and synovial fluid culture (if effusion is present) are negative.

VIII. FEVER AND NEUTROPENIA:

A. Definition:

1. Definition of fever varies; however, temperature clearly greater than the usual for the patient constitutes a febrile state. In general, if a patient has a single oral temperature ≥38.5°C or two recordings ≥38.0°C obtained at least 2 hours apart, the patient is considered to have a fever.
2. Neutropenia is defined strictly as an absolute neutrophil count (ANC) <1,000/mm^3. However, ANCs <200/mm^3

are particularly significant in that the risk of serious infection increases dramatically at this level.

3. Fever and neutropenia are an increasingly common clinical situation, with increasing use of aggressive cancer chemotherapy and immunosuppression for other diseases and organ transplantation.

B. **Etiology:**

1. Infections in neutropenic patients are caused most frequently by aerobic gram-negative bacilli (*E. coli, Klebsiella pneumoniae,* and *Pseudomonas aeruginosa*) and gram-positive cocci (especially coagulase-negative staphylococci, α-hemolytic streptococci, and *S. aureus*).
2. Fungi are also common causes of infections, especially in neutropenic patients who have received courses of broad-spectrum antibiotics and/or have had invasive procedures and lines.
3. The portals of infection are primarily the alimentary tract in which chemotherapy-induced mucosal damage (mucositis) occurs and the integument that is breached by procedures such as placement of vascular access devices and other tubes.
4. Particularly in children, many febrile neutropenic episodes are not proved to have a bacterial or fungal etiology; a large portion of these may represent viral infections.

C. **Evaluation:**

1. A thorough history should be taken, and the patient should be examined carefully.
2. Specimens for culture should be collected before institution of antibiotic therapy:
   a. At least two sets of blood cultures for bacterial and fungal agents should be obtained.
   b. If a central venous catheter is in place, blood cultures should be obtained from each lumen, as well as from a peripheral vein.
   c. Localized lesions should be cultured and examined by Gram's stain.
   d. Stool and urine cultures (and cerebrospinal fluid if clinically indicated) should be obtained.
   e. Routine cultures of the anterior nares and oropharynx

are of low yield but may provide clues to possible causative agents.

3. Chest radiograph should be performed.
4. CBC with differential, platelet count, electrolyte concentrations, blood urea nitrogen level, creatinine, and serum transaminase levels should be obtained.
5. Imaging techniques (ultrasound, CT, magnetic resonance imaging) of the abdomen, for example, should be performed if specific clinical indications are present or if fever continues despite therapy.

D. Antibiotic therapy:

1. Cancer patients with fever and ANC $<500/\text{mm}^3$ or those with ANC of 500 to $1{,}000/\text{mm}^3$ in whom a decrease in neutrophils is anticipated (e.g., in response to chemotherapy) should be considered to have a potentially life-threatening bacterial infection and therefore should be treated empirically with broad-spectrum antibiotics.
2. Several acceptable antibiotic regimens are available. Most commonly used schemes include coverage for staphylococci and gram-negatives, such as one of the following:
   a. Imipenem-cilastatin.
   b. Cefadyl or nafcillin plus an aminoglycoside (e.g., gentamicin) and an antipseudomonal penicillin (e.g., ticarcillin).
   c. Vancomycin plus ceftazidime.
3. When an etiologic agent is identified by culture, antibiotics should be changed to cover a narrower antimicrobial spectrum. Antibiotics should be continued until cultures are negative, the patient is afebrile, all sites of infection have resolved, and preferably when the ANC is $>500/\text{mm}^3$.
4. If the patient defervesces and appears well but no organism is isolated, we recommend discontinuing antibiotics and observing the patient closely. Others, however, recommend continuing antibiotics for at least 7 days.
5. If fever persists >3 days despite antibiotics and the patient is still neutropenic, the scheme in Table 2–4 should be used.
6. The empiric use of antiviral drugs in patients without clear evidence of viral disease is not generally recommended.

TABLE 2–4.
Scheme for Persistent Fever (>3 Days)

Reevaluate: Perform careful physical examination, reculture; consider diagnostic imaging.
- Doing well: Continue antibiotics.
- Condition deteriorating: Change antibiotics; add vancomycin if patient is not receiving it previously. Consider amphotericin B.
- If patient is febrile despite 1 week of antibiotics: Start amphotericin B intravenously.

7. Granulocyte transfusions are not generally recommended in febrile neutropenic patients because they have not been demonstrated to be effective.

IX. FEVER AND PETECHIAE:

A. The management of fever and petechiae in children is challenging because these findings may be present in a variety of illnesses that range from self-limited viral illnesses to life-threatening conditions. Petechiae also may be seen after prolonged coughing, crying, or other Valsalva maneuvers (usually present only on the upper body) or after compression of a limb by a blood pressure cuff or tourniquet.

B. Etiology:

1. **Meningococcemia** (see Chapter 7, section A, 9): Meningococcemia is the most important illness to consider, because often it is rapidly fatal if untreated. Patients may initially have fever and a few petechiae and appear well. Their condition deteriorates rapidly, and often septic shock and/or disseminated intravascular coagulation (DIC) develops. Meningococcemia can occur with or without meningitis.
2. **Rocky Mountain spotted fever (RMSF)** (see Chapter 11, section C): Patients with RMSF typically have fever, chills, headache, and a history of exposure to wood ticks or dog ticks. The rash, which may be macular and/or petechial, occurs several days after the onset of illness, and is noted first on the extremities.

3. **Streptococcal pharyngitis** (see Chapter 6, section B, 4): Group A streptococcal pharyngitis is a common cause of petechiae and fever. Patients usually have exudative pharyngitis and do not appear systemically ill.
4. **Infective endocarditis** (see Chapter 6, section F): Infective endocarditis may present with fever and petechiae. However, these patients usually have underlying heart disease as well as other findings, such as splenomegaly, new heart murmur, and hematuria.
5. **Other viral infections:** Other infectious causes of fever and petechiae include infectious mononucleosis, atypical measles, CMV infection, and enterovirus infection.
6. Noninfectious causes of fever and petechiae in children include drug reactions, Henoch-Schönlein purpura, hemolytic uremic syndrome, and leukemia.

C. **Evaluation:**

1. History: Duration of illness, degree of fever, associated symptoms (e.g., headache, sore throat, diarrhea), current or recent medications, travel history, exposure to ill contacts.
2. Physical examination: General appearance of the child ("toxic" vs benign), vital signs, mental status, severity and distribution of rash, meningeal signs, heart murmur, splenomegaly.
3. Laboratory data:
   a. CBC with differential, platelet count. Peripheral leukocyte count and band forms usually are higher with invasive bacterial disease than with nonbacteremic disease.
   b. Throat culture to test for group A streptococci.
   c. Blood culture to test for endocarditis, meningococcemia (or rarely *H. influenzae* type b or pneumococcal bacteremia).
   d. Lumbar puncture to test for Gram's stain, latex agglutination test, culture, cell count, protein, and glucose.
   e. Febrile agglutinins (Proteus OX2 and OX19 for RMSF).

D. Management:

1. The following patients should be hospitalized immediately and given intravenous antibiotics:
   a. Any patient who appears "toxic."
   b. Children with fever and petechiae on the lower half of the body.
   c. Patients with abnormal CSF findings and/or meningeal signs.
   d. Patients suspected to have RMSF on clinical grounds.
2. The older patient with an obvious focus of infection elsewhere (e.g., pharyngitis, upper respiratory tract infection, otitis media) who appears well and has completely normal clinical findings may be discharged with good follow-up and therapy with oral antibiotics as indicated.
3. Patients who do not fall into any of the above categories probably should be hospitalized or observed closely in a holding area for at least 12 to 24 hours.

NEONATAL INFECTIONS

3

I. RELATIVE DEFICIENCIES OF IMMUNE SYSTEM PREDISPOSING NEONATE TO INFECTION:

A. Antibody-mediated (B-cell) immunity:

1. Minimal fetal immunoglobulin synthesis occurs, with the exception of IgM in some congenital infections.
2. IgG is the only immunoglobulin transferred across the placenta to the fetus. Term infants have 100% to 110% of maternal IgG concentrations in serum, reflecting active transport. However, because >50% of transplacental IgG transport takes place after 32 weeks' gestation, premature infants are usually markedly deficient in IgG.
3. Neonatal B lymphocytes generate impaired antibody responses to antigenic challenge compared with adults, with delay in the normal switch from IgM to IgG production. This reflects delayed development of IgG-secreting lymphocytes and a lack of T-helper augmentation of IgM synthesis.
4. B-cell numbers in neonates are equal to adult values.

B. Cell-mediated (T-cell) immunity:

1. Neonates have a decreased percentage of T cells but a normal absolute number of T cells compared with adults.
2. Neonates have more immature T cells in circulation than do adults.
3. Neonatal T cells have a higher level of spontaneous (unstimulated) activity, with good responses to mitogen stimulation.
4. Neonatal T cells have diminished cytotoxic activity.
5. Stimulated neonatal T cells appear to release lower amounts of lymphokines.

6. Neonatal T cells release suppressor factors that impair other immune responses.
7. Skin test (tuberculin-type) reactivity is impaired in neonates, but this probably is a result of a poor cutaneous inflammatory response rather than a T-cell defect.

C. Complement-mediated immunity:

1. Although serum levels of individual components are lower than adult values, the classical complement pathway is fully functional in term infants but requires antigen-specific antibody. Therefore, it is of value only if the neonate has acquired specific antibody transplacentally. In addition, premature neonates have even further decreased serum concentrations of C1q, C4, C3, and CH_{50} activity.
2. The alternate pathway is relatively more important in the neonate because preexisting antibody is not required for activation. However, neonatal factor B levels are significantly lower than adult values and do not vary with gestational age. Properdin concentrations are also much lower than in adults but do vary directly with gestational age.

D. Neutrophil (polymorphonuclear neutrophil [PMN]):

1. The peripheral PMN count is related to gestational age. Although term neonates actually undergo a transient neutrophilia (>7,500 PMNs/mm^3) in the first day of life, extremely small healthy prematures may be neutropenic (<1,000 PMNs/mm^3).
2. Neonates have a decreased number of PMN precursors in their bone marrow, which, in turn, may have diminished ability to proliferate in response to infection. In addition, the PMN storage pool is relatively small in neonates and is rapidly depleted by stress or infection.
3. Neonatal PMNs have a number of relative functional defects, including diminished chemotaxis, abnormal adhesion and aggregation, decreased cell deformability, and decreased intracellular bactericidal capacity.

II. MANIFESTATIONS OF INFECTION IN THE NEONATE:

A. In utero infections:

1. In utero TORCHES (toxoplasmosis, rubella, cytomegalovirus, herpes simplex, and syphilis) infections all produce

similar signs and symptoms. These findings include intrauterine growth retardation, jaundice, hepatosplenomegaly, intracranial calcifications, microcephaly, chorioretinitis, cataracts, thrombocytopenia, hemolytic anemia, pneumonitis, and cardiac abnormalities.

2. Individual agents may produce characteristic clusters of physical findings, which are discussed in Chapter III. (See Table 3–1.)

B. Neonatal sepsis and meningitis:

1. Initial signs and symptoms are fairly nonspecific and include lethargy, irritability, poor feeding, emesis, abdomi-

TABLE 3–1.
Features of Torches Infections

	Rubella	CMV	Toxoplasmosis	Syphilis	Herpes
Microcephaly	1+	3+	2+	0	1+
Meningoencephalitis	2+	1+	2+	1+	4+
Intracranial calcifications	0	3+	3+	0	0
Hydrocephalus	1+	1+	3+	0	1+
Deafness	4+	3+	0	3+ (late)	0
Chorioretinitis	4+	2+	4+	2+	2+
Cataract	4+	0	1+	0	1+
Microphthalmia	3+	0	1+	0	0
Keratoconjunctivitis	0	0	0	1+	3+
Glaucoma	3+	0	0	1+	0
Optic atrophy	1+	2+	2+	1+	0
Petechiae, purpura	3+	4+	1+	2+	2+
Vesicular rash	0	1+	0	0	3+
Maculopapular rash	0	0	1+	4+	1+
Hepatosplenomegaly	3+	3+	3+	3+	3+
Jaundice	3+	3+	3+	3+	3+
Bone lesions	3+	0	1+	4+	0
Intrauterine growth retardation	4+	4+	2+	1+	0
Congenital heart disease	4+	0	0	0	0
Myocarditis	2+	0	1+	0	1+
Pneumonia	1+	3+	1+	1+	1+

0 = Rarely present, 1+ = occasionally present, 2+ = often present, 3+ = frequently present, 4+ = characteristic.

nal distention, and temperature instability (fever or hypothermia).

2. Tachypnea, cyanosis, apnea, tachycardia or bradycardia, and hypotension are later signs.
3. Jaundice may occur, especially with gram-negative sepsis.

C. **Laboratory aids to diagnosis:**

1. Peripheral white blood cell (WBC) counts:
   a. Septic neonates may demonstrate leukopenia, leukocytosis, or normal WBC counts. The total WBC count and the absolute neutrophil count (ANC = WBC × % neutrophils) are not highly reliable indicators of infection, especially in preterm infants.
   b. The best indicator of bacterial infection is an elevated immature/total neutrophil ratio, which rarely exceeds 0.4 in full-term, noninfected infants. However, the applicability of this index to the premature infant is not established.
2. Thrombocytopenia may occur but is not a sensitive indicator of infection.
3. Evidence of hemolysis on the peripheral blood smear is consistent with neonatal sepsis but is not sensitive or specific for infection.
4. Gram's stain of the buffy coat from a blood specimen has a predictive value of about 50% for bacterial sepsis and may indicate the degree of bacteremia.
5. The erythrocyte sedimentation rate (ESR) is elevated in most neonates with bacterial infection but has a delayed rate of rise and is falsely positive in Coombs'-positive hemolytic disease. Normal values during the first 2 weeks of life are up to the age in days plus 2.
6. Other acute-phase reactants such as C-reactive protein have not been found helpful in the diagnosis of neonatal sepsis.
7. Elevated serum IgM levels (>15–20 mg/dL) in the first week of life suggest congenital or perinatal infection. However, maternofetal bleeding can cause falsely elevated IgM levels, and overwhelming infection may be associated with normal levels.
8. Latex agglutination tests, usually performed on urine or cerebrospinal fluid (CSF), may assist diagnosis of infec-

tions with group B streptococci, *Escherichia coli* K1, or, rarely, *Hemophilus influenzae* type b, pneumococcus, or meningococcus.

9. TORCHES titers must be interpreted carefully in cases of suspected congenital infection with one of the TORCHES agents (see Table 3–1). Organism-specific IgM titers are usually helpful in establishing a diagnosis but are not always available. Organism-specific IgG titers in the newborn are reflective only of maternal titers. If serial IgG titers are followed in the neonate, initial maternal titers must be known to provide a point of comparison. Failure of neonatal IgG titers to fall below maternal values after several weeks may establish a diagnosis.

III. CONGENITAL (IN UTERO) INFECTIONS:

A. Congenital rubella:

1. **Epidemiology and pathogenesis:**
   a. Presumed route of infection: Maternal viremia leading to placental infection, which then results in fetal infection.
   b. Fetal infection can occur at any stage of pregnancy, with highest infection rates during the first trimester and after 30 weeks gestation. Fetal infection rates approach 100% if maternal rubella is contracted during the last month of pregnancy.
   c. Many clinical findings in congenital rubella result from vascular damage; inflammation is not a prominent finding.
   d. The timing of fetal infection determines the consequences. Sensorineural hearing loss and cardiovascular abnormalities occur only in neonates infected during the first trimester. Congenital defects are not seen in fetuses infected after the fifth month.
2. **Clinical findings:**
   a. General: Intrauterine growth retardation, hepatosplenomegaly, jaundice, and chemical evidence of hepatitis.
   b. More than one half of all infected neonates appear normal at birth, but most later develop signs of disease.
   c. The most common finding is sensorineural hearing loss, which may be progressive.

   d. Central nervous system: Mental retardation, behavioral disorders, hypotonia, seizures, transient electroencephalogram abnormalities, and elevated CSF protein level.
   e. Cardiac: Patent ductus arteriosus, peripheral and valvar pulmonary stenosis, aortic stenosis, and ventricular septal defect.
   f. Ocular: Cataracts, "salt-and-pepper" retinopathy, corneal clouding, and glaucoma (less common).
   g. Orthopedic: Radiographic lucencies in long bone metaphyses.
   h. Hematologic: Transient thrombocytopenia with purpura.
   i. Dermatologic: Dermatoglyphic abnormalities, "blueberry muffin" spots representing dermal erythropoiesis (classic but uncommon).
   j. Endocrine: Diabetes is a common finding in the second or third decade of life.
   k. Pulmonary: Interstitial pneumonitis.
3. **Laboratory aids to diagnosis:**
   a. Documented maternal rubella immunity before conception virtually excludes the diagnosis. Rubella-specific IgM in cord or neonatal blood is a reliable indicator of infection. Rubella-specific IgG in the neonate reflects only maternal immune status.
   b. The virus can usually be isolated from the nasopharynx for the first 6 months of life and may also be cultured from the urine, removed lens tissue, and CSF.
4. **Therapy and prevention:**
   a. No specific therapy exists.
   b. The only means of prevention is maternal avoidance of sources of infection. Immune serum globulin given after exposure does not prevent maternal or fetal infection. Rubella vaccination is contraindicated during pregnancy but is important pre-pregnancy.
   c. Ultimate prevention depends on herd immunity among preschool and school-aged children.

B. Congenital cytomegalovirus (CMV):

1. **Epidemiology and pathogenesis:**
   a. Transplacental infection is common, occurring in 50% of mothers with primary CMV infection but only 1%

of those with recurrent CMV infection. Congenital CMV infection occurs in 1% to 2% of all pregnancies.

b. Fetal damage occurs in 10% to 15% of all congenital CMV infections, nearly always as a result of **primary** maternal infection.
c. In mothers with primary CMV infection, the rate of **symptomatic** fetal infection is highest during the first 6 months of gestation. However, the overall fetal infection rate is highest when the maternal infection occurs near term.
d. CMV infection may interfere with organogenesis early in pregnancy or infect fully formed tissues later in gestation.

2. **Clinical findings:**
   a. Sensorineural hearing loss is most common and occurs in 10% to 15% of **all** children with congenital infection, often as an isolated finding.
   b. More severe congenital CMV infection, termed cytomegalic inclusion disease, may manifest with any combination of the following: intrauterine growth retardation, jaundice, hepatosplenomegaly, chorioretinitis, petechiae secondary to thrombocytopenia, microcephaly, periventricular calcifications, and mental and motor retardation.
3. **Laboratory aids to diagnosis:**
   a. A urine culture for CMV is the gold standard for diagnosis, with CMV usually cultivable from the urine of symptomatic infected neonates in 2 to 3 days. A negative urine culture, if properly performed, virtually excludes congenital CMV infection.
   b. CMV-specific IgM titers may be of value but are of variable reliability and are unnecessary if the urine is properly cultured for CMV.
4. **Therapy and prevention:**
   a. No effective therapy currently exists, but ganciclovir, an antiviral agent used to treat other forms of CMV infection, is presently being evaluated as a treatment for congenital CMV infection.
   b. Efforts to develop a CMV vaccine have not yet succeeded.

C. **Herpes simplex virus (HSV):**
  1. **Epidemiology and pathogenesis:**
     a. The majority of neonatal HSV infection is caused by HSV-2. Incidence is 1 in 2,000 to 5,000 deliveries.
     b. Intrapartum infection is by far the most common form of neonatal HSV infection, but in utero fetal infection, although rare, is well described.
     c. Intrapartum infection results from contact with infective maternal lesions and secretions during labor and passage through the birth canal. The eyes may frequently be the initial portal of infection. Infections in utero may occur transplacentally with maternal viremia or may represent ascending infection across intact membranes.
     d. Intrapartum and in utero infection are most often caused by primary maternal HSV but can also occur with recurrent maternal infection.
  2. **Clinical findings:**
     a. HSV infection in utero typically involves skin (vesicles, bullae, scarring), eye (chorioretinitis, microphthalmia), and CNS (microcephaly, brain atrophy, and hydranencephaly). Cutaneous scarring is not seen in other TORCHES infections and may be a valuable diagnostic clue. Other organs (liver, spleen, lungs, and adrenal glands) may also be involved. Most survivors of in utero HSV infections have severe neurologic deficits.
     b. Intrapartum HSV infections may be divided into three clinical classes:
        1) Disease limited to skin (vesicles and bullae), eye (keratoconjunctivitis and chorioretinitis), and mucous membranes (vesicles and ulcerations) that manifests at about 10 to 11 days of age: Mortality is low in this group, but 25% later develop neurologic abnormalities despite absence of initial CNS involvement.
        2) Localized CNS disease with or without mucocutaneous or ocular involvement, usually manifested by encephalitis (lethargy, irritability, and seizures) manifesting at about 2 weeks of age: Mortality is

15% to 20% in treated and 50% in untreated patients; 40% of survivors have long-term neurologic sequelae.

3) Disseminated disease with or without CNS involvement, usually manifesting in the first week of life with the usual signs and symptoms of sepsis. The liver (hepatomegaly and hepatitis) and adrenals are primarily involved, but many other organs may also be affected, including the lung (pneumonitis) and heart (myocarditis). Few infants initially have obvious manifestations of herpetic disease, such as skin vesicles. Mortality is 15% to 20% in treated and 80% in untreated patients; 40% to 50% of survivors have long-term neurologic sequelae.

3. **Laboratory aids to diagnosis:**
   a. Viral cultures are very useful, but a single negative culture does not exclude infection. Sites for culture include skin vesicles, throat, nasopharynx, conjunctivae, CSF, and urine.
   b. Serology is of limited value. Anti-HSV IgM titers are useful if available. Anti-HSV IgG titers are of little value.
4. **Therapy and prevention:**
   a. Isolation of infected neonates is essential because the virus is excreted in large quantities.
   b. Intravenous (IV) acyclovir, 10 mg/kg q8h for 21 days, is the drug of choice for treatment. Topical ophthalmic therapy is probably also advisable regardless of symptomatic ocular involvement. Suitable agents for ophthalmic therapy include trifluorothymidine, vidarabine, or idoxuridine ophthalmic ointment.
   c. Avoidance of vaginal delivery in mothers who are shedding HSV is an obvious means of preventing intrapartum infection but may be difficult, because 70% of infected newborns are born to mothers who are asymptomatic at delivery. Weekly viral cultures in high-risk women during the last 4 to 8 weeks of pregnancy are not useful for identifying those shedding virus at the time of delivery. Therefore, women with a history of

genital herpes who are asymptomatic and have no lesions on examination at the time of delivery should probably be allowed to deliver vaginally. Cesarean section is indicated for mothers with symptomatic or clinically apparent genital HSV at onset of labor, provided that the membranes have been ruptured <12 hours and ideally <4 hours.

d. Infants born to mothers with active genital HSV should be isolated and cultures done of exposed mucous membranes at 1 to 2 days of age. If cultures are positive, the infant should be treated as outlined above, regardless of symptoms.

e. There is no effective means of preventing in utero HSV infection.

D. Congenital toxoplasmosis:

1. **Epidemiology and pathogenesis:**

a. Intrauterine infection occurs virtually only with primary maternal infection.

b. One half to two thirds of U.S. women of childbearing age are susceptible. Primary infection during pregnancy carries a 60% overall risk of fetal infection. In the United States, the incidence of congenital toxoplasmosis is about 1 per 1,000 live births; 20% of infected infants are symptomatic at birth.

c. Primary maternal infection early in pregnancy uncommonly results in fetal infection, but severe congenital disease results when fetal infection does occur. Primary infection late in pregnancy frequently results in fetal infection but rarely produces symptomatic congenital disease.

d. Placental and fetal infections are caused by the circulating tachyzoite form of the organism.

2. **Clinical findings:**

a. Infection early in gestation can result in fetal death.

b. Chorioretinitis is the most common manifestation of congenital infection. Other features include microcephaly or hydrocephaly, intracranial calcifications, seizures, jaundice, hepatosplenomegaly, rash, cataracts, optic atrophy, pneumonitis, and anemia.

3. **Laboratory aids:**

a. No useful methods of culturing the organism exist, so diagnosis relies on serology.
b. Because the majority of mothers and their newborns are not immune to toxoplasma, antitoxoplasma IgG titers are of value. Negative titers exclude the diagnosis of congenital toxoplasmosis. A positive IgG titer requires confirmatory IgM titers.
c. Anti-*Toxoplasma* IgM is best detected by enzyme-linked immunosorbent assay (ELISA), with 80% sensitivity. Therefore, a negative IgM titer does not totally rule out infection.

4. **Therapy and prevention:**
   a. Treatment is indicated for any symptomatic neonate or any neonate with a positive anti-*Toxoplasma* IgM result.
   b. The infected infant is treated with oral pyrimethamine and sulfadiazine for 21 to 30 days, with supplemental folinic acid.
   c. Treatment of primary maternal infection reduces the incidence of fetal infection. Maternal therapy consists of a 28-day course of pyrimethamine and sulfadiazine with folinic acid. Pyrimethamine is avoided during the first trimester (potential teratogenicity), and sulfadiazine is avoided near term (possible bilirubin displacement).
   d. Isolation is not required; those infected do not excrete the organism.
   e. Prevention: Avoidance of close contact with cat feces and ingestion of raw meats by pregnant women.

E. Congenital syphilis:

1. **Epidemiology and pathogenesis:**
   a. The incidence of congenital syphilis has been increasing since 1980, with an increase from 111 reported cases in the United States in 1980 to 691 reported cases in 1988. In areas of high prevalence, the present incidence of congenital syphilis is about 1 per 1,000 live births; in New York City alone, estimates indicate roughly 1,000 cases for 1989.
   b. The disease typically occurs in infants of mothers with inadequate prenatal care and no serologic testing early in pregnancy.

c. Pathology is a result of the host inflammatory response to *Treponema pallidum*. Thus, symptomatic fetal infection occurs only after the fetus is able to mount an inflammatory response (16–18 weeks gestation), although the treponeme can probably cross the placenta at any time during gestation.
d. Nearly all infants born to women with untreated primary or secondary syphilis are congenitally infected, and 50% are symptomatic. Congenital infection is rare in infants of mothers with latent syphilis.
e. Fetal mortality is highest in untreated first and second trimester infections but is uncommon in third trimester infections. Overall fetal and neonatal mortality may reach 50%.

2. **Clinical findings:**
   a. Clinical features differ for early (<2 years of age) and late (>2 years of age) congenital syphilis.
   b. Common features in neonates: Hepatomegaly, jaundice, and osteochondritis; other findings include nonimmune hydrops, lymphadenopathy, pneumonitis, myocarditis, pseudoparalysis, and anemia.
   c. Infants >1 month of age: Periostitis, rhinitis ("snuffles"), and joint swelling.
   d. Late congenital syphilis: Peg-shaped, notched permanent upper central incisors ("Hutchinson's teeth"), "mulberry molars," interstitial keratitis, eighth nerve deafness, saddle nose, and various neurologic deficits.
3. **Laboratory aids to diagnosis:**
   a. Definitive diagnosis is possible only in rare instances when the organism is directly visualized.
   b. A higher VDRL (Venereal Disease Research Laboratory) titer in the neonate than in the mother indicates probable infection. However, serologic results can be negative in neonates with perinatally acquired infection. Total neonatal IgM and specific antitreponemal IgM titers are **not** reliable indicators of infection.
   c. Long bone radiographs will show osteochondritis and/or periostitis in more than 95% of infected neonates.
   d. CSF examination is essential in neonates with suspected infection and may show elevated protein levels

and pleocytosis. A positive CSF VDRL result is presumptive evidence for congenital neurosyphilis.

4. **Therapy and prevention:**
   a. Neonatal treatment is indicated if maternal treatment for syphilis was inadequate, occurred late in gestation, or did not include penicillin; if neonatal quantitative VDRL result is higher than maternal VDRL result; or when CSF VDRL result is positive.
   b. Neonatal treatment consists of 10 to 14 days of parenteral aqueous penicillin G (100,000–150,000 U/kg/d). This regimen is indicated regardless of CSF VDRL results, because spirochetes have been cultured from otherwise normal CSF.
   c. Prevention includes maternal serologic screening at the first prenatal visit, with additional screening at 28 weeks and at delivery in high-risk populations. Treatment of early maternal syphilis with a single dose of intramuscular (IM) benzathine penicillin G (treatment regimens differ for late and neurosyphilis) prevents 98% of congenital infections.
   d. Follow-up titers are necessary to ensure efficacy of therapy.

F. **Congenital parvovirus B19:**

1. **Epidemiology and pathogenesis:**
   a. The frequency of this infection is low.
   b. Fetal damage results from parvovirus infection of erythroid cell precursors in the bone marrow, causing severe anemia and nonimmune hydrops.
   c. The risk of fetal death secondary to transplacental infection is at least 5% among all infected women and is highest during the first 20 weeks of pregnancy. Fetal death may occur 1 to 10 weeks after maternal infection.
2. **Clinical findings:**
   a. To date, no congenital anomalies are attributable to congenital parvovirus B19 infection.
   b. Infected liveborn infants are usually asymptomatic.
   c. Fetal death from nonimmune hydrops fetalis is usual in symptomatic congenital infection.

3. **Laboratory aids to diagnosis:**
   a. Parvoviral DNA has been demonstrated in tissues of stillborn hydropic fetuses, and assays for virus-specific IgM and IgG exist. These studies may establish congenital parvovirus infection as a cause of death in hydropic stillborns.
4. **Therapy and prevention:**
   a. No specific antiviral therapy exists.
   b. In utero blood transfusions may benefit fetuses with severe anemia from congenital parvovirus B19 infection.
   c. In mothers with acute parvovirus B19 infection (usually manifested by erythema infectiosum, aplastic crisis, or acute arthritis), fetal monitoring with serial ultrasounds and maternal α-fetoprotein (AFP) levels is indicated. Maternal AFP level is elevated in most women with symptomatic fetal infection.

G. Congenital tuberculosis (TB):

1. **Epidemiology and pathogenesis:**
   a. Congenital TB is rare but well described, with >200 reported cases.
   b. Infection may occur in the fetus of any mother with active TB and may result from:
      1) Hematogenous spread via the umbilical vein, resulting in primary liver and lung involvement.
      2) In utero aspiration or swallowing of infected amniotic fluid, resulting in primary lung or gastrointestinal (GI) involvement.
   c. Neonatally acquired TB results from aspiration of infective material during birth or from early postpartum exposure. The manifestations, treatment, and prognosis are similar for congenital and neonatally acquired TB.
   d. The mortality rate is very high in undiagnosed infection but is low if diagnosis is made and treatment is promptly begun.
   e. The severity of neonatal TB is probably related to relative impairments in neonatal T-cell function (see section I, B.).
2. **Clinical findings:**
   a. Hepatosplenomegaly from primary liver involvement is most common, along with respiratory distress (most

have an abnormal chest x-ray film, often with a miliary infiltrate). Fever is common. Neonatal fever and pneumonia unresponsive to antibiotics should strongly suggest the possibility of TB.

b. Other findings include poor feeding, lethargy or irritability, lymphadenopathy, ear discharge, and skin lesions. CNS involvement is less common.

3. **Diagnosis:**
   a. The Beitzke criteria, established in 1935 from autopsy cases, have been used to establish a diagnosis of congenital TB:
      1) Culture-proved *Mycobacterium tuberculosis* infection.
      2) Demonstration of a primary liver complex.
      3) Lesions present in the first days of life.
      4) Exclusion of extrauterine infection if conditions (2) and (3) do not apply.

      These criteria are now less widely used because survival rates are higher, and distinguishing congenital from neonatal TB is of only epidemiologic importance.
   b. The organism is best cultured from early morning gastric aspirates, liver, skin, and lymph node biopsy specimens. Acid-fast bacilli (AFB) may be seen on smears of tracheal aspirates, skin lesion biopsy specimens, bone marrow, and middle ear fluid.
   c. Tuberculin skin test results are rarely positive initially but become positive 2 to 4 months later.
4. **Prevention and therapy:**
   a. Prevention: Prompt diagnosis and treatment of infected mothers. Fetal and neonatal risk is minimal if the mother has a negative sputum culture and has completed chemotherapy. If the mother has not been adequately treated, daily isoniazid (INH) prophylaxis should be initiated for the uninfected infant. Bacille Calmette-Guérin (BCG) vaccination might be considered for the infant in an unreliable home situation with a high risk of infection.
   b. Infected infants should be treated daily with INH, rifampin, and pyrazinamide for 2 months, followed by

4 months of INH and rifampin, if drug resistance is not documented.

c. Isolation is **not** indicated for infected neonates.

IV. PERINATAL INFECTIONS:

A. Enteroviruses (Coxsackie B viruses and echoviruses):

1. **Epidemiology and pathogenesis:**
   a. Coxsackie B virus serotypes 1 to 5 and echovirus serotypes 5, 7, 9, 11, 17, 18, 19, and 22 cause the majority of perinatal enteroviral infections.
   b. Intrauterine transmission of enteroviruses occurs, but most neonatal infections occur intrapartum or immediately postpartum. The mechanism of mother-infant transmission is unknown.
   c. Maternal enterovirus infection is common but is usually asymptomatic in both mother and infant. Symptomatic maternal illness, with fever and abdominal pain, occurs in about 60% of cases of severe neonatal infection.
   d. Symptomatic neonatal infection is most likely if maternal infection occurs within 1 week of delivery. Maternal infection before that time leads to production of IgG, which crosses the placenta and protects the neonate.
   e. Sporadic outbreaks of enteroviral infections have been reported in several nurseries.
2. **Clinical findings:**
   a. Echovirus (especially echovirus 11) produces two distinct neonatal syndromes:
      1) Meningitis/meningoencephalitis, sometimes with pneumonia or myocarditis. CNS infection is usually self-limited but may produce long-term neurologic sequelae.
      2) Primary liver involvement with massive hepatic necrosis, coagulopathy, and hemorrhage. Other organs are relatively spared. Mortality is >80%.
   b. Coxsackie B virus may cause mild, nonspecific febrile illness or severe meningoencephalitis and/or myocarditis.
   c. Enteroviruses are not known to be teratogens.

3. **Laboratory aids to diagnosis:**
   a. Enteroviruses grow readily in culture and may be isolated from nose, throat, stool, blood, urine, and CSF.
   b. Serologic testing is impractical because enteroviruses do not share a common group antigen, and a number of different serotypes cause infection.
4. **Therapy and prevention:**
   a. No effective antiviral chemotherapy exists.
   b. In nursery outbreaks, cohorting infected infants and good handwashing are probably adequate control measures.

B. Listeriosis (*Listeria monocytogenes*):
1. **Epidemiology and pathogenesis:**
   a. Neonatal listeriosis represents one half of all human listerial infections.
   b. Most cases are "early-onset" infections resulting from in utero infection of the fetus and membranes, which precipitates abortion, stillbirth, or preterm delivery a few days to weeks after infection. Fetal infection may involve hematogenous spread via the placenta or ascending infection from the maternal genital tract.
   c. About 20% of cases are "late-onset" infections, manifested by meningitis and sepsis a few days to weeks after delivery. Epidemiology and pathogenesis are uncertain, but the mothers of these infants frequently are genital carriers of *Listeria*.
   d. Early-onset listeriosis is associated with serovars Ia and IVb; late-onset disease is associated with the IVb serovar.
   e. *Listeria* is an intracellular pathogen.
2. **Clinical findings:**
   a. Early-onset listeriosis manifests with stillbirth or with the typical findings of neonatal sepsis (see section II.B.) and often with pneumonia. Early-onset listeriosis is termed "granulomatosis infantiseptica," with widespread microabscesses and granulomas ("listeriomas"), especially in the liver, spleen, and lungs. Characteristic cutaneous and posterior pharyngeal listeriomas may be seen.

b. Late-onset listeriosis is typically manifested by meningitis and sepsis, occurring a few days to weeks after birth in an initially well-appearing neonate.

3. **Laboratory aids to diagnosis:**
   a. Culture of *Listeria* from body fluids or infected tissues is the definitive diagnostic test. Because the organism is a gram-positive to gram-variable coccobacillus, it may be confused on Gram's stain with other organisms.
   b. Serologic testing is not widely available in the United States, but antibody titers by agglutination or complement fixation may be helpful.
4. **Therapy and prevention:**
   a. High-dose parenteral ampicillin for 7 to 10 days is the preferred therapy; longer courses are indicated if widespread granulomas or CNS infection are present. Concomitant use of an aminoglycoside may provide synergism.
   b. Lack of knowledge regarding perinatal transmission makes preventive strategies difficult to devise.

C. Group B streptococcus (GBS) (***Streptococcus agalactiae***):

1. **Epidemiology and pathogenesis:**
   a. GBS is the most common cause of neonatal sepsis and meningitis in most areas.
   b. Two forms of neonatal GBS disease exist:
      1) **Early-onset,** manifested in the first few days of life, results from perinatal mother-infant transmission.
      2) **Late-onset,** manifested after 1 week of age, usually results from nosocomial or community acquisition of GBS.
   c. 30% to 40% of pregnant women are vaginally and/or rectally colonized with GBS, and 40% to 70% of those colonized will vertically transmit GBS to the neonate. About 1% of colonized neonates develop invasive GBS disease, giving an incidence for early-onset GBS sepsis of about 2 to 3 per 1,000 live births. The incidence for late-onset disease is 0.5 to 1.0 per 1,000 live births. Incidence is increased among premature infants.
   d. Invasive GBS disease occurs mainly in neonates, who

do not transplacentally acquire specific antibody because of prematurity or lack of maternal immunity.

e. Two thirds of all GBS sepsis (early and late onset) and nearly all GBS meningitis is caused by serotype III.

2. **Clinical findings:**
   a. Early-onset disease manifests often in the first hours of life with the typical findings of fulminant neonatal sepsis. Pneumonia is often present and indistinguishable from hyaline membrane disease (HMD) on chest x-ray. About 30% of infants with early-onset GBS sepsis develop meningitis.
   b. Late onset disease manifests after the first week of life with meningitis and often with sepsis. Late-onset GBS infection has a more insidious onset and is usually less severe than early-onset infection.
   c. Neonatal skin infections, septic arthritis, and osteomyelitis are often caused by GBS.
3. **Laboratory aids to diagnosis:**
   a. GBS is readily cultured from blood, CSF, urine, or endotracheal tube aspirates.
   b. Rapid antigen detection by latex agglutination or counterimmunoelectrophoresis (CIE) of urine or CSF is a reliable and efficient diagnostic tool.
4. **Therapy and prevention:**
   a. Treatment of choice for established GBS infection is parenteral aqueous penicillin G (150,000–200,000 units/kg/day if meningitis is not present; the dose is doubled if meningitis is present). Duration of treatment is 14 to 21 days, depending on clinical response.
   b. An effective maternal GBS vaccine will not be available in the near future.
   c. Studies have indicated that parenteral ampicillin given at the onset of labor to women heavily colonized with GBS is effective in preventing neonatal GBS infection. Rapid antigen detection methods enable prompt identification of heavily colonized mothers.
   d. Neonatal immunoprophylaxis with IV immunoglobulin (IVIG) may be effective, but proof of efficacy is presently lacking.
   e. Immunotherapy using hyperimmune IVIG with a high

concentration of specific anti-GBS antibody is a promising but unproved treatment modality.

D. *E. coli:*

1. **Epidemiology and pathogenesis:**
   a. **E. coli** is the second most common cause of neonatal sepsis and meningitis.
   b. Three fourths of neonatal *E. coli* meningitis and 40% of neonatal *E. coli* sepsis are caused by strains with the K1 capsular antigen.
   c. 20% to 30% of infants are colonized with *E. coli* K1 as a result of perinatal mother-infant transmission; 0.3% to 0.5% of colonized infants develop invasive *E. coli* disease.
   d. Enteropathogenic *E. coli* (EPEC) is a cause of neonatal gastroenteritis. Infection with EPEC is by the fecal-oral route and can result in nursery epidemics. The pathogenesis of EPEC gastroenteritis involves adherence to intestinal mucosa with disruption of microvilli and possibly toxin production.
2. **Clinical findings:**
   a. Invasive *E. coli* infection manifests with the usual findings of neonatal sepsis. A distinctive clinical syndrome does not exist.
   b. *E. coli* causes a variety of localized infections, including urinary tract infections and ascending cholangitis (especially in infants receiving prolonged parenteral hyperalimentation following biliary tract surgery).
   c. Neonatal gastroenteritis caused by EPEC manifests with emesis and diarrhea of variable severity, beginning 2 to 12 days after exposure. Fever is not always present. Stools are rarely bloody.
3. **Laboratory aids to diagnosis:**
   a. *E. coli* is reliably cultured from blood, CSF, and urine.
   b. K1 antigen is reliably detected by latex agglutination or CIE in urine and CSF.
   c. It is very difficult for clinical laboratories to differentiate EPEC from normal fecal flora, except in nursery epidemics. No convenient methodology for detection currently exists.
4. **Therapy:**

a. Treatment of invasive *E. coli* infections: Parenteral ceftriaxone or ampicillin, with or without an aminoglycoside. Treatment is continued for a minimum of 3 weeks in cases of *E. coli* meningitis and for 2 to 3 weeks for sepsis without meningitis.
b. Treatment of EPEC gastroenteritis is primarily supportive. The value of antibiotic therapy is uncertain.

V. POSTNATAL AND NOSOCOMIAL INFECTIONS:

A. Coagulase-negative staphylococci (CNS):

1. **Epidemiology and pathogenesis:**
   a. Neonatal sepsis caused by CNS is seen chiefly in long-term neonatal intensive care unit (NICU) patients, particularly premature infants with indwelling vascular catheters or those subjected to invasive procedures.
   b. *Staphylococcus epidermidis* is the species most commonly isolated, but other species are seen, including *Staphylococcus hominis, Staphylococcus warneri,* and *Staphylococcus saprophyticus.*
   c. CNS are the most common nosocomial pathogens in many NICUs, causing sepsis in up to 3% to 10% of all NICU admissions and accounting for at least 10% of all septic episodes in most NICUs.
   d. The source of the organism is usually skin, but contaminated hyperalimentation solutions may be implicated.
2. **Clinical findings:**
   a. CNS sepsis is usually of subacute onset, manifesting with apnea, bradycardia, lethargy, temperature instability, and feeding intolerance. Osteomyelitis may occur.
   b. Mortality rates are relatively low in CNS sepsis.
3. **Laboratory aids to diagnosis:**
   a. CNS are reliably recovered from infected body fluids.
   b. CNS in blood cultures are sometimes dismissed as skin contaminants. They should be considered pathogens if they grow from aerobic and anaerobic bottles in ≤ 72 hours, are grown from a second site (e.g., repeat blood culture or CSF), or if they are recovered from a septic-appearing NICU patient who has indwelling vascular

catheters or has undergone invasive procedures. They are also likely to be significant in infants with indwelling prosthetic devices such as CSF shunts or reservoirs.

4. **Therapy and prevention:**
   a. Because of high rates of methicillin resistance among CNS, parenteral vancomycin is the treatment of choice and should be given for a minimum of 10 days. Many CNS isolates appear sensitive to cephalothin in vitro, but this may not be a suitable drug, particularly for methicillin-resistant strains or central nervous system infections.
   b. Removal or replacement of indwelling vascular catheters is indicated when possible.
   c. Minimizing invasive procedures and limiting the use of indwelling vascular catheters are useful but often impractical preventive strategies in the ill NICU patient.

B. *Candida:*

1. **Epidemiology and pathogenesis:**
   a. Four forms of neonatal candidal infections exist: oral candidiasis (thrush), cutaneous (diaper area) candidiasis, systemic candidiasis, and congenital candidiasis (rare).
   b. *Candida albicans* is the main species causing neonatal disease, but other species occasionally infect infants.
   c. *Candida* is acquired during passage through the birth canal or postnatally during breast-feeding, from contaminated bottle nipples, or other sources in the environment. Congenital candidiasis presumably results from ascending infection with amnionitis.
   d. *Candida* is normally a commensal organism but becomes pathogenic when the normal host-organism relationship is disrupted. Such disruptions include host immunosuppression, antibiotic use that alters normal bacterial flora and allows candidal overgrowth, and disruption of normal tissue barriers. These contribute to the high prevalence of systemic candidiasis in premature infants, who are relatively immunosuppressed, frequently receive antibiotic therapy, and usually have indwelling vascular catheters.

e. Oral and cutaneous candidiasis are common throughout the neonatal period. Systemic candidiasis occurs sometime after the first week in the premature, long-term NICU patient and may occur in up to 2% to 4% of all very low birth weight (VLBW) infants. Congenital candidiasis is rare and manifests at birth.

2. **Clinical findings:**
   a. Oral candidiasis manifests with adherent white mucosal plaques. It is usually asymptomatic but may produce irritation interfering with feeding.
   b. Cutaneous candidiasis in the diaper area manifests as coalescent erythematous vesiculopapular lesions accompanied by satellite lesions encircled by a fine, scaling collarette. It is most prominent in intertriginous areas.
   c. Congenital candidiasis typically manifests at birth with an extensive maculopapular rash, sometimes with vesicles or pustules, maximal in intertriginous areas. Candidal pneumonia may also be present and carries a grave prognosis. Hematogenous spread does not occur; infection is limited to the skin, lungs, and GI tract.
   d. Systemic candidiasis is defined as candidal infection of a normally sterile body site. Candidemia is usual. Sites of involvement may include eyes (endophthalmitis), urinary tract (renal parenchymal or bladder infection), CNS (meningitis), liver (usually asymptomatic), lungs, bones and joints, occasionally skin (rash, abscess), and, rarely, the heart (endocarditis). Thrombocytopenia may be present. Clinical onset may be somewhat subtle, but infected infants usually appear septic, with a predominance of GI and respiratory symptoms.
3. **Laboratory aids to diagnosis:**
   a. In oral and cutaneous candidiasis, potassium hydroxide preparations of scrapings from lesions frequently demonstrate the organism.
   b. Systemic candidiasis is definitively diagnosed by culturing the organism from a normally sterile body site. *Candida* grows well in routine blood cultures but may require several days. Blood cultures may be intermittently positive.

c. There are no useful serologic or rapid antigen detection tests for candidiasis.

4. **Therapy:**

a. Oral candidiasis is treated with nystatin solution. Topical 1% gentian violet may be used in persistent or severe cases. Cutaneous candidiasis is treated with topical antifungals containing nystatin, clotrimazole, or a related agent.

b. The cornerstone of therapy for systemic candidiasis is IV amphotericin B, beginning at a dose of 0.1 to 0.25 mg/kg/day and increasing in increments of 0.25 mg/kg/day as tolerated to a maximum dose of 0.5 to 1.0 mg/kg/day. The drug is given once daily over 4 to 6 hours. The maximum daily dose and duration of therapy are controversial and may be limited by patient tolerance. Treatment is for at least 4 weeks and longer if candidemia is persistent. It is common to change to alternate-day therapy after clearance of infection is demonstrated and the patient has stabilized. Side effects that may require limitation of dosage or temporary cessation of therapy are nephrotoxicity with hypokalemia, hepatotoxicity, and bone marrow suppression.

c. For systemic candidiasis, flucytosine (5-FC) may be given orally, 100 to 150 mg/kg/day in three to four divided doses in conjunction with amphotericin B. It provides better central nervous system penetrance and may be synergistic with amphotericin.

VI. EVALUATION AND TREATMENT OF THE FEBRILE NEONATE AND YOUNG INFANT (<2 MONTHS):

A. Definition of fever:

1. Rectal temperatures **must** be taken; surface (axillary) temperatures are poor indicators of core temperatures.
2. A single rectal temperature >38.5°C definitely constitutes having a fever; many define having a fever as a rectal temperature >38.0°C, especially if present on two readings at least 1 hour apart.

B. Identification of the febrile neonate at risk for sepsis:

1. Febrile prematures and neonates <30 days of age who have perinatal risk factors for sepsis (e.g., maternal fever,

prolonged rupture of membranes) are at increased risk for sepsis.

2. The single most useful predictor of sepsis or bacteremia is the infant's overall clinical appearance (activity, responsiveness, consolability, feeding pattern), especially if confirmed by more than one observer. Laboratory tests should be used to confirm clinical impressions and should not be the sole basis for decision making.
3. A total WBC count $<5{,}000/mm^3$, a total band count of $>1{,}500/mm^3$, and an immature/total neutrophil ratio >0.4 appear to indicate a greater likelihood of sepsis.
4. Latex agglutination or CIE of urine or CSF to detect bacterial antigens may be of value in identifying the bacteremic neonate.
5. Nonspecific indicators of inflammation such as the ESR and C-reactive protein (see section II.C.5–6) are of limited value by themselves but may be useful in conjunction with other diagnostic tests.

C. Initial diagnostic evaluation:

1. Overall clinical assessment with a thorough physical examination looking for foci of infection is essential.
2. Minimum laboratory evaluation includes a CBC, with differential, urinalysis, urine culture (via suprapubic aspiration or urethral catheterization), chest x-ray, and at least one blood culture with a minimum of 0.5 mL of blood/bottle. Lumbar puncture is usually indicated unless the clinical suspicion for sepsis or meningitis is extremely low and the child will be under close observation.
3. Other diagnostic tests (latex agglutination or CIE, ESR, C-reactive protein) may be performed at the physician's discretion.

D. Treatment options:

1. Ill-appearing infants or those with confirmed meningitis or other serious focal bacterial infections should be admitted to the hospital for appropriate parenteral antibiotic therapy.
   a. Initial empiric therapy before availability of culture results include ampicillin; in addition, an aminoglycoside is typically used; ampicillin plus ceftriaxone or cefotaxime is an acceptable alternative and is preferred in

neonates >1 month of age. Ceftriaxone may be used alone in young infants >1 month of age. In the older NICU patient who becomes febrile, empiric penicillinase-resistant penicillin (e.g., nafcillin) and an aminoglycoside are recommended.

b. If no organisms are isolated from cultures after 72 hours and no focus of infection is apparent, antibiotics may be stopped. In the persistently febrile, ill-appearing neonate with negative bacterial cultures, systemic viral infection must be considered, especially HSV-2.

2. The well-appearing neonate with no focus of infection may be admitted for observation without antibiotic therapy until all cultures are negative. Observation at home is an option only when the care providers are extremely reliable and can easily return to the hospital if the infant's condition worsens.
3. These are only general guidelines; tailoring of treatment decisions to the clinical situation at hand is essential.

4 DISEASES IN IMMUNOCOMPROMISED HOST

I. PRIMARY IMMUNE DEFICIENCY STATES:

A. Disorders of Antibody-Mediated Immunity:

1. Transient hypogammaglobulinemia of infancy:
   a. **Definition:**
      1) Exaggerated physiologic hypogammaglobulinemia.
      2) Results from delayed onset of immunoglobulin synthesis.
      3) Onset between 4 and 9 months of age, after most maternal IgG has been catabolized, and lasts 6 to 18 months.

   b. **Epidemiology:** Occasional familial occurrence; affects both males and females. Premature infants are particularly susceptible.

   c. **Clinical course:**
      1) Usually manifests after 6 months of age with recurrent viral and/or bacterial infections, most frequently of the respiratory tract.
      2) Many infants with transient hypogammaglobulinemia have no significant infections.
      3) IgG level is usually greater than 200 mg/dL but less than normal for age.

   d. **Treatment:** Usually no therapy is required. Occasionally, immune serum globulin (ISG) is indicated in patients with severe recurrent infections.

2. X-linked agammaglobulinemia:
   a. **Definition:**
      1) Also called Bruton's, or congenital, hypogammaglobulinemia.
      2) These patients have virtually no circulating B cells, low to absent serum immunoglobulin levels, and no

plasma cells or germinal centers in lymphoid tissues.
3) T cells are normal both qualitatively and quantitatively.
4) This B-cell defect is probably secondary to a maturational block in early B-cell development from pre-B-cells to B-cells.

b. **Epidemiology:** Transmitted in an X-linked recessive pattern.

c. **Clinical course:**
1) Affected individuals after 6 months of age have recurrent infections, most often with encapsulated bacteria.
2) Most common sites of infection are the upper and lower respiratory tracts, and the patient has meningitis, sepsis, and osteomyelitis/septic arthritis as well.
3) Gastrointestinal (GI) tract is usually free of disease.
4) Chronic inflammation and swelling of joints similar to juvenile rheumatoid arthritis develop frequently.
5) These patients have a severe to absolute deficiency of all immunoglobulin classes; cellular immunity is intact.

d. **Treatment:**
1) Periodic (q3–4wk) immune serum globulin or intravenous γ-globulin (IVGG) replacement therapy is effective in preventing severe recurrent infections.
2) Prophylactic antibiotics are not recommended.
3) Without replacement therapy, many develop chronic progressive bronchiectasis and ultimately die of pulmonary insufficiency.

3. Common variable hypogammaglobulinemia (acquired or late-onset hypogammaglobulinemia):

a. **Definition:**
1) Represents many separate disorders, with heterogeneous features.
2) Most probably have an intrinsic defect in B-cell differentiation; many defects are described.

   b. **Epidemiology:** Both sexes are affected equally; familial occurrences are reported.
   c. **Clinical course:**
      1) Symptoms rarely begin before 6 years of age; in most patients, the disease begins in the second or third decade of life.
      2) Recurrent and chronic sinopulmonary infections are the most common manifestations.
      3) Chronic progressive bronchiectasis frequently develops.
      4) Other manifestations:
         a) Sprue-like syndrome, occurring in up to 60% of patients.
         b) Pernicious anemia, autoimmune hemolytic anemia, leukopenia, and thrombocytopenia.
         c) Polyarthritis/polyarthralgias.
         d) Rheumatoid arthritis, systemic lupus erythematosus (SLE), idiopathic thrombocytopenic purpura (ITP), and other autoimmune disorders.
         e) Sarcoid-like noncaseating granulomas of the lungs, spleen, liver, and skin.
      5) **Laboratory abnormalities:**
         a) IgG levels usually <300 mg/dL; IgA and IgM levels are frequently undetectable.
         b) Many have or later develop T-cell abnormalities.
      6) **Treatment:** ISG is effective both for control of recurrent infections and for other associated manifestations. Chronic sinopulmonary disease can slowly progress.
4. Selective IgA deficiency:
   a. These patients have absent or markedly reduced levels of serum IgA (<5 mg/dL), with normal or elevated levels of IgG or IgM. Secretory IgA is usually absent also.
   b. This is the most common form of immunodeficiency; incidence is between 1 in 400 and 1 in 700.
   c. This disorder appears to be inherited as autosomal recessive or dominant.
   d. Some patients remain healthy throughout life; others have recurrent infections or an increased risk for al-

lergy, sinopulmonary infections, GI tract disease, and autoimmune disease.

e. Patients with IgA deficiency and recurrent upper and lower respiratory tract infections often have associated deficiency of IgG2, IgG3, or IgG4.

f. ISG or IVGG should not be used because they contain only IgG. To avoid anaphylaxis, only IgA-free preparations of IVGG should be used only in cases with severe recurrent infections and associated IgG subclass deficiency.

B. Cellular Immunodeficiency Disorders:

1. Severe combined immunodeficiency disease (SCID):
   a. **Epidemiology:** Can be inherited as an autosomal recessive (adenosine deaminase [ADA] deficient) or an X-linked recessive trait.
   b. **Clinical features:**
      1) Infants usually are sick early in life with recurrent infections with fungi, *Pneumocystis carinii,* viruses, and bacteria.
      2) These patients are susceptible to graft-vs-host disease (GVH) after transfusions or attempts to reconstitute them.
      3) Physical examination reveals absence of tonsils and lymph nodes; oral thrush and wasting are usually present.
      4) Laboratory data include lymphopenia, diminished serum immunoglobulin levels, anemia, negative intradermal skin tests, and impaired in vitro proliferative responses to mitogens and antigens.
   c. **Management:**
      1) Care must be taken to limit exposure to infection.
      2) Use irradiated blood to prevent GVH.
      3) Histocompatible bone marrow transplantation is the treatment of choice. ADA-deficient patients can be treated with red blood cell (RBC) transfusions or gene replacement therapy.
      4) Fetal tissue (liver or thymus) transplants have had limited success.
   d. **Prognosis:** Without a bone marrow transplant, the majority of patients die of infection before 1 to 2 years of age.

2. DiGeorge syndrome:
   a. **Epidemiology:** Dysmorphogenesis of the third and fourth pharyngeal pouches results in aplasia or hypoplasia of the thymus and of parathyroid glands, as well as abnormalities of the great vessels.
   b. **Clinical features:**
      1) These infants have a characteristic facies with short philtrum, mandibular hypoplasia, hypertelorism, and low-set notched ears.
      2) Patients may be seen for hypocalcemic seizures or for evaluation of cardiac disease.
      3) Severity of thymic hypoplasia is extremely variable. Most patients have partial or complete absence of T-cell function, which may improve with time, with normal to near-normal B-cell function.
   c. **Treatment:**
      1) Must be individualized based on severity of the disease.
      2) Immunologic defect can be corrected by fetal thymic implant.
3. Chronic mucocutaneous candidiasis (CMC):
   a. **Epidemiology:** A collection of related syndromes in which patients may have limited local disease or extensive cutaneous and mucosal involvement.
   b. **Clinical features:**
      1) Cell-mediated immunity is most frequently impaired, with nonreactive skin test to *Candida* antigens despite candidiasis.
      2) Cellular immunity to other organisms is normal.
      3) The antibody, complement, and phagocytic systems are intact, thereby protecting the patient from overwhelming *Candida* sepsis.
      4) CMC may be associated with autoimmune polyendocrinopathy, including hypoparathyroid, hypothyroid, hypoadrenal, and hypogonadism. Autoimmune chronic active hepatitis, renal tubular acidosis, or chronic pulmonary disease may develop.
      5) Patients with this disorder should receive a complete endocrinologic and hepatic evaluation.
   c. **Treatment:** Topical antifungal agents; IV amphotericin B, oral ketoconazole or fluconazole may be necessary

in more severe disease. (See Table A–18.) Endocrinopathies must be treated by replacement therapy. Chronic active hepatitis responds to corticosteroids or cytotoxic drugs.

4. Wiskott-Aldrich syndrome:
   a. **Definition:** X-linked recessive disease with recurrent infection, eczema, thrombocytopenia, and inability to form specific antibody to carbohydrate antigens. The basic defect is unknown.
   b. **Clinical manifestations:**
      1) Affected boys may as newborns have bleeding and petechiae secondary to thrombocytopenia.
      2) Recurrent infections, especially with encapsulated organisms, begin in infancy.
      3) Eczema may become very extensive.
      4) As cellular immune function decreases with age, the incidence of viral, fungal, and protozoal infections increases.
      5) These patients are predisposed to malignancies.
   c. **Laboratory manifestations:**
      1) Platelets are diminished in number and one half the normal size.
      2) IgG levels are normal or slightly low; IgM level is usually low; IgA and IgE levels are markedly elevated.
      3) Isohemagglutinin levels and responses to polysaccharide antigens are diminished.
      4) T-cell responses to antigens and mitogens are impaired.
   d. **Treatment:**
      1) Splenectomy may improve thrombocytopenia.
      2) Bone marrow transplantation from an HLA/MLC identical donor is the optimal treatment.
   e. **Prognosis:**
      1) Without transplantation, mean age at death is approximately 3 to 4 years.
      2) Early deaths are usually secondary to massive hemorrhage.
      3) Older children usually die of an overwhelming infection or lymphoid malignancy.

5. Ataxia-telangiectasia:
   a. **Definition:** Autosomal recessive syndrome characterized by progressive cerebellar ataxia, increasing telangiectasia, recurrent sinopulmonary infections, and a propensity to develop malignancies.
   b. **Clinical manifestations:**
      1) Ataxia is often the first manifestation and usually becomes evident when the infant begins to sit or stand.
      2) Telangiectasias, which usually appear later than ataxia, initially develop on the bulbar conjunctivae, later on skin.
      3) Initially patients may have normal antibody-mediated and cell-mediated immunity; however, both deteriorate with time.
      4) Numerous malignancies occur in these patients; lymphosarcoma is the most common. Others include Hodgkin's disease, leukemia, adenocarcinoma, dysgerminoma, and medulloblastoma.
   c. **Treatment:** No satisfactory therapy is currently available.
   d. **Prognosis:** Tumors and chronic sinopulmonary infections are the most common causes of death. Life expectancy is variable; it may range from several years after manifestation to as long as 40 years.
6. Acquired immunodeficiency syndrome (see chapter 5).

C. Disorders of the Complement System:

1. Clq, Clr, Cls, C2, and C4 deficiencies:
   a. These disorders are associated with an increased susceptibility to bacterial infection, as well as to development of collagen vascular diseases, especially SLE.
   b. In addition to SLE, Henoch-Schönlein purpura, dermatomyositis, vasculitis, inflammatory bowel disease, glomerulonephritis, mild urticaria, common variable hypogammaglobulinemia, and Hodgkin's disease have been reported in these patients.
2. C3 deficiency:
   a. C3 plays an important role in opsonization.
   b. Patients with this deficiency frequently have recurrent severe encapsulated bacterial infections.

3. Deficiency of the terminal complement components (C5, C6, C7, C8, and C9).
   a. These patients may be healthy.
   b. Some individuals with these deficiencies have increased susceptibility to systemic neisserial infections (gonococcal, meningococcal).
   c. These patients manifest abnormal bacteriolysis for *Neisseria*.

D. Disorders of the Phagocytic System:

1. Chronic granulomatous disease (CGD):
   a. **Definition:** CGD is associated with several distinct defects in intracellular killing of bacteria after opsonization and phagocytosis, resulting in chronic, granulomatous deep-seated infections.
   b. **Epidemiology:** The most common forms are inherited as X-linked recessives, although autosomal recessive forms exist.
   c. **Clinical features:**
      1) Organisms that cause infections are those that do not produce hydrogen peroxide and/or do produce catalase (i.e., primarily staphylococci, *Klebsiella, Serratia, Salmonella, Aspergillus,* and *Candida*).
      2) Patients usually have staphylococcal skin infections or lymphadenitis.
      3) Pulmonary disorders (e.g., pneumonia, hilar lymphadenopathy, empyema, and lung abscess) occur in most affected children.
      4) GI disorders are also common in patients with CGD, including gastric outlet obstruction, malabsorption, and perianal fistula. Liver abscesses are common.
      5) Hepatosplenomegaly is a frequent finding, probably secondary to the spread of bacteria to the reticuloendothelial system.
   d. **Diagnosis:** Made by demonstration of the inability of leukocytes to reduce nitroblue tetrazolium (NBT) from colorless to deep blue during phagocytosis (NBT test) and confirmed by showing impaired killing after phagocytosis.

e. **Treatment:**
   1) Long-term prophylactic antibiotics (usually trimethoprim-sulfa) decrease the number of infections.
   2) Bone marrow transplantation has been successful in a few patients.
   3) Recombinant interferon-γ is effective in reducing the frequency and severity of infections.

2. Chediak-Higashi syndrome:
   a. Characterized by frequent bacterial infections, partial oculocutaneous albinism, and giant cytoplasmic granules in peripheral leukocytes.
   b. It is inherited in an autosomal recessive manner.
   c. Intracellular bacterial killing is defective secondary to impaired lysosomal fusion with phagocytic vacuoles.
   d. Neutropenia may be present.
   e. Lymphocyte natural killer cell activity is decreased.
   f. Infections are treated with appropriate antibiotics. Ascorbic acid may improve neutrophil function.
3. Job syndrome (Hyper-IgE syndrome):
   a. Etiology is unknown.
   b. These patients have repeated episodes of skin abscess formation associated with otitis, chronic eczema, mucocutaneous candidiasis, and serum levels of IgE $> 2,000$ μg/dL.
   c. Abscesses typically do not manifest warmth, redness, or swelling.
   d. The organism most frequently isolated is *Staphylococcus aureus*.
4. Myeloperoxidase deficiency:
   a. There is a complete absence of peroxidase-positive granules in monocytes and neutrophils.
   b. Affected patients are at risk for opportunistic bacterial and fungal infections; *Candida albicans* poses the greatest threat to these patients.

II. SECONDARY IMMUNODEFICIENCIES:

Secondary immunodeficiencies are more common than primary immunodeficiencies and refer to impaired host defenses (transiently or permanently) as a result of a primary disease.

A. Malnutrition:

1. This is the most common form of secondary immunodeficiency worldwide.
2. Malnutrition, especially at an early age, results in severe immunologic impairment.
3. Malnutrition markedly increases susceptibility to infections.
   a. Almost 50% of children with protein-calorie malnutrition (PCM) who require hospital admission do so because of acute infection.
   b. Bacterial infections, especially pneumonias, are very frequent in these patients.
   c. Measles is a major cause of morbidity and mortality in these patients.
   d. The immunodeficiency of PCM includes numerous defects of the immune system.
      1) Cell-mediated immunity is most commonly impaired in PCM:
         a) Malnourished patients have thymic atrophy, depletion of paracortical cells in peripheral lymphoid tissue, and varying degrees of lymph node germinal center depletion.
         b) Lymphopenia occurs in one fourth of children who die from malnutrition.
         c) The absolute T-cell number is diminished.
         d) Cutaneous delayed hypersensitivity reactions are impaired.
      2) Several defects of polymorphonuclear neutrophil (PMN) function have been described:
         a) Diminished migration of PMNs in response to bacterial chemotactic factors.
         b) Decreased adherence of PMNs.
         c) Diminished bactericidal and candidicidal activity.
      3) Decreased serum levels of complement components have been found.
      4) Serum immunoglobulin concentrations are normal to increased.

B. Thermal Burns:

1. Burns are a major cause of acquired immunodeficiency.
2. Septicemia is a common complication.
3. *Pseudomonas, Proteus,* streptococci, and *S. aureus* are the major offenders.
4. Burn patients are also at risk for viral infections, such as *herpes simplex* and varicella.
5. The immune system is affected in the following ways:
   a. With injury to the skin, a primary barrier to infection is compromised.
   b. Impaired PMN margination and phagocytic function occur.
   c. Serum immunoglobulin levels fall during the first few days after thermal injury and return to normal over the next several weeks.
      1) IgG is the major immunoglobulin affected.
      2) Lowest immunoglobulin levels occur 2 days after injury.
   d. C3 and C4 deficiencies have been reported.
   e. Lymphopenia occurs promptly after thermal injury, and counts return to normal levels within the first week.
   f. Delayed hypersensitivity skin reactions are depressed.

C. Lymphoid Malignancies:

1. Hodgkin's disease and other lymphomas:
   a. The degree of immunologic defect may be related to the clinical stage and the histologic type of the disease, as well as to therapy.
   b. Lymphocytosis is more commonly seen, but lymphopenia may develop as the disease progresses.
   c. Leukocyte chemotaxis is abnormal.
   d. Defects of cell-mediated immunity are frequent:
      1) The majority of patients show a loss of cutaneous reactivity.
      2) Many patients have decreased in vitro lymphocyte responses to mitogens such as phytohemagglutinin (PHA), as well as impaired synthesis of lymphokines and macrophage aggregation factor.
   e. Serum immunoglobulin levels are usually normal.
   f. Total serum complement is normal or elevated in most patients.

2. **Leukemia:**
   a. Increased susceptibility to infections occurs particularly in patients with neutropenia; however, infections may also occur when the leukocyte count is normal.
   b. Local leukocyte mobilization is markedly decreased.
   c. In contrast to patients with lymphomas, patients with leukemia usually have normal humoral and cell-mediated immunity until they receive chemotherapy or are terminal.

D. Immunosuppressive Agents:

1. **Radiation therapy:**
   a. Lymphopenia and impaired lymphocyte responses to mitogens may persist for more than 1 year.
   b. T-helper cells (CD4+ cells) are most drastically affected.
   c. Humoral immunity (antibody responses) is relatively radioresistant.
2. **Corticosteroids:**
   a. Corticosteroids cause lymphopenia and monocytopenia.
   b. Antibody-mediated immunity:
      1) Large doses of corticosteroids can decrease serum immunoglobulin levels.
      2) Low to moderate doses do not affect antibody synthesis.
   c. Cell-mediated immunity:
      1) Transient panlymphopenia occurs hours after high-dose IV glucocorticoids; CD4+ (helper) cells are more severely depressed than CD8+ (suppressor) cells.
      2) In patients receiving alternate-day prednisone therapy, lymphocyte numbers and responses are normal on the off-day of therapy.
      3) Cutaneous delayed hypersensitivity responses are suppressed; however, this is thought to actually result from impaired macrophage function.
   d. Phagocytic system:
      1) Corticosteroids suppress the accumulation of PMNs at a site of inflammation.
      2) Bactericidal and fungicidal activity of monocytes is reduced.

3. Cyclophosphamide:
   a. Cyclophosphamide decreases immunoglobulin production and impairs both B- and T-cell function.
   b. Large doses effectively suppress antibody responses.
   c. Lymphopenia may develop, especially of CD4+ (helper) cells.
   d. Even low doses can impair cutaneous delayed hypersensitivity.
   e. This agent is anti-inflammatory, as well as immunosuppressive.

E. Sickle Cell Disease (SCD):

1. Patients with SCD manifest an increased incidence of meningitis and septicemia.
2. Serious infections are more common in SCD (homozygous hemoglobin S) than in patients with other hemoglobinopathies.
3. *Streptococcus pneumoniae* is the most common offending organism; *Hemophilus influenzae* type b is the other common offender.
4. Both splenic hypofunction and tissue hypoxia related to microvascular sludging by sickled erythrocytes contribute to the increased susceptibility to infections.
   a. The spleen, in addition to the liver, helps in the clearance of microorganisms from the bloodstream and is particularly important in the nonimmune individual.
   b. As a major lymphoid organ, the spleen also plays an important role in the synthesis of antibodies.
5. Sera from patients with SCD have a deficiency of opsonic activity against *S. pneumoniae;* however, the deficient factor has not been identified.
6. These patients have normal to elevated levels of serum immunoglobulins.
7. Patients with SCD should receive chronic oral penicillin prophylaxis and pneumococcal and *Hemophilus* vaccines, in addition to routine vaccinations. Antibody responses to pure polysaccharide agents are very limited before 18 to 24 months of age. (See Chapter 1.)

PEDIATRIC AIDS: HIV INFECTION IN CHILDREN

5

I. DEFINITION:

Human immunodeficiency virus (HIV) infection covers a spectrum ranging from apparently healthy to critically ill. The most severe HIV-related disease is acquired immune deficiency syndrome (AIDS). Summary of the revised 1987 CDC Surveillance case definition for pediatric AIDS is as follows:

A. **Without laboratory evidence of HIV infection** (i.e., not done or inconclusive), a patient with AIDS:
   1. Does not have another cause of immunodeficiency.
   2. Has one of the following AIDS indicator diseases definitively diagnosed:
      a. Candidiasis of the esophagus, trachea, bronchi, or lungs.
      b. Extrapulmonary cryptococcosis (e.g., meningitis).
      c. Cryptosporidiosis, with diarrhea persisting > 1 month.
      d. Cytomegaloviral disease other than of liver, spleen, or lymph nodes in a patient >1 month.
      e. Herpes simplex of the mouth of >1 month duration, bronchitis, pneumonitis, or esophagitis in a patient >1 month.
      f. Primary brain lymphoma in a patient < 60 years.
      g. Lymphoid interstitial pneumonia (LIP) in a child < 13 years old.
      h. Atypical mycobacterial disease disseminated to sites other than lungs, skin, or cervical/hilar lymph nodes.
      i. *Pneumocystis carinii* pneumonia (PCP).
      j. Progressive multifocal leukoencephalopathy.
      k. Toxoplasmosis of the brain in a patient >1 month.

B. **With laboratory evidence of HIV infection,** a patient with AIDS:

1. Has one of the AIDS indicator diseases listed previously or one of the following AIDS indicator diseases definitively diagnosed:
   a. Multiple or recurrent (at least two within 2 years) serious bacterial infections in a child < 13 years old.
   b. Disseminated coccidiomycosis or histoplasmosis to site other than to lungs or cervical/hilar lymph nodes.
   c. HIV encephalopathy.
   d. Isosporiasis with diarrhea persisting > 1 month.
   e. Kaposi's sarcoma.
   f. Primary brain lymphoma or other non-Hodgkin's lymphoma.
   g. Disseminated atypical mycobacterial disease involving a site other than lungs, skin, or lymph nodes.
   h. Tuberculosis involving at least one site other than lungs.
   i. HIV wasting syndrome.
2. Or has one of the following AIDS indicator diseases presumptively diagnosed:
   a. Esophageal candidiasis.
   b. Cytomegalovirus (CMV) retinitis with loss of vision.
   c. Kaposi's sarcoma.
   d. LIP or lymphoid hyperplasia in a child < 13 years old.
   e. Disseminated mycobacterial infection to a site other than lungs or lymph nodes.
   f. PCP.
   g. Toxoplasmosis of the brain in a patient >1 month old.

C. **With laboratory evidence against HIV infection** (negative test results), a patient with AIDS does not have another cause of underlying immunodeficiency *and:*

1. Has had PCP definitively diagnosed.
2. Or has had definitive diagnosis of one of the AIDS indicator diseases listed under section A. plus a CD4+ lymphocyte count <400/mm^3.

D. **Asymptomatic HIV-infected children** are considered seropositive.

E. **Symptomatic children not meeting the CDC criteria for AIDS** are classified as having AIDS-related complex (ARC).

F. **CDC classification schema for pediatric HIV infection** is as follows:

1. P-0: Indeterminate infection in children <15 months old with antibody to HIV.
2. P-1: Asymptomatic infection with:
   - P-1 A: Normal immune function.
   - P-1 B: Abnormal immune function.
   - P-1 C: Immune function not tested.
3. P-2: Symptomatic infection with:
   - P-2 A: Presence of nonspecific findings (i.e., fever, failure to thrive, >10% weight loss, hepatomegaly, splenomegaly, lymphadenopathy, parotitis, or persistent/recurrent diarrhea).
   - P-2 B: Progressive neurologic disease.
   - P-2 C: LIP.
   - P-2 D: Secondary infectious diseases:
     - D1: Those listed in CDC definition of AIDS.
     - D2: Recurrent serious bacterial infections.
     - D3: Other infections (i.e., persistent oral candidiasis, recurrent herpes stomatitis, or multidermatomal or disseminated herpes zoster).
   - P-2 E: Presence of secondary cancers:
     - E1: Kaposi's sarcoma, B-cell non-Hodgkin's lymphoma, or primary brain lymphoma.
     - E2: Other.
   - P-2 F: Other diseases probably caused by HIV infection (i.e., hepatitis, cardiomyopathy, nephropathy, anemia, thrombocytopenia, or dermatologic disorders).

II. EPIDEMIOLOGY:

A. **In 1990, > 1 million people in the United States were infected with HIV:** As of January 1992, approximately 3,000 children < 13 years old had a diagnosis of AIDS. AIDS is most frequently urban, with nearly three fourths of childhood cases from New York, New Jersey, California, and Florida. Racial distribution of pediatric AIDS is 57% black, 22% Hispanic, and 20% white.

B. **Sources of infection in pediatric AIDS:** 80% perinatally; 12% via transfusion; 5% through hemophilia therapy; 3% indeterminate. Perinatal acquisition usually represents maternal-child transmission, with three fourths having at least one parent who is an intravenous (IV) drug abuser. Other mothers have histories of sexual contact with a bisexual, hemophiliac, or otherwise infected man; multiple sexual partners or history of prostitution; or recipient of a contaminated transfusion.

C. **Mother-to-child transmission of HIV:**

1. One half of mothers of perinatally affected children are asymptomatic at delivery; however, virtually all are positive for HIV antibody.
2. The risk of a seropositive woman transmitting HIV to her offspring is about 30%.
3. The mechanism and timing of transmission are unknown. Virus can be acquired either in utero, during delivery from infected maternal blood, or postnatally. HIV has been isolated from a second trimester abortus, amniotic fluid, vaginal secretions, cord blood, and breast milk. HIV has also been isolated from infants delivered by cesarean section. Transmission from an infected mother to her infant after birth, other than perhaps by breast-feeding, is highly unlikely.

III. CLINICAL MANIFESTATIONS OF HIV INFECTION IN CHILDREN:

A. **HIV is diagnosed during the first year of life** in 50% and by 3 years in 82%. Children infected perinatally have a mean age at diagnosis of 17 months and a median age of 9 months. Mean interval between transfusion and HIV diagnosis in those infected by transfusion is 24 months (median 17 months).

B. **Most young children with HIV infection** have nonspecific **findings:** failure to thrive, developmental delay, hepatosplenomegaly, diarrhea, weight loss, oral candidiasis, fever, and lymphadenopathy.

C. **Most common opportunistic infections in pediatric AIDS:**

1. PCP
2. Candidal esophagitis
3. Disseminated CMV
4. Disseminated *Mycobacterium avium-intracellulare*
5. Cryptosporidiosis
6. Chronic herpes simplex

D. **Recurrent or serious bacterial infections** are also common: Most frequent organisms are *Streptococcus pneumoniae, Hemophilus influenzae* type b (Hib), *Salmonella,* and *Staphylococcus aureus*.

E. Lymphocytic interstitial pneumonitis: LIP is characteristic of HIV infection in children. A variant with lymphoid nodule formation is termed pulmonary lymphoid hyperplasia:

1. LIP occurs in approximately one half of children with AIDS.
2. LIP is characterized by diffuse peribronchial and interstitial infiltration of lung by lymphocytes, plasma cells, and immunoblasts.
3. Because interstitial pneumonitis may be caused by either opportunistic infections (especially PCP and CMV) or by LIP, definitive diagnosis requires biopsy. However, clinical findings may enable presumptive diagnosis of LIP without histologic confirmation:
   a. PCP usually presents more acutely with some fever, tachypnea, retractions, and hypoxemia; there are few auscultatory findings despite rapid and shallow respirations. (PCP is discussed in Chapter 6.)
   b. Children with LIP frequently have generalized lymphadenopathy, salivary gland enlargement, and digital clubbing.
   c. Patients with LIP more often have elevated serum immunoglobulin levels.
   d. Judicious use of corticosteroids has been beneficial in children with LIP.

e. The prognosis for children with LIP is much better than that of children with PCP, with median survival times of 91 months and 14 months, respectively.

F. **Encephalopathy** is a frequent manifestation of HIV infection:

1. Neurologic dysfunction occurs in up to 50% of HIV-infected children and probably represents HIV infection of the brain.
2. Manifestations: Lack of achieving milestones, loss of milestones, intellectual deterioration, paresis, ataxia, abnormal muscle tone, or seizures. Microcephaly is common among younger children.
3. Electroencephalograms show diffuse slowing; cerebrospinal fluid can be normal or show mild protein elevation or pleocytosis; computed tomography scans typically reveal cerebral atrophy.

G. **Kaposi's sarcoma** (the most common malignancy with AIDS in adults) is uncommon in children, reported in 4%. HIV-associated lymphoma, especially intracranial, is seen rarely. A polyclonal, polymorphic B-cell lymphoproliferative disorder and leiomyomas also occur.

H. **A specific craniofacial dysmorphism related to HIV** does not exist.

I. **Abnormalities of almost any organ system** can occur with HIV infection. Other manifestations of HIV infection in children include:

1. Chronic parotid swelling, which occurs in about 10%;
2. hematologic abnormalities such as thrombocytopenia (usually immune-mediated), anemia, neutropenia, or coagulopathy;
3. hepatitis without evidence of the usual infectious etiologies;
4. HIV-associated renal disease, most commonly presenting as nephrotic syndrome;
5. cardiomyopathy, manifested by CHF which can be fatal;
6. pancreatitis;
7. ophthalmologic disorders, including perivasculitis of the retinal vessels; and
8. mononucleosis-like syndrome with malaise, lymphade-

nopathy, myalgia, arthralgia, pharyngitis, fever, and rash (particularly shortly after infection).

J. Laboratory abnormalities may include:

1. Anemia, lymphopenia, neutropenia, thrombocytopenia.
2. Elevated quantitative immunoglobulin levels.
3. Depressed numbers of CD4+ lymphocytes (< 200/mm^3 correlates with high risk for opportunistic infections).
4. Reversal of the 2:1 helper/suppressor ratio.

IV. PATHOPHYSIOLOGY OF HIV INFECTION:

A. Etiology: HIV, previously called human T-cell lymphotropic virus type III (HTLV-III), or lymphadenopathy-associated virus (LAV), is the cause of AIDS. It is a retrovirus, consisting of an RNA genome, reverse transcriptase (to make DNA copies), a core protein (p24), and a glycoprotein envelope. HIV-2, which is endemic to West Africa, has not been reported to cause pediatric AIDS in the U.S.

B. Pathogenesis: HIV preferentially infects cells by interacting with the cell surface CD4 molecule, which serves as its receptor, on helper/inducer lymphocytes (T4 or CD4), macrophages, and monocytes.

1. Infected CD4+ cells function abnormally, may undergo syncytia formation and eventual cell lysis.

C. HIV infection causes many abnormalities of the immune system, including:

1. Decreased response to mitogens.
2. Impaired cytotoxic activity.
3. Decreased chemotaxis/phagocytosis.
4. Decreased specific antibody production.
5. Impaired feedback control of the immune response.

V. DIAGNOSIS:

Diagnosis of pediatric HIV infection is made by clinical presentation and confirmation by serologic tests.

A. Serodiagnosis:

1. Enzyme-linked immunosorbent assay (ELISA) to detect anti-HIV. This test is simple, inexpensive, sensitive, and therefore useful for screening. Confirmatory testing is needed because false positives occur.

2. In the **Western blot,** serum reacts with electrophoretically separated HIV antigens to determine the banding pattern of serum with specific viral proteins. This confirmatory test is more specific, but it is also more expensive and subject to laboratory variability.
3. Children exposed to HIV postnatally generally are anti-HIV positive within 6 to 12 weeks after infection.

B. **Other methods of laboratory diagnosis:**
1. Viral culture of peripheral lymphocytes or plasma: This is expensive, laborious, and insensitive.
2. p24 core antigen: This may be simpler and less expensive; however, many HIV-infected children lack detectable p24 antigen.
3. Polymerase chain reaction (PCR) for detecting HIV DNA in lymphocytes:
   a. Advantages: Provides direct evidence of infection. Is extremely sensitive and specific.
   b. Disadvantage: Is not yet widely available.

C. **Diagnosis of HIV infection in infants <15 months old** is difficult:
1. Maternal antibodies may persist in infant sera for 15 to 18 months.
2. Some infected infants become anti-HIV negative and then later become positive.
3. Presence of IgM anti-HIV is unreliable.
4. p24 antigen is often negative in infants.
5. Polymerase chain reaction (PCR) shows great promise.
6. For now, serial clinical follow-up and antibody assay every 2 to 4 months may be necessary.

VI. PROGNOSIS

A. **Median survival is 9 months** after diagnosis of AIDS is made. 75% are dead within 2 years of diagnosis.

B. **Poor prognostic factors** include:
1. Depressed CD4+ lymphocyte count.
2. Other immunologic abnormalities, such as lymphopenia, impaired T-cell responses to mitogens, hypogammaglobulinemia, and elevated HIV antigen levels.
3. Diagnosis <1 year of age.
4. *P. carinii* or other fungal infections.
5. Disseminated *M. avium-intracellulare*.

VII. MANAGEMENT:

A. General management: Multidisciplinary approach with excellent general medical and supportive care, as well as psychosocial support, is crucial for these often multisocial-problem families.

B. Nutrition: Nutrition is a serious problem in HIV-infected children, especially those with diarrhea. Some require chronic nasogastric feedings or IV alimentation.

C. Immunizations: The Advisory Committee for Immunization Practices recommends:

1. In patients with HIV infection:
   a. Live vaccines, in general, should not be given; however, measles-mumps-rubella (MMR) is recommended.
   b. Inactivated vaccines, i.e., diphtheria-tetanus-pertussis (DTP), inactivated poliomyelitis vaccine (IPV), Hib, influenza, and pneumococcal polysaccharides should be given.
   c. Passive immunization: Immune serum globulins and varicella-zoster immunoglobulin should be given after measles exposure and varicella exposure, respectively.
2. For household contacts of children with AIDS:
   a. MMR should be given; oral poliomyelitis vaccine (OPV) and (BCG) bacille Calmette-Guérin should be withheld.
   b. DTP, IPV, and Hib should be given; influenza and pneumococcal vaccines are not required.
   c. Passive immunization is not necessary.

D. Therapy for any suspected infection should begin promptly: Specific therapies are discussed elsewhere.

E. IV immunoglobulin (IVIG) may be beneficial in preventing bacterial infections in HIV-infected children with recurrent infections:

1. Recent studies show decreased incidence of bacterial infections in HIV infected children with CD4 counts > 200/mm.[3]
2. The long-term prognosis may be unaffected by IVIG.
3. Adverse reactions are rare; however, HIV patients are more prone to such reactions.

F. **Antiretroviral therapy:** Most promising to date is 3-azido-3-deoxythymidine (azidothymidine, AZT). AZT is thought to work by inhibiting reverse transcriptase and/or by chain termination:

1. Preliminary results in adults suggest that AZT:
   a. Slows the progression of disease.
   b. Reduces the risk of opportunistic infections.
   c. Reduces viral shedding.
   d. May lead to neurologic improvement in infants and children.
2. Major side effects include anemia and neutropenia. Studies of AZT with granulocyte colony-stimulating factor (G-CSF) are underway in an attempt to prevent dose-limiting neutropenia of AZT.

G. Trials of recombinant CD4, dideoxyinosine (DDI), dideoxycytidine (DDC) and α-interferon are in progress in the United States.

VIII. PSYCHOSOCIAL ISSUES:

A. HIV-infected children frequently have families with few resources.

1. Parent(s) often are poor and uneducated.
2. Parents often are IV drug abusers.
3. Most have an HIV-infected mother, who may be ill, dying, or dead, and other family members (e.g., father, siblings) who also may be ill, dying, or dead.

B. The diagnosis of HIV infection poses a great burden on the family:

1. Taking care of a sick child is emotionally and financially demanding.
2. Coping with the guilt of having transmitted the infection to the child.
3. Coping with a diagnosis that ultimately is fatal.
4. Dealing with adverse reactions from other family members and the community.
5. Dealing with the possibility of the parents' death.

C. Therefore children and families with HIV infection have **many needs** that are best met by a multidisciplinary team, usually consisting of physicians, nurses, social workers, psychologists, dieticians, occupational and physical therapists, teachers, and clergy.

D. Important issues that must be addressed include:
1. Patient and parental understanding of the diagnosis of HIV infection.
2. Psychosocial evaluation.
3. Counseling for the child and family.
4. Referrals to deal with issues such as child care, foster care, home health care, school arrangements, and finances.
5. Referral of family members for drug abuse treatment.

IX. PREVENTION:

A. Because the majority of pediatric HIV infection is acquired perinatally, prevention will occur by decreasing the number of births to HIV-infected women.
1. The woman who already is infected should be counseled:
   a. To consider delaying or avoiding pregnancy.
   b. To modify sexual practices to avoid transmission of the virus.
   c. To refer her sexual partner(s) for testing and counseling.
   d. To avoid use of IV drugs and shared needles.
   e. To avoid breast-feeding.
   f. Not to donate blood or organs.
2. The woman who is not HIV-infected but is at high risk of acquiring the virus should be counseled:
   a. To be aware of the risk factors for contracting HIV.
   b. To be aware of the value of using condoms.
   c. To delay pregnancy until she no longer is considered at risk.
   d. To avoid donating blood or organs.
   e. To seek treatment for IV drug abuse.

B. Because sexual contact and needle sharing are the primary routes of HIV transmission among adolescents and adults, education regarding safe sex practices and the dangers of sharing needles is crucial.

C. Since serologic screening of blood donors began in March 1985, the risk of transfusion-associated HIV infection has decreased markedly. Similarly, heat-treated, donor-screened factor VIII products have greatly reduced new infections in patients with hemophilia.

INFECTIONS BY ORGAN SYSTEM 6

I. BACTEREMIA AND SEPTIC SHOCK:

A. Definitions:

1. **Bacteremia** refers to the presence of bacteria in the blood without evidence of hemodynamic instability or organ system failure and without appearing seriously ill.
2. **Septic shock** connotes a complex series of metabolic and hemodynamic changes that lead to reduced tissue oxygen consumption relative to actual metabolic needs, with the potential for multiple organ system failure. This is a possible but not inevitable consequence of bacteremia and rarely may occur in the absence of bacteremia if toxic substances are absorbed systemically.
3. **Sepsis** and **septicemia** refer to systemic illness directly resulting from microbial invasion of the bloodstream but do not necessarily imply the presence of septic shock.

B. Epidemiology:

1. Bacteremia without an infectious focus ("occult bacteremia") occurs predominantly in children <5 years of age and is particularly common in the 6-to 24-month age group. The risk of bacteremia is higher in children with higher fevers, particularly those without a focus of infection or with a known serious infection. Children with mild, localized infections such as otitis media or pharyngitis are rarely bacteremic.
2. The incidence of septic shock in children is unknown. It is more common in those with systemic infections caused by gram-negative organisms, especially enteric organisms, *Pseudomonas aeruginosa, Hemophilus influenzae* type b (Hib) and *Neisseria meningitidis*. Children with asplenia or other immunodeficiency states are more prone to septic shock.

C. **Etiology and pathogenesis:**

1. Bacteremia:
   a. Beyond the neonatal period, *Streptococcus pneumoniae,* Hib, *Salmonella* species (spp.) and *N. meningitidis* are the most common causes of childhood bacteremia. The first three organisms, particularly *S. pneumoniae,* are the most common causes of occult bacteremia. Meningococcal bacteremia is not usually occult.
   b. The polysaccharide capsules of the organisms listed earlier are largely responsible for their virulence, because polymorphonuclear neutrophils (PMNs) complement, and specific anticapsular antibodies contribute to host defense against such encapsulated organisms. PMN function and complement activity are adequate throughout childhood, but antibody responses to polysaccharides are suboptimal during infancy and early childhood.
2. Septic shock:
   a. Septic shock results from the systemic release of microbial toxins, most commonly endotoxin (lipopolysaccharide), a constituent of the gram-negative bacterial cell wall. However, gram-positive bacteria, viruses, rickettsiae, and fungi all have been associated with septic shock on occasion.
   b. The pathogenesis of septic shock is quite complex and incompletely understood. The following are some basic mechanisms that appear important:
      1) Endotoxin stimulates production of humoral mediators, which are, in turn, responsible for the pathophysiologic manifestations of gram-negative sepsis. The most important of these mediators are tumor necrosis factor (TNF) and interleukin 1 (IL-1) produced by macrophages.
      2) Direct inhibition of mitochondrial respiration results in a shift to anaerobic metabolism with lactic acid production and metabolic acidosis.
      3) Activation of endothelial lipoxygenase and cyclo-oxygenase pathways of arachidonic acid metabolism leads to platelet aggregation, vasodilata-

tion, increased vascular permeability, and PMN adherence to endothelial cells.

4) Endotoxin-mediated activation of the classical and alternate complement pathways leads to complement consumption, neutrophil activation, and chemotaxin production. Activated neutrophils, in turn, release substances that result in tissue injury, particularly in the lung.

5) TNF and IL-1 induce fever by stimulation of hypothalamic prostaglandin synthesis.

c. These and other mechanisms result in the characteristic physiologic alterations of septic shock, which include:

1) Diffuse capillary leak.
2) Lowered systemic vascular resistance.
3) Depressed myocardial function.
4) Respiratory compromise secondary to pulmonary edema and surfactant deficiency.

D. Clinical and laboratory findings:

1. Bacteremia:

a. High fever (temperature ≥ 39°C rectally) is a sensitive but not specific indicator of bacteremia.

b. Patients with occult bacteremia may be relatively well appearing. Those with bacteremia secondary to a focal infection usually have findings typical for that infection.

c. Assessment of clinical variables such as level of activity, feeding, and degree of irritability is of uncertain value in selecting those febrile children who are most likely to be bacteremic.

d. Leukocytosis (usually white blood cell [WBC] count $>15{,}000/mm^3$) is a sensitive but not specific indicator of bacteremia. Leukopenia (WBC count $<5{,}000/mm^3$) in a febrile child is a sensitive and specific indicator of bacteremia and is usually a poor prognostic sign.

2. Septic shock:

a. The early, or "warm," phase of septic shock results from marked reduction in systemic vascular resistance and impaired mitochondrial respiration. It is characterized by tachycardia, warm, well-perfused extremities, and bounding pulses. Hypotension is **not** present, but the pulse pressure is widened. Mild respiratory alkalosis may be seen. Irritability, listlessness, and poor feeding may be present.

b. With increasing tissue injury and capillary leak, progression from "warm" to "cold" shock occurs. Cold shock is characterized by tachycardia, cold, clammy extremities, and hypotension, with a narrow pulse pressure. Metabolic acidosis is present. Unless aggressive medical management is promptly initiated, cold shock quickly progresses to multiple organ system failure, cardiovascular collapse and death.

c. In early septic shock, elevated mixed venous Po_2 may indicate impaired oxygen extraction. Activation of the coagulation system can produce a picture of disseminated intravascular coagulation (DIC).

d. Septic shock is a clinical diagnosis based on the previously mentioned signs and symptoms. There are no pathognomonic laboratory tests.

E. Evaluation and therapy:

1. Bacteremia:

a. A seriously ill-appearing, highly febrile child with no focus of infection should have blood cultures drawn, should have a lumbar puncture performed, and should be hospitalized. Serious consideration should be given to empiric parenteral antibiotic therapy with ceftriaxone or cefotaxime pending culture results.

b. Blood cultures and CBC should be considered in a relatively well-appearing child < 24 months of age with a high fever (temperature ≥39°C rectally). If the WBC count is >15,000/mm^3, the incidence of bacteremia is about 10%. In such children, close observation either at home or in the hospital is indicated.

c. Empiric antibiotic therapy is not recommended at this time for febrile children <24 months of age with no focus of infection who are not ill appearing, but this is controversial.

d. A child with an initially positive blood culture should be reexamined and repeat blood culture obtained. If the initial blood culture yielded *S. pneumoniae* and the child is afebrile and well appearing on follow-up without a focus of infection, treatment is not necessary if the second culture is negative. If the initial culture is positive for *H. influenzae, N. meningitidis,* or *Salmonella,* antibiotic therapy should be instituted. Likewise, therapy should be instituted in any child who is ill appearing or has a focal infection on follow-up examination or who has a blood culture persistently positive for *S. pneumoniae*.

2. Septic shock:
   a. Prompt establishment of the diagnosis early in the disease process is critical to the successful management of septic shock.
   b. Management is best carried out in an intensive care unit capable of invasive continuous hemodynamic monitoring.
   c. Restoration of hemodynamic stability is the primary goal of management. To this end, aggressive fluid resuscitation is indicated until optimal cardiac preload is established. Because myocardial function is typically depressed and systemic vascular resistance is low in early septic shock, dopamine, epinephrine, and/or norepinephrine is indicated to improve cardiac function and elevate systemic vascular resistance. If epinephrine or norepinephrine is used, low-dose dopamine should be concomitantly infused to enhance renal blood flow. If systemic vascular resistance is elevated, as in late septic shock, dobutamine may be the preferred inotrope.
   d. Aggressive support of systemic oxygenation is essential, frequently with endotracheal intubation and ventilation.
   e. Empiric antibiotic therapy directed against the most likely pathogens should be initiated promptly.
   f. The use of corticosteroids in septic shock is controversial and is not recommended on a routine basis.

g. Various therapeutic modalities directed at disruption of the metabolic cascade of septic shock, including arachidonic acid inhibitors and oxygen radical scavengers, are under investigation but are not recommended for routine use at present. Some studies in adults have suggested the possible value of monoclonal antibody to endotoxin, and studies of this and of antibody to TNF are in progress.

II. UPPER RESPIRATORY TRACT INFECTION (URI):

A. Common cold:

1. **Definition:** An acute viral infection associated with low-grade fever, coryza, sneezing, rhinorrhea, nasal stuffiness, and throat irritation.
2. **Etiology:** More than 100 different viral agents cause the common cold, including more than 90 rhinoviruses, parainfluenza viruses, respiratory syncytial virus (RSV), coronaviruses, and reoviruses.
3. **Epidemiology:** The average number of colds in children is 4 to 8/year, with about one half of them transmitted to adults within the family. Maximal transmission of colds occurs in schools and day-care centers, with introduction into families by young children. Colds tend to occur more frequently in the winter. Transmission occurs predominantly by sneezing, nose blowing, and contamination of hands with nasal secretions, with acquisition occurring by infection of the nose and/or conjunctivae.
4. **Clinical features:** The usual incubation period is 2 to 3 days, and acute symptoms last 3 to 7 days. Common symptoms include low-grade fever, nasal symptoms, and coryza. In infants and young children, irritability and restlessness, feeding difficulties, and vomiting and diarrhea may occur.
5. **Treatment:** No specific therapy is beneficial. Symptomatic therapy includes antipyretics, analgesics, local decongestants, saline solution nose drops, and humidification of air. Salicylates should be avoided in children because of the risk of Reye syndrome.
6. **Prevention:** No true effective prophylaxis exists.

B. Sinusitis:

1. **Definition:** Infection of the mucosal lining of the paranasal sinuses.
2. **Etiology:** Acute sinusitis is most often caused by *S. pneumoniae* and *H. influenzae,* with *Streptococcus pyogenes, S. aureus,* and *Moraxella catarrhalis* also implicated. Chronic sinusitis is caused by these same organisms with the addition of anaerobic bacteria. Inflammatory obstruction of the sinus ostia contributes to the development of sinusitis.
3. **Pathogenesis:** At birth, ethmoid and small maxillary sinuses are present. The sphenoid sinuses begin to develop at 2 years of age but are not well developed until about age 6. Frontal sinuses begin to develop after 2 years of age, are quite small until about 6 years, and are fully developed by the late teens. Sinusitis results when the normal nasal flora extend into the sinuses or when there is dysfunction of the normal defenses (i.e., ciliary function, ostial patency, mucosal immunoglobulins, and lysozyme). Contributors to this dysfunction include allergy, nasopharyngitis, the common cold, and foreign bodies.
4. **Epidemiology:** Sinusitis is not contagious and occurs with increased frequency in certain populations of children, such as those who are atopic, are immune deficient, have cystic fibrosis, or have chronic ear infections.
5. **Clinical features:** Acute sinusitis is most often associated with fever, rhinorrhea, and cough, with headache, sore throat, periorbital swelling, vomiting, sinus tenderness, and otitis media also sometimes present. Chronic sinusitis is associated with the same signs and symptoms but with a lower frequency of fever. Radiographic evidence of sinus mucosal thickening and/or opacification is usually present. Leukocytosis and elevated sedimentation rate are often present in acute sinusitis.
6. **Treatment:** Empiric oral antibiotic therapy (usually amoxicillin, 50 mg/kg/day) and local and/or systemic vasoconstrictive agents are used. Chronic or recurrent

sinusitis should be treated with amoxicillin/clavulante or TMP-SMX for 3 to 4 weeks. Surgical drainage of the sinuses is occasionally needed.

7. **Prevention:** No effective prophylaxis exists except for allergic therapy in atopic children.

C. **Otitis media:**

1. **Definition:** Inflammation of the middle ear cavity; this process can be acute or chronic; **serous otitis media** refers to nonpurulent, frequently sterile fluid collections in the middle ear space.
2. **Etiology:** Acute and chronic otitis media are generally bacterial infections caused by organisms that comprise the normal nasopharyngeal flora, particularly *S. pneumoniae, H. influenzae* (nontypable), and *M. catarrhalis;* chronic otitis media alternatively may be caused rarely by *S. aureus* or gram-negative enteric bacilli.
3. **Pathogenesis:** Otitis media occurs primarily as a result of eustachian tube dysfunction (i.e., lack of the normal ventilatory, protective, and drainage functions of the eustachian tube) as a consequence of allergy, viral infection, or blockage by hypertrophied adenoids.
4. **Epidemiology:** Otitis media occurs with increased frequency in young children, in atopic or immune-deficient individuals, and in those with cleft palate or other craniofacial abnormalities; increased incidence occurs during the colder months, corresponding with acute viral colds and during the "allergy season."
5. **Clinical features:** Fever, earache, and irritability are common features of acute otitis media, with otoscopic examination demonstrating decreased mobility, erythema, bulging, and/or loss of landmarks of the tympanic membrane; chronic otitis may be manifested primarily by a dull, thickened appearance of the tympanic membrane with poor mobility.
6. **Treatment:** Oral antibiotic agents are useful in acute and chronic otitis media, with frequent choices being amoxicillin/clavulanate, amoxicillin, cefaclor, or trimethoprim-sulfamethoxazole (TMP-SMX); careful follow-up is indicated to ensure response and resolution of the

middle ear effusion; decongestants are of little value; recurrent or chronic infections refractory to therapy may require surgical intervention with placement of tympanostomy tubes.

7. **Prevention:** There is no evidence that prophylactic decongestant therapy during colds prevent otitis media or that pneumococcal vaccine is beneficial in this regard. In children who have had frequent recurrences of acute otitis media, prophylaxis with TMP-SMX or amoxicillin given as half the daily therapeutic dose qhs is frequently successful.

D. **Pharyngitis and tonsillitis:**

1. **Definition:** Inflammation of the tonsillopharyngeal region, generally of viral or bacterial origin.
2. **Etiology:** Most episodes of pharyngitis are a result of viral infections with agents such as Epstein-Barr virus (EBV), adenovirus, influenza, enteroviruses, and herpes simplex virus; the most important bacterial agent by far is group A streptococcus, with other causes including *Archanobacterium (Corynebacterium) hemolyticum, N. gonorrhoeae, C. diphtheriae* (diphtheria), *Francisella tularensis,* and non–group A streptococci.
3. **Epidemiology:** Group A streptococcal pharyngitis occurs most often in children between 5 and 11 years of age, with peak incidence in the late winter and early spring. As with many other respiratory pathogens, crowded living conditions (e.g., large families, barracks) facilitate transmission. Many of the other agents also most commonly cause infection during the winter months.
4. **Clinical features:** Acute streptococcal pharyngitis ("strep throat") is classically characterized by abrupt onset of headache, fever, sore throat, abdominal pain, nausea, and vomiting. Examination frequently demonstrates tender anterior cervical nodes, tonsillar hypertrophy, pharyngeal erythema sometimes with exudates, and palatal petechiae. Cough, rhinorrhea, and hoarseness are notably absent in acute strep throat but are quite common in viral illnesses.

5. **Diagnosis:** It is difficult to diagnose streptococcal pharyngitis accurately solely on clinical grounds. Therefore, diagnostic tests such as rapid antigen detection tests and throat cultures are widely employed to distinguish strep throat from other forms of pharyngitis. Rapid tests are highly specific (very few false positives) but generally lack high sensitivity (frequent false negatives). Throat cultures plated on sheep blood agar usually demonstrate β-hemolysis (clear) with inhibition surrounding a bacitracin disk when group A streptococci are present. Normal pharyngeal flora are present on throat cultures in those with viral pharyngitis.
6. **Treatment:** Although streptococcal pharyngitis is self-limited, therapy with an appropriate agent hastens resolution of signs and symptoms by about 18 to 24 hours. Treatment is indicated primarily to prevent acute rheumatic fever. Penicillin is the treatment of choice, with oral penicillin V tid or qid used most often, and erythromycin is given to penicillin-allergic patients. More expensive agents such as ampicillin, amoxicillin, and cephalosporins are effective but not indicated because of cost. TMP-SMX is definitely **not** effective for strep throat.

E. Mastoiditis:

1. **Definition:** Inflammation of the mastoid air cells, usually as an extension of otitis media.
2. **Etiology and pathogenesis:** Flora similar to those that cause otitis media and sinusitis are responsible for acute mastoiditis. The most common agents are *S. pneumoniae* and group A streptococci, with *S. aureus* also involved. Chronic mastoiditis in children is frequently associated with anaerobes, *Proteus,* and *P. aeruginosa*. The mastoid air cells directly communicate with the middle ear cavity and become inflamed frequently as an extension of otitis media.
3. **Epidemiology:** Mastoiditis most often develops in children with history of recurrent or chronic middle ear infections, although an occasional child without apparent previous ear infections may have acute mastoiditis.
4. **Clinical features:** Fever with tenderness and/or swell-

ing behind the ear is typical. Frequently the pinna is pushed down and out. The tympanic membrane is usually inflamed. A subperiosteal abscess is sometimes palpable over the mastoid region.

5. **Diagnosis:** The clinical features are highly suggestive. Plain x-ray studies usually show opacification (decreased aeration) of the mastoid region. Computed tomography (CT) may show fluid and/or bony destruction of the air cells. Typanocentesis may be useful to indicate the major causative organism.
6. **Therapy:** Acute mastoiditis requires surgical drainage only if central nervous system (CNS) spread is suspected or when the patient fails to respond to appropriate therapy, such as parenteral cefuroxime. Chronic mastoiditis more frequently requires surgical drainage in addition to aggressive antibiotic therapy for the specific pathogens.
7. **Complications:** The proximity to the intracranial venous sinuses and to CNS structures occasionally results in venous sinus thrombosis, epidural, subdural, or intracerebral abscess. Petrous pyramid inflammation (petrositis) can lead to sixth nerve dysfunction (Gradenigo's syndrome).
8. **Prevention:** Prompt therapy of acute and chronic otitis media generally prevents extension of infection to the mastoid air cells.

F. Epiglottitis:

1. **Definition:** Inflammation and swelling of the epiglottis and other supraglottic structures, which can lead to fatal airway obstruction.
2. **Etiology:** In contrast to most other respiratory tract infections in children, the majority of epiglottitis cases are caused by a single bacterium, Hib. Bacteremia is present very commonly (75%–90%). Other bacteria or viruses are rarely involved.
3. **Epidemiology:** This is almost exclusively a disease of young children, with 75% between 1 and 5 years old. However, the median age of 3 to 4 years is substantially greater than for other bacteremic *H. influenzae* infections.

4. **Clinical features:** Patients have abrupt onset of fever, systemic toxicity, and stridorous respirations, with drooling and abnormal phonation. Dysphagia, respiratory distress, and anxiety are present. Examination shows respiratory distress, stridor, and a swollen cherry-red epiglottis; airway obstruction can be precipitated by examination with a tongue depressor, and therefore caution is necessary.
5. **Diagnosis:** Careful examination with characteristic lateral neck radiographic appearance establish the diagnosis. Leukocytosis is the rule.
6. **Therapy:** Airway management with elective nasotracheal intubation (rather than tracheostomy), coupled with intravenous (IV) antibiotic therapy with ampicillin and chloramphenicol or a cephalosporin such as ceftriaxone, cefotaxime, or cefuroxime.
7. **Prevention:** As with other hematogenous infections caused by Hib, Hib vaccination usually prevents epiglottitis.

III. PERITONSILLAR ABSCESS:

A. **Definition:** Localized suppuration lateral to the tonsil; also known as **quinsy.**

B. **Etiology and pathogenesis:** Group A streptococci are most common, with *S. aureus,* anaerobes *(Fusobacterium, Bacteroides),* and *H. influenzae* also implicated occasionally. Most peritonsillar infections occur as a result of direct extension from the tonsil through the fibrous tonsillar capsule.

C. **Clinical features:** Unilateral throat pain, fever, dysphagia, trismus, and a muffled voice are often presenting symptoms. Examination shows toxicity, drooling, and shift of the uvula and soft palate away from the affected side, with swelling around the tonsil and ipsilateral cervical adenitis.

D. **Laboratory features:** Leukocytosis is common. CT scan is very useful to define the anatomic relationships and to differentiate between cellulitis and frank abscess formation.

E. **Treatment:** IV penicillin is usually adequate, with surgical drainage of an abscess and/or tonsillectomy. Needle aspiration of the peritonsillar region is frequently attempted.

F. **Complications:** Destruction or invasion of adjacent structures, with involvement of the pterygomaxillary space, and thence involvement of the carotid sheath structures, cranial nerves IX to XII, and the cervical sympathetic chain.

IV. RETROPHARYNGEAL ABSCESS:

A. **Definition:** Localized infection confined to the retropharyngeal space, most often secondary to suppuration of lymph nodes in this space that drain the pharynx, nasopharynx, and adenoids.

B. **Etiology and pathogenesis:** These are frequently mixed aerobic-anaerobic infections. The most common aerobes are group A streptococci, *S. aureus,* and less commonly non–group A β-streptococci, viridans streptococci, and gram-negative enterics. Anaerobes include *Bacteroides fragilis, Bacteroides melanogenicus,* and *Fusobacterium*. Infection of the pharynx and/or adenoids may result in direct extension to the retropharyngeal space or in lymphangitic spread to the lymph nodes in that space, with suppuration and abscess formation.

C. **Clinical features:** Patients may manifest symptoms of airway obstruction, dysphagia, drooling, and nuchal rigidity related to paraspinal muscle spasm. A fluctuant mass may be visable or palpable behind the posterior pharyngeal wall.

D. **Laboratory features:** Leukocytosis is common. Lateral neck radiographs may show convexity or straightening of the cervical vertebrae and a widened posterior pharyngeal space, occasionally with gas. CT scans more precisely define the extent of involvement and better differentiate cellulitis from a defined abscess that requires surgical drainage.

E. **Treatment:** IV antibiotic therapy with nafcillin, cephapirin sodium (Cefadyl), or clindamycin is appropriate, as is surgical drainage if a well-defined abscess is demonstrated.

F. **Complications:** Inadequately treated retropharyngeal abscess has the potential to extend inferiorly to the posterior mediastinum or posteriorly to the prevertebral space.

V. CROUP:

A. **Definition:** Laryngotracheobronchitis (LTB) most characteristically manifested by inspiratory stridor and barky cough.

B. Etiology and pathogenesis:

1. Croup is almost always viral in origin, with multiple agents capable of producing the syndrome, particularly parainfluenza 1 to 3 and influenza A and B. These and other agents cause inflammation of the larynx, trachea, and/or bronchi, resulting in combinations of hoarseness, stridor, and/or cough, respectively.
2. Epithelial cell infection leads to ciliary dysfunction, submucosal edema, and inflammatory infiltration.
3. Bacterial tracheitis is a recently rediscovered entity caused usually by *S. aureus, S. pneumoniae* or *H. influenzae*. This may represent bacterial superinfection of viral croup.

C. Clinical features:

1. Croup occurs predominantly in the 6 to 36-month-old age range, peaks in the fall months, and is twice as common in boys than girls.
2. LTB generally manifests initially with URI symptoms that typically progress after 12 to 48 hours to obstructive upper airway signs and symptoms, most characteristically a barky cough (like a barking seal) and inspiratory stridor. Hoarseness and prolonged expiratory phase are very common. Progression to severe respiratory distress and hypoxia can occur. This illness must be distinguished from acute epiglottitis.

D. Laboratory features:

1. Mild leukocytosis is common. Lateral neck radiograph demonstrates subglottic narrowing that can be distinguished from the swollen epiglottis of epiglottitis.

E. Therapy:

1. Supportive care includes administration of mist with humidified air (or oxygen, if needed) to prevent desiccation of secretions and epithelium.
2. The role of corticosteroids remains unclear, without a clearly demonstrable benefit in most studies.
3. Nebulized racemic epinephrine may be of benefit and may prevent need for tracheotomy or intubation in more severe cases.
4. Nasotracheal intubation is the preferred form of airway management in severe cases of croup.
5. Antibiotics are generally not indicated in croup.

F. Complications:

1. Airway obstruction and hypoxia occur in severe cases of croup.
2. Bacterial superinfection leading to bacterial tracheitis may occur occasionally.

VI. LOWER RESPIRATORY TRACT INFECTIONS:

A. Bronchitis:

1. **Definition:** Acute or chronic inflammation of the major bronchi, manifested by fever and cough (acute bronchitis) or by cough and wheezing (chronic bronchitis).
2. **Etiology:**
   a. Acute bronchitis is predominately viral or mycoplasmal, with adenovirus, influenza A and B, parainfluenza 1–3, RSV, rhinoviruses, and *Mycoplasma pneumoniae* most common.
   b. Chronic bronchitis is associated with the same agents and with asthma and pulmonary irritants such as pollution and cigarette smoke.
3. **Clinical features:**
   a. Acute bronchitis is characterized initially by low grade fever and URI symptoms, then by fever and loose cough; posttussive emesis is common in young children. Examination of the chest yields rhonchi and coarse rales.
   b. Chronic bronchitis is manifested by little or no fever, chronic cough, and sometimes wheezing.
4. **Laboratory features:**
   a. Laboratory tests are of limited value in bronchitis. Chest x-ray studies are usually normal unless there is pulmonary involvement.
5. **Therapy:**
   a. Hydration, judicious use of cough suppressants, and acetaminophen are helpful. Antibiotics are not useful unless high fever and toxicity suggest bacterial superinfection.
   b. Removal from smoke and pollutants hastens recovery.
   c. Bronchodilator therapy is useful in chronic bronchitis with wheezing.

6. **Complications:**
    a. Persistant chronic bronchitis may lead to chronic pulmonary disease.

B. Bronchiolitis:

1. **Definition:** An acute illness of infants that is characterized by coryza, fever, cough, respiratory distress, prolonged expiratory phase, and wheezing.
2. **Etiology and pathogenesis:**
    a. Respiratory syncytial virus is clearly the most common agent, with parainfluenza and other respiratory viruses also implicated but less commonly.
    b. The pathogenesis of bronchiolitis is complex and incompletely understood, probably involving both an inherited predisposition to hyperreactive airways and IgE-mediated hypersensitivity to viral antigens.
3. **Epidemiology:**
    a. Bronchiolitis typically affects infants 2 to 12 months of age with history of exposure to URI. Peak incidence is at 1 to 3 months.
    b. The large majority of cases are observed from January to May; very few occur from August to October. Male/female ratio is 1.5:1.
    c. Incubation period is 3 to 6 days.
4. **Clinical features:**
    a. Nasal discharge is followed by fever (mean temperature 39°C), cough, irritability, anorexia, and gradual onset of respiratory distress, with tachypnea, flaring, retracting, and wheezing that is often audible. Prolonged expiration is typical.
    b. Symptoms progress over 3 to 7 days and occasionally become severe enough to necessitate oxygen supplementation and mechanical ventilation. Hypoxia is more common than hypercarbia except when patients develop respiratory failure.
    c. Children at particularly high risk for severe bronchiolitis are those with preexisting cardiac or pulmonary disease.
5. **Laboratory features:**
    a. Chest x-ray shows hyperinflation, flattening of the diaphragms, and areas of atelectasis.

b. Most patients have normal WBC counts, and some increase in the number of neutrophils and bands is common.
c. Specific diagnosis can be confirmed by viral culture or (more conveniently) by RSV enzyme immunoassay of upper respiratory (nasal) secretions.

6. **Therapy:**
   a. Supportive care with humidity and oxygen is important. Mechanical ventilation is necessary for particularly severe cases.
   b. Antiviral therapy with nebulized ribavirin is not indicated for those with routine cases but appears to benefit severely affected patients significantly by shortening their time of ventilation and oxygen requirement.
   c. Children with cardiac or pulmonary disease should be treated with ribavirin to minimize morbidity and mortality.
7. **Complications:**
   a. Secondary bacterial infection is very rare.
   b. Episodes of wheezing subsequent to an episode of bronchiolitis more than likely reflect primary hyperreactive airways rather than the result of previous bronchiolitis.

C. **Lung Abscess:**

1. **Definition:** A localized area of suppuration involving the lung parenchyma caused by pyogenic bacteria.
2. **Etiology and pathogenesis:**
   a. The bacterial agents recovered from lung abscesses depend on the quality of anaerobic culture techniques. When specimens are handled optimally (with minimal exposure to oxygen), anaerobes such as *Bacteroides, Peptococcus,* and *Peptostreptococcus* species are almost always found, together with aerobes such as *S. pneumoniae,* group A streptococcus, viridans streptococci, *Staphylococcus aureus* and enteric bacilli. An average of five to six different organisms can be recovered.
   b. Lung abscess frequently develops after aspiration or after an unresolved pyogenic pneumonitis. Impaired

ciliary function (e.g., with anesthesia, sedation, viral infection, aspiration of gastric contents or vascular and/or airway obstruction), ineffective cough, and/or deficient alveolar macrophage function can predispose to liquefaction necrosis and abscess formation.

3. **Clinical features:**
   a. Onset may be insidious (with fever, cough, anorexia and weakness) or abrupt (with fever, rigors, prostration, and sometimes pleuritic pain).
   b. Rupture into the pleural space may occur, leading to empyema, especially with *S. aureus* infection.
   c. Rupture into a bronchus is associated with foul breath and/or bloody sputum.
4. **Diagnosis:**
   a. Leukocytosis with predominance of neutrophils is typical.
   b. Chest x-ray studies show a dense parenchymal lung lesion with surrounding pulmonary inflammation, occasionally an air-fluid level within an abscess cavity, and often pleural reaction or effusion.
   c. CT scan usually shows a well-defined mass within the lung parenchyma, with contrast enhancement surrounding the mass.
5. **Therapy:**
   a. Aggressive IV antibiotic therapy, usually with penicillin or clindamycin, is important.
   b. Percutaneous aspiration under CT guidance is useful diagnostically and therapeutically. Drainage by bronchoscopy is an alternate approach. Surgical resection of a lung abscess is occasionally necessary, particularly with very large lesions.
   c. The presence of empyema indicates the need for chest tube drainage. Decortication of the peel on the surface of the lung is frequently necessary.
6. **Prognosis:**
   a. In children pulmonary abscesses heal remarkably well, with most leaving no residua or impaired pulmonary function.

D. Pneumonia:

1. Nonbacterial pneumonia:

a. Etiology and pathogenesis:

1) These comprise the majority of pneumonic infections in otherwise healthy infants and children.
2) The agents commonly responsible include *M. pneumoniae, Chlamydia trachomatis,* and *C. pneumoniae* (TWAR), RSV, parainfluenza virus (especially type 3), influenza A and B, adenoviruses, cytomegalovirus (CMV), and rhinoviruses. Less common are enteroviruses, coronavirus, measles, rubella, varicella, herpes simplex virus (HSV), EBV, other mycoplasmas, *Ureaplasma urealyticum, Chlamydia psittaci,* and *Pneumocystis carinii.*
3) Particularly common in immunocompromised hosts are CMV, varicella, and *Pneumocystis carinii.*
4) The majority of these agents reach the lungs from the upper respiratory tract, although varicella, measles, rubella, EBV, CMV and herpes simplex are hematogenously disseminated.

b. Epidemiology:

1) Nonbacterial pneumonia in neonates and young infants is usually caused by RSV, *C. trachomatis,* and CMV, with parainfluenza 3 and influenza A and B also seen with some frequency.
2) Older infants and preschool children most often are infected with RSV, parainfluenza 1 or 3, influenza A or B, probably *C. pneumoniae,* or adenovirus.
3) In school-aged children, the most common agents are *M. pneumoniae,* parainfluenza 3, influenza A, and adenovirus.
4) The precise roles of *C. pneumoniae, P. carinii,* and *U. urealyticum* still need to be clarified.
5) RSV, parainfluenza viruses, *M. pneumoniae,* and influenza A and B generally cause well-defined seasonal outbreaks during the colder

months. Transmission is most often by droplet spread related to relatively close contact with an infected source.

c. **Clinical features:**
   1) Infants may have an afebrile pneumonitis, caused most commonly by *C. trachomatis,* with staccato cough, diffuse rales, and interstitial infiltrates on x-ray film. However, most nonbacterial pneumonias manifest with low-grade fever, early URI symptoms, and gradual onset of cough, increased respiratory effort, anorexia, and posttussive emesis. Wheezing may be present, as well as hyperresonance, grunting, and fine rales.
   2) Older children typically have malaise, myalgia, anorexia, URI symptoms, nonproductive cough, and mild tachypnea.

d. **Diagnosis:**
   1) Peripheral WBC counts are highly variable in nonbacterial pneumonia.
   2) X-ray features are highly variable but are more likely to demonstrate interstitial rather than lobar infiltrates, as well as air trapping.
   3) Viral isolation from respiratory secretions or specific serum antibody responses (acute compared with convalescent) are helpful in confirming a specific etiologic diagnosis. Enzyme assays are available for rapid diagnosis of RSV infection. Cold agglutinin titers may be positive in acute mycoplasmal but also some acute viral infections.
   4) *P. carinii* generally requires bronchoscopic or lung biopsy demonstration of organisms.

e. **Therapy:**
   1) Most nonbacterial pneumonias are not amenable to specific therapy, and supportive care is essential.
   2) RSV can be treated with aerosolized ribavirin, but this should be limited to severely ill patients or to those with underlying cardiac or pulmonary disease.

3) *M. pneumoniae* infections respond to erythromycin or tetracycline (>7 years old) therapy.
4) Chlamydial infections are treated with erythromycin, tetracycline (>7 years old), or TMP-SMX.

f. **Prognosis and prevention:**
1) The majority of these infections resolve without sequelae. Occasional patients develop chronic pulmonary changes.
2) Nosocomial transmission of these agents can be prevented by appropriate use of universal precautions. Vaccines are available for prevention of influenza virus infections.

2. **Bacterial pneumonias:**

a. **Etiology and pathogenesis:**
1) *S. pneumoniae* is the leading bacterial cause of pneumonia in children, with Hib and *S. aureus* also relatively common. Group A streptococci, group B streptococci in neonates, and enteric gram-negative rods also cause these infections. Other agents including *Legionella pneumophila*, are rare.
2) The potential role of antecedent viral respiratory tract infections in bacterial pneumonia is unproved. Most of these bacterial infections extend from the upper respiratory tract and may be associated with secondary bacteremia. Occasionally *S. aureus* pneumonia results from hematogenous spread from an extrapulmonary site of infection.

b. **Epidemiology:**
1) Most of the common agents are normal inhabitants of the upper respiratory tract.
2) These infections occur sporadically year round but are most frequent during winter and spring, with males affected twice as often as females.
3) Epidemics are quite rare in children.

c. **Clinical features:**
1) General manifestations include fever, toxic appearance, headache, malaise, anorexia, and rigors. Respiratory signs and symptoms include

tachypnea, grunting, dyspnea, cough (often productive in older children), and use of accessory muscles of respiration.

2) Auscultation may yield rales and rhonchi and decreased breath sounds, percussion may show dullness (particularly with a pleural effusion), and palpation may show decreased fremitus.
3) Extension to the pleura is often accompanied by pleuritic pain, a friction rub, and dyspnea.
4) Abdominal pain with lower lobe pneumonia may resemble appendicitis.

d. **Diagnosis:**

1) Radiologic features more often include lobar consolidation and pleural effusion compared with nonbacterial pneumonia.
2) Etiologic diagnosis can be established by recovery of an organism on culture of blood or pleural fluid (Table 6–1) or by demonstration of specific bacterial antigen (e.g., *H. influenzae* or *S. pneumoniae*) in urine or serum or pleural fluid. Culture of throat or upper airway secretions is highly unreliable. Sputum is generally not obtainable from young children; when it is available, Gram's stain examination is more valuable than culture to indicate the likely cause of pneumonia.

TABLE 6–1.
Pleural Fluid Evaluation

	Transudate	Exudate
Gross appearance	Clear	Clear/cloudy
Protein content (g/dL)	<3.0	>3.0
Pleural fluid/serum protein (%)	<50	>50
Lactic dehydrogenase (IU/L)	<200	>200
Pleural fluid/serum LDH (%)	<60	>60
Glucose (mg/dL)	>60	Often <60
Leukocyte count (per mm^3)	$<1,000$	$>1,000$
Polymorphonuclear neutrophils (%)	<50	>50
pH (highly variable)	>7.2	<7.2

3) Leukocytosis with predominance of neutrophils is quite common in bacterial pneumonia.

e. **Therapy:**

1) Supportive measures such as maintenance of adequate hydration, humidification, oxygen when required, and antipyretics are useful.
2) Empiric antibiotic therapy before identification of the specific agent should encompass the most likely agents:
   a) *Neonatal pneumonia:* Ampicillin or nafcillin plus an aminoglycoside or broad-spectrum cephalosporin such as ceftriaxone.
   b) *Pneumonia from 1 month to 5 years:* Coverage for *H. influenzae* and *S. pneumoniae,* as with cefuroxime.
   c) *Pneumonia after age 5 years: S. pneumoniae* is most important and *H. influenzae* uncommon, so penicillin can be used.
3) Drainage of empyema with a chest tube facilitates recovery when thick exudate is present.

f. **Prognosis:**

1) Childhood bacterial pneumonia is generally associated with complete recovery without long-term impairment of pulmonary function.

g. **Prevention:**

1) *H. influenzae* pneumonias will be prevented substantially by use of the conjugate Hib vaccines.
2) Patients with sickle cell disease or asplenia can be prevented from developing pneumococcal pneumonia by use of prophylactic oral penicillin V and pneumococcal vaccine.

E. Tuberculosis:

1. **Definition:** Infection by *M. tuberculosis,* almost always involving the lungs, with or without spread to other tissues.
2. **Etiology and pathogenesis:**

a. **Primary childhood TB** occurs when viable *M. tuberculosis* are inhaled by a previously uninfected individual and deposit in alveoli where a nidus of infection forms, with a resultant host inflammatory response. Some organisms are carried to regional (hilar) lymph nodes by the lymphatics, and a bacillemic phase occurs, with potential spread to distant sites, particularly CNS, bone, liver, and spleen. During the subsequent 2 to 6 weeks, cell-mediated (T-cell) hypersensitivity to tuberculoprotein develops, with formation of granulomas at sites of replication of *M. tuberculosis*. Most often, fibrosis and calcification develop at the pulmonary and hilar node sites, leading to a Ghon complex, and the illness is self-limited.

   b. **Reactivation (adult) TB** represents reactivation of a previously inactive fibrotic and/or calcific lesion (usually at the apices of the lungs) and rarely occurs in children.

3. **Epidemiology:**
   a. *M. tuberculosis* is almost always acquired by inhalation of droplet nuclei that contain a small number of viable organisms. Droplet nuclei are produced when an adult with active TB coughs, sneezes, or talks.
   b. In the United States, rates of childhood TB are highest in urban, nonwhite populations and in immigrant families from high-risk countries. TB cases in human immunodeficiency virus (HIV)–infected adult populations are recognized increasingly and serve as new sources of infection of children.
4. **Clinical features:**
   a. Primary TB is most often manifested by nonspecific, usually mild, signs and symptoms that resolve without specific therapy. Mild cough, low-grade fever, and anorexia are common.
   b. Occasional children, particularly very young infants or immunocompromised hosts, develop symptomatic disseminated primary infection ranging from a relatively mild illness to overwhelming rapidly fatal infection (miliary tuberculosis) before their development of cell-mediated immunity.

5. **Laboratory features:**
   a. Chest x-ray studies in primary childhood TB may be normal, may show a nonspecific patchy area of pneumonitis, or may demonstrate more advanced disease, with pleural effusion and/or extensive infiltration. Prominant hilar adenopathy is common.
   b. Diagnosis can be established by culture and/or demonstration of acid-fast mycobacteria in early-morning gastric aspirates or in tracheal aspirate specimens. Tuberculin skin test reactivity reflects cell-mediated immunity to tuberculoprotein and implies infection with *M. tuberculosis* at some time (except in those who have received bacille Calmette-Guérin (BCG) immunization).
6. **Therapy** (see Table A–21 for dosages):
   a. Asymptomatic infection (skin test positive without disease):
      1) Isoniazid (INH) for 9 months.
      2) Consider substituting rifampin for 9 months if INH-resistant TB is documented. Efficacy of this and other regimens is unproved.
   b. Pulmonary TB (including hilar adenopathy):
      1) Standard 6-month regimen: 2 months of INH, rifampin, and pyrazinamide, followed by 4 months of INH and rifampin daily or twice weekly.
      2) Alternate 9-month regimen: 9 months of INH and rifampin daily **or** 1 month of INH and rifampin daily, followed by 8 months of INH and rifampin twice weekly.
   c. TB meningitis, bone or joint infection, or disseminated disease.
      1) 2 months of INH, rifampin, pyrazinamide, and possibly streptomycin, followed by 10 months of INH and rifampin daily or twice weekly.
   d. Other forms of extrapulmonary TB: Same as for pulmonary disease.
   e. Pubertal or post-pubertal patients receiving INH also should be given pyridoxine, 5 to 10 mg/day.

VII. EYE INFECTIONS:

A. Conjunctivitis:

1. **Etiology:**
   a. Nontypable *H. influenzae* are the most common cause of bacterial conjunctivitis in children. *S. pneumoniae* is also a common etiologic agent.
   b. *Neisseria gonorrhoeae* may cause conjunctivitis in neonates (acquired from an infected maternal genital tract) or in sexually active adolescents (autoinoculation). Gonococcal conjunctivitis in other pediatric age groups should raise suspicion of sexual abuse.
   c. *S. aureus* may cause some cases of bacterial conjunctivitis, but its role is uncertain, because it is often recovered from the conjunctivae of asymptomatic individuals.
   d. Adenovirus is the most common cause of viral conjunctivitis in childhood. Enteroviruses also cause conjunctivitis; enterovirus type 70 has been associated with epidemics of hemorrhagic conjunctivitis.
   e. HSV may cause conjunctivitis in a neonate born to an infected woman, generally as part of a systemic infection.
   f. *C. trachomatis* is a common cause of neonatal conjunctivitis, occurring in 20% to 50% of neonates born to vaginally infected women.
   g. Several systemic infections may manifest with conjunctivitis (Table 6–2).
2. **Clinical findings:**
   a. Specific signs and symptoms depend on etiology.
   b. *H. influenzae* conjunctivitis manifests with conjunctival inflammation and purulent discharge; otitis media may also be present ("otitis-conjunctivitis syndrome").
   c. Adenoviral conjunctivitis manifests with conjunctival erythema and often follicular hyperplasia. An associated pharyngitis is often present ("pharyngoconjunctival fever").
   d. Enteroviral conjunctivitis usually occurs in association with other manifestations of enteroviral infection such as rash or aseptic meningitis. Enterovirus

TABLE 6–2.
Systemic Infections Associated With Conjunctivitis or Conjunctival Injection

Infection	Key Features
Varicella	Typical vesicular rash
Measles	Cough, coryza, rash, Koplik's spots
Kawasaki disease	Fever >5 days, cervical adenopathy, oral mucositis, rash, extremity changes, no eye discharge
Leptospirosis	Jaundice, history of rat exposure
Rocky Mountain spotted fever	Fever, headache, peripheral rash spreading centripetally
Cat-scratch disease (Parinaud's syndrome)	Conjunctivitis and preauricular adenopathy, history of cat exposure

70 may produce severe conjunctivitis with bulbar conjunctival hemorrhages.

e. Gonococcal conjunctivitis classically manifests with marked conjunctival hyperemia and copious purulent discharge. In neonates, it usually is apparent in the latter half of the first week of life. If untreated, this infection can produce serious ocular damage.

f. Neonatal chlamydial conjunctivitis usually manifests during weeks 1 to 4 of life. Involvement is often unilateral with purulent discharge. Chlamydial pneumonitis subsequently occurs in some infected infants.

g. Neonatal herpes conjunctivitis usually occurs in association with systemic infection but may be the only apparent manifestation of HSV infection. Vesicles may develop on the eyelids and around the eyes.

3. **Evaluation:**

a. Careful history and physical examination often suggest the etiology; exclusion of noninfectious processes that cause conjunctival erythema is important (Table 6–3).

b. Gram's stain and culture of conjunctival exudate are usually the only necessary laboratory studies. In neonates, chlamydial culture must be done, and rapid

TABLE 6–3.
Noninfectious Causes of Ocular Injection

Cause	Distinguishing Features
Silver nitrate prophylaxis	Occurs first 1–2 days of life
Corneal abrasions	History of trauma; eye pain
Allergic conjunctivitis	Eye itching; presence of other allergic symptoms
Stevens-Johnson syndrome	Severe rash, mucositis
Glaucoma	Eye pain, corneal haze, corneal enlargement, excess tearing
Collagen-vascular disease (scleritis)	Arthritis, rash, vasculitis

antigen detection tests for *Chlamydia* using conjunctival swabs may be helpful.

c. Fluorescein dye application to the eye and examination with a Woods lamp is helpful in excluding corneal abrasion if this is believed to be a diagnostic possibility.

4. **Therapy:**
   a. Therapy of choice for gonococcal conjunctivitis is now single-dose parenteral ceftriaxone or cefotaxime because of the prevalence of penicillinase-producing *N. gonorrhoeae* in many areas. Topical therapy is not necessary.
   b. Chlamydial conjunctivitis should be treated with oral erythromycin, 40 to 50 mg/kg/day for 2 weeks. Topical therapy is not reliably effective.
   c. Other forms of bacterial conjunctivitis may be treated with topical antibiotics.
   d. Therapy of adenoviral and enteroviral conjunctivitis is supportive.
   e. Neonatal herpetic conjunctivitis should be treated with parenteral acyclovir, as well as topical antiviral therapy.

B. **Orbital Cellulitis:**

1. **Definition, etiology, and pathogenesis:**
   a. Orbital cellulitis is defined as infection and inflammation of the orbital tissues posterior to the orbital

septum (the tarsal plate of the upper and lower eyelids).

b. Pathogenetic mechanisms:
   1) Two thirds of the orbital wall is formed by the very thin bony plates of the paranasal sinuses, and direct two-way communication exists between the veins of the sinuses and orbit. Therefore, sinusitis may lead to orbital infection by rupture through the orbital walls or by phlebitic spread.
   2) Orbital trauma or skull fracture is a less common cause of orbital cellulitis.
   3) Hematogenous spread is an uncommon cause of orbital cellulitis, except in neonates.
c. Etiologic agents:
   1) Coagulase-positive staphylococci are most common in neonates.
   2) Coagulase-positive staphylococci, streptococci, and anaerobes are the predominant organisms in older children.

2. **Clinical findings and complications:**
   a. Proptosis, limitation of eye movement, and pain with eye movement are the cardinal signs of orbital cellulitis and must be carefully sought in any child with eye or periorbital swelling. Chemosis may also be present. Diminished or absent pupillary light response indicates significant optic nerve compromise. Fever is common.
   b. Sinusitis is present in most cases, although preexisting symptoms to suggest sinusitis are often absent.
   c. Orbital or periosteal abscess occurs in 5% to 10% of cases. Meningitis occurs in 2% to 3% of cases as a result of spread posteriorly from the orbit.
   d. Blood cultures are rarely positive.
3. **Evaluation:**
   a. Correct initial diagnosis by physical examination as described in section VII, B, 2, a, is crucial.
   b. CT scan of the sinuses and orbits is generally indicated to confirm (or to rule out) orbital cellulitis and to evaluate any coexistent sinusitis.

4. **Therapy:**
   a. Surgical decompression of the orbit is frequently necessary, particularly if a subperiosteal or orbital abscess is present. Advanced sinusitis may also require surgical drainage of the sinuses.
   b. IV antibiotic therapy is mandatory. Initial antibiotic therapy should include nafcillin, vancomycin, or clindamycin (if anaerobes are suspected). Treatment usually is for 2 to 3 weeks.

C. **Periorbital Cellulitis:**

1. **Definition, etiology, and pathogenesis:**
   a. Periorbital (preseptal) cellulitis is defined as inflammation and infection of the soft tissues anterior to the orbital septum (the tarsal plate of the upper and lower eyelids).
   b. Pathogenetic mechanisms:
      1) Sinusitis may result in periorbital cellulitis because of direct two-way venous communications between the face, nasal cavity, and paranasal sinuses.
      2) Local trauma (bites, lacerations) may disrupt skin integrity, giving rise to periorbital cellulitis.
      3) Bacteremia/septicemia, particularly with *H. influenzae,* may result in seeding of infection in the periorbital soft tissues.
   c. Etiologic agents:
      1) *H. influenzae* and *S. pneumoniae* are most common in children < 5 years of age.
      2) Gram-positive cocci are most common in children > 5 years of age; *H. influenzae* is rarely seen in this age group.
      3) *S. aureus* and streptococci are most common in patients with periorbital cellulitis secondary to local trauma or styes.
2. **Clinical findings and complications:**
   a. Involvement is nearly always unilateral, with left-sided involvement slightly more common.
   b. Swelling and erythema of the lids and periorbital tissues is always seen; violaceous discoloration may also be present. Fever is common.

c. Blood cultures are positive in 20% to 30% of patients, particularly in children <3 years old with no history of antecedent local trauma. Leukocytosis is usually present.
d. Meningitis is present in 2% to 3% of cases. Development of a lid abscess that requires drainage occurs in up to 2% to 3% of cases, particularly when *S. aureus* is the offending organism.

3. **Evaluation:**
   a. Thorough examination of the affected eye is essential to exclude orbital involvement. CT scan is highly effective for this purpose.
   b. Complete blood count (CBC) and blood cultures are essential. Culture of wound drainage in trauma or sty-associated cases is indicated; culture of conjunctival exudate is not helpful. Urine counterimmunoelectrophoresis (CIE) or latex agglutination may be helpful in cases with no apparent etiology.
   c. Sinus x-ray studies may be helpful in establishing a predisposing condition.
   d. Lumbar puncture should be considered in children < 18 months of age to exclude meningitis.
4. **Therapy:**
   a. In children < 5 years of age with no antecedent local trauma or sty, IV cefuroxime is recommended in meningitic doses (240 mg/kg/day) as initial therapy. If blood and cerebrospinal fluid (CSF) cultures are negative, the dose can be lowered to 100 mg/kg/day.
   b. Patients > 5 years of age or with cellulitis secondary to local trauma should be treated with an IV penicillinase-resistant penicillin such as nafcillin or a first-generation cephalosporin such as cephapirin sodium.
   c. IV antibiotic therapy is continued at least until substantial clinical improvement is seen, usually 3 to 5 days. Oral antibiotics, usually cefaclor, should then be started to finish a 7- to 10-day course of treatment (3 weeks if sinusitis is present). In patients proved to be bacteremic, 7 to 10 days of IV venous treatment is indicated.

VIII. DENTAL INFECTIONS:

A. Dental Caries:

1. **Definition:** Progressive tooth destruction that is primarily the result of organic acids produced by glycolytic activity of bacteria present in dental plaque.
2. Caries is the most important cause of tooth loss in the child and young adult. Newly erupted teeth are most susceptible to caries.
3. **Bacteriology:** The viridans streptococci, most importantly *S. mutans,* as well as some lactobacilli and actinomyces, are cariogenic organisms found in plaque. These must have access to dietary monosaccharides and disaccharides as substrates for glycolysis with organic acid production.
4. **Clinical features:** Erosive lesions that extend inward from the tooth surface, either the enamel-coated crown or the cementum of the exposed root surface.
5. **Complications:** Extension of dental caries into the pulp chamber of the tooth and through the root canal to the periapical area can lead to a periapical abscess or to a chronic periapical granuloma or sinus tract. Further extension can lead to alveolar osteomyelitis, to cervical adenitis or cellulitis, and, rarely, to septic thrombophlebitis. Bacterial endocarditis is a potential complication, particularly if bacteremia develops in a patient with underlying heart disease (e.g., associated with dental manipulation).
6. **Prevention:** Fluoride, administered systemically or topically, greatly reduces caries by producing a more acid-resistant tooth structure resulting from incorporation of fluoride rather than hydroxyl ions into the hydroxyapatite mineral structure of the tooth. Frequent removal of plaque and reduction of dietary intake of monosaccharides and disaccharides contribute to caries prevention.

B. Acute necrotizing ulcerative gingivitis:

1. **Definition:** Also known as Vincent's infection, fusospirochetal disease, or trench mouth, this is an acute painful infection of the gingiva.
2. **Bacteriology:** A variety of fusiform bacteria and spirochetes have been implicated.

3. **Clinical features:** Rapidly progressing ulcerative lesions of the interdental areas of the gingiva leading to foci of frank bleeding and formation of a pseudomembranous necrotic exudate; foul breath and taste, pain, and thick saliva; malaise and some fever may be present; patients should be evaluated for possible leukocyte adhesion defect (CD11/CD18 deficiency).
4. **Complications:** Destruction of the interdental papillae and pathologic bone resorption may develop.
5. **Therapy:** Localized curettage and rinses with hydrogen peroxide or chlorhexidine; systemic penicillin may also be of benefit.

IX. CARDIAC INFECTIONS:

A. Infective Endocarditis

1. **Epidemiology and pathogenesis:**
   a. Infective endocarditis (IE) occurs in 0.1% to 0.3% of all pediatric hospital admissions. Children comprise about 20% of all patients with IE.
   b. IE usually results from hematogenous infection of a preexisting fibrin-platelet thrombus that formed in an area of endocardium or vascular endothelium damaged by abnormally turbulent blood flow. Therefore, the main group of children at risk for IE are those with congenital heart disease and particularly those with prosthetic valves, patches, and conduits. The decline in incidence of rheumatic fever has lessened its importance as a risk factor for development of IE.
   c. The long-term presence of a central venous catheter is an important risk factor for development of IE.
   d. IV drug use, a very important risk factor for IE in adults, is an uncommon risk factor in the pediatric population.
   e. Occasionally IE occurs in children with structurally normal hearts; the pathogenesis of these infections is obscure.
   f. The bacteremia that is a prerequisite for the development of IE does not result from common events such as adjustment of orthodontic braces and shedding of teeth. However, oral surgery and GI and

genitourinary (GU) procedures carry a significant risk of bacteremia and require antibiotic prophylaxis in patients at risk for IE.

2. **Etiologic organisms:**
   a. Streptococci and staphylococci together account for 80% of pediatric IE.
   b. Staphylococci are an increasingly common cause of pediatric IE and are the leading cause in some centers. *S. aureus* is the most common cause of IE in children with structurally normal hearts; *S. aureus* and coagulase-negative staphylococci are frequent causes of postoperative IE. Less common organisms include *Hemophilus* (non-*influenzae* spp.), diphtheroids, and miscellaneous gram-negative bacilli.
   c. Neonatal IE is mainly caused by staphylococci, especially *S. aureus*. Group B streptococci are a rare cause of neonatal IE.
   d. Enterococcal IE, common in elderly adults and difficult to treat, is rare in children.
   e. Fungal IE, usually caused by *Candida* or *Aspergillus,* is rare but often lethal despite therapy. Surgical resection is usually necessary.
3. **Clinical and laboratory findings:**
   a. Persistent fever in a child with heart disease or in a child with a new or changing cardiac murmur strongly suggests IE. IE may rarely manifest as fever of unknown origin in a patient with a structurally normal heart.
   b. Extracardiac manifestations of IE (splinter hemorrhages, Roth spots, splenomegaly, significant renal disease, etc.) are less common in children than in adults. Nonspecific symptoms such as headache and malaise may occur. Signs of congestive heart failure may be one of the initial manifestations of IE.
   c. Neonatal IE manifests in a nonspecific manner, often with signs and symptoms of sepsis. It typically occurs in neonates with indwelling central venous catheters and structurally normal hearts.
   d. The blood culture is the cornerstone of diagnosis of IE and is ultimately positive in 90% to 95% of pa-

tients. Because the bacteremia of IE, although low grade, is continuous, blood cultures do not have to be obtained only with fever spikes. Collection of three sets of blood cultures in 24 hours is generally adequate for diagnosis. The blood volume per culture should be as large as is reasonable, although this is clearly limited by patient size. Patients with fungal IE are only intermittently fungemic and are therefore less likely to have positive blood cultures. In these patients, the diagnosis is most often established by echocardiogram, at surgery, or at autopsy.

e. Echocardiography, when positive, is of great importance in diagnosis of IE; however, failure to demonstrate a vegetation on echocardiogram does not exclude the diagnosis.

f. Other laboratory findings frequently associated with IE include elevated erythrocyte sedimentation rate (ESR), anemia, and microscopic hematuria. Leukocytosis is infrequently seen.

4. **Therapy and prophylaxis:**

   a. Therapy requires a prolonged course of parenteral antibiotics because bacteria are present at very high densities within vegetations and are relatively protected from host defense mechanisms at these sites.

   b. The American Heart Association has recently provided guidelines for therapy of streptococcal, staphylococcal, and enterococcal IE; these guidelines are summarized in Tables 6–4 to 6–6. Duration of therapy is generally 2 weeks longer for patients with intracardiac prosthetic material. Note that dosage of certain drugs (e.g., gentamicin) may need modification in patients with renal insufficiency.

   c. Fungal endocarditis usually requires surgical excision of the infected valve or vegetation, together with at least 6 weeks of IV amphotericin B therapy.

   d. Treatment of culture-negative endocarditis should include a penicillinase-resistant penicillin such as nafcillin plus gentamicin. Penicillin-allergic patients or postoperative patients with intracardiac prosthetic

TABLE 6–4.
Treatment of Infective Endocarditis Caused by Streptococci or Enterococci in Non-Penicillin-Allergic Patients

Highly penicillin-sensitive streptococci (MIC up to 0.1 μg/mL)

1. Penicillin G 200,000 u/kg/day IV (up to 20 million units/day) × 4 wk, **or**
2. Penicillin G 200,000 u/kg/day IV (up to 20 million units/day) × 2 wk **plus** gentamicin 2.0–2.5 mg/kg/dose IV (up to 80 mg) q8h × 2 wk, **or**
3. Penicillin G 200,000 u/kg/day IV (up to 20 million units/day) × 4 wk **plus** gentamicin 2.0–2.5 mg/kg/dose IV (up to 80 mg) q8h × 2 wk.

Relatively penicillin-resistant streptococci (MIC > 0.1 μg/mL, < 0.5 μg/mL)

Penicillin G 300,000 u/kg/day IV (up to 20 million units/day) × 4 wk **plus** gentamicin 2.0–2.5 mg/kg/dose IV (up to 80 mg) q8h × 2 wk.

Enterococci or penicillin-resistant streptococci

1. Penicillin G 300,000 u/kg/day IV (up to 30 million units/day) × 4–6 wk **plus** gentamicin 2.0–2.5 mg/kg/dose IV (up to 80 mg) q8h × 4–6 wk, **or**
2. Ampicillin 300 mg/kg/d IV (up to 12 g/day) × 4–6 wk **plus** gentamicin 2.0–2.5 mg/kg/dose IV (up to 80 mg) q8h × 4–6 wk.

material should be treated with vancomycin plus gentamicin. If there is a marked response to therapy, the gentamicin may be discontinued after 2 weeks. Total duration of treatment should be 6 weeks.

TABLE 6–5.
Treatment of Streptococcal or Enterococcal IE in Penicillin-Allergic Patients

Highly penicillin-sensitive streptococci (MIC up to 0.1 μg/mL)

1. Cephalothin 100–150 mg/kg/day IV (up to 12 g/day) × 4 wk. **or:**
2. Vancomycin 40 mg/kg/day IV in 2–4 divided doses (up to 2 g/day) × 4 wk.

Relatively penicillin-resistant streptococci (MIC > 0.1 μg/mL, < 0.5 μg/mL)

1. Cephalothin 100–150 mg/kg/day IV (up to 12 g/day) × 4 wk **plus** gentamicin 2.0–2.5 mg/kg/dose IV (up to 80mg) q8h × 2 wk, **or:**
2. Vancomycin 40 mg/kg/d IV in 2–4 divided doses (up to 2 g/day) × 4 wk **plus** gentamicin 2.0–2.5 mg/kg/dose IV (up to 80 mg) q8h × 2 wk.

Enterococci or penicillin-resistant streptococci

Vancomycin 40 mg/kg/day IV in 2–4 divided doses (up to 2 g/day) × 4–6 wk, **plus** gentamicin 2.0–2.5 mg/kg/dose IV (up to 80 mg) q8h × 4–6 wk.

TABLE 6–6.
Treatment of Staphylococcal IE

Methicillin-susceptible staphylococci in absence of prosthetic valve or material

1. Nafcillin or oxacillin 150–200 mg/kg/day IV (up to 12 g/day) × 4–6 wk **with or without** gentamicin 2.0–2.5 mg/kg/dose (up to 80 mg) q8h × 5 days.
2. **For penicillin-allergic patients:** Cefazolin 80–100 mg/kg/day IV (up to 6 g/day) × 4–6 wk **with or without** gentamicin 2.0–2.5 mg/kg/dose IV (up to 80 mg) q8h times 5 days, OR:
3. For Penicillin-allergic patients: Vancomycin 40 mg/kg/day IV in 2–4 divided doses (up to 2 g/day) × 4–6 wk.

Methicillin-resistant staphylococci in absence of prosthetic valve or material

Vancomycin 40 mg/kg/day IV in 2–4 divided doses (up to 2 g/day)× 4–6 wk.

Methicillin-susceptible staphylococci in presence of prosthetic valve or material

1. Nafcillin or oxacillin 150–200 mg/kg/day IV (up to 12 g/day) × 6–8 wk **plus** rifampin 20 mg/kg/d po (up to 900 mg/day) × 6–8 wk **plus** gentamicin 2.0–2.5 mg/kg/dose (up to 80 mg) q8h × 2 wk.
2. For penicillin-allergic patients: Vancomycin 40 mg/kg/day, IV in 2–4 divided doses (up to 2 g/day) × 6–8 wk **plus** rifampin and gentamicin as above.

Methicillin-resistant staphylococci in presence of prosthetic valve or material

Vancomycin 40 mg/kg/day IV in 2–4 divided doses (up to 2 g/day) × 6–8 wk **plus** rifampin and gentamicin as above.

e. Antibiotic prophylaxis for prevention of IE is indicated for patients with any of the following: intracardiac prosthetic material, acquired valvular disease, structural heart disease (except atrial septal defect [ASD]), idiopathic hypertrophic subaortic stenosis, mitral valve prolapse with mitral insufficiency, and previous heart surgery (except ASD or patent ductus arteriosus [PDA] repair). A summary of the American Heart Association's current recommendations for prophylaxis is presented in Table 6–7.

B. Infective Myocarditis

1. Epidemiology, etiology, and pathogenesis:

a. Infective myocarditis (IM) is an uncommon disease in pediatrics, although prevalence data are not available. IM may be subclinical and may occur as a component of pancarditis, as in acute rheumatic fever.

TABLE 6–7.
Antibiotic Regimens for Infective Endocarditis Prophylaxis

For oral surgery, dental procedures causing gingival bleeding, and upper respiratory tract procedures

1. Standard regimens:
   a. Amoxicillin 50 mg/kg (up to 3 g) po 1 hr before the procedure and one half the initial dose 6 hr after the first dose.
   b. For children unable to take oral medications, parenteral ampicillin 50 mg/kg (up to 2 g) 30 min before the procedure and one half the initial dose 6 hr after the first dose.
2. Regimen for those with intracardiac prosthetic valves or systemic-pulmonary shunts: parenteral ampicillin 50 mg/kg (up to 2 g) **plus** parenteral gentamicin 2.0 mg/kg (up to 80 mg), given 30 min before the procedure. Oral amoxicillin 25 mg/kg (up to 1.5 g) is given 6 hr after the initial antibiotics, or the parenteral regimen can be repeated 8 hr after the first dose. Many authorities recommend the above standard regimen for this high risk group.
3. Regimen for penicillin-allergic patients:
   a. Oral: Erythromycin ethylsuccinate or stearate 20 mg/kg (up to 800 mg of erythromycin ethylsuccinate or $\leq$ 1 g of erythromycin stearate) 2 h before the procedure, followed by one half the initial dose 6 hr after the first dose. Alternative regimen: Clindamycin 10 mg/kg (up to 300 mg) po 1 hr before the procedure, followed by one half the initial dose 6 hr after the first dose.
   b. Parenteral: Clindamycin 10 mg/kg IV (up to 300 mg) 30 min before the procedure, followed by one half the initial dose 6 hr after the first dose.
   c. Parenteral for patients with intracardiac prosthetic material or systemic-pulmonary shunts: Vancomycin 20 mg/kg IV (up to 1 g) given over 1 hr, starting 1 hr before the procedure.

For GI/GU procedures

1. Standard regimen: Parenteral ampicillin and gentamicin 30–60 min before the procedure and again 8 hr after the first dose. Alternatively, oral amoxicillin may be given 6 hr after the initial antibiotics. Dosages are the same as given earlier.
2. Oral regimen for minor procedures in a low-risk patient: Amoxicillin 50 mg/kg (up to 3 g) 1 hr before the procedure and one half the initial dose 6 hr after the initial dose.
3. Regimen for penicillin-allergic patients: IV vancomycin and gentamicin 1 hr before the procedure, with a repeat dose 8 hr after the first dose. Dosages are the same as given earlier.

b. Viruses are the most common cause of IM in children. Implicated viruses include Coxsackie A virus, Coxsackie B virus, echovirus, influenza, mumps, measles, and varicella virus. Coxsackie B virus has been associated with nursery epidemics of IM.
c. Various bacteria, including staphylococci, streptococci, meningococci, *Klebsiella,* and *H. influenzae* have been implicated as causes of IM. Bacterial myocarditis most often occurs as part of a myopericarditis.
d. Diphtheria toxin is a well-described but now rare cause of myocarditis.
e. *Borrelia burgdorferii,* the causative agent of Lyme disease, causes a myocarditis that is one of the key features of the disease. Myocarditis may also occur in cases of syphilis.
f. Myocarditis may complicate several parasitic diseases including trichinosis, American trypanosomiasis (Chagas' disease), toxoplasmosis, and malaria.
g. The pathogenesis and pathologic findings of myocarditis depends on the class of infecting organism:
    1) Viruses may infect myocytes and either cause direct cytolysis or incorporate viral antigen into the myocyte cell membrane, leading to immune-mediated myocyte destruction.
    2) Bacterial myocarditis, often manifesting as myopericarditis, typically produces microabscesses and focal suppuration. Myocardial abscesses may complicate bacterial endocarditis.
    3) Myocardial involvement in trichinosis may be indicated by an eosinophilic infiltrate. Cysts do not form in the myocardium. Trypanosomal infection causes an intense myocarditis resulting from rupture of intracellular cysts. Myocardial capillary occlusion is sometimes seen in malaria.

2. **Clinical and laboratory findings:**
    a. Myocarditis may be subclinical, or it may occur as a component of pancarditis, with the clinical findings dependent on the layer of the heart most severely involved.

b. Neonates with myocarditis typically manifest with nonspecific symptoms such as fever, cyanosis, tachycardia, and tachypnea.
c. Older infants and children with myocarditis usually present with signs of low-output cardiac failure: pallor, cool extremities, tachypnea, tachycardia, thready pulse and hepatomegaly. Murmurs are usually absent.
d. Electrocardiogram (ECG) findings include low-voltage QRS complexes, low-amplitude or inverted T waves, and ST-segment elevation in the precordial leads. Various conduction disturbances, both bradycardias and tachycardias, may be seen.
e. The echocardiogram is extremely valuable for assessing ventricular function in myocarditis and helps to exclude pericardial effusion as a source of cardiac dysfunction.
f. Laboratory findings include elevated ESR, leukocytosis, and sometimes elevated creatine phosphokinase (CPK) and lactic dehydrogenase (LDH) levels. Blood cultures may be positive in cases of bacterial myocarditis. Specific IgM assays are available for several of the viruses implicated in myocarditis.

3. **Therapy:**
   a. The cornerstone of treatment is intensive supportive therapy, including bedrest and inotropic drugs if needed. Arrhythmias should be promptly recognized and treated.
   b. Antibiotics should be given if bacterial infection is suspected. No specific antiviral therapy is available for the viruses commonly thought to cause myocarditis.
   c. The role of immunosuppressive therapy in treatment of viral myocarditis is still controversial.
   d. Cardiac transplantation may be an option in cases of myocarditis that result in intractable, end-stage cardiac failure.

C. **Infective pericarditis:**

1. **Epidemiology, etiology, and pathogensis:**
   a. Infective pericarditis (IP) is an uncommon disease but is more frequent in children than adults.

b. Bacteria, mycobacteria, and fungi are the best-documented causes of IP. Certain viruses are generally believed to be causes of IP but often cannot be documented as etiologic agents.
   1) The bacteria most commonly causing IP are *S. aureus* (40%–50% of bacterial pericarditis), Hib (20%–25%), *N. meningitidis* (10%–15%), and *S. pneumoniae* (5%–10%)
   2) *M. tuberculosis* is an uncommon cause of acute IP but may cause chronic constrictive pericardial disease. Tuberculous pericarditis occurs in 0.5% to 5% of all children with TB.
   3) Fungal pericarditis is rare. Known causative agents include *Aspergillus, Blastomyces, Coccidioides, Histoplasma,* and *Candida.*
   4) Viruses documented to cause IP include coxsackie, adenovirus, echovirus, varicella, mumps, and influenzae.

c. IP usually represents spread from a primary site of infection.
   1) *S. pneumoniae, S. aureus,* and *H. influenzae* may produce primary pulmonary infection that can spread to the pericardium via the bronchial circulation, direct extension, or hematogenous spread. Osteomyelitis, septic arthritis, or impetigo may be caused by *S. aureus,* which then reaches the pericardium hematogenously. *H. influenzae* and *N. meningitidis* may produce a primary meningitis or septic arthritis with bacteremia that results in pericardial infection.
   2) Tuberculous pericarditis usually occurs in association with miliary tuberculosis. It may result from either hematogenous spread or direct extension from infected mediastinal lymph nodes.

2. **Clinical findings:**
   a. Fever, tachypnea, and tachycardia are the most common findings in IP; however, these are common findings in any serious infection.
   b. More specific signs and symptoms include precordial pain (infrequent in young children), a pericardial friction rub, and muffled heart sounds.

c. Evidence of cardiac tamponade may be present and is an indication for emergent pericardiocentesis. Signs of tamponade include a narrow pulse pressure, pulsus paradoxus > 10 mm Hg, jugular venous distention, hepatomegaly, and, in severe cases, frank hypotension. Tamponade is most likely when pericardial fluid accumulation has been rapid. It is rare in viral pericarditis.
d. Because IP is usually a secondary infection, a thorough search should be made for a site of primary infection (pneumonia, meningitis, osteomyelitis, etc.)
e. Viral pericarditis is usually associated with an antecedent URI. Patients with viral pericarditis are usually less ill than those with purulent pericarditis.

3. **Laboratory evaluation:**
   a. An enlarged cardiac silhouette on chest x-ray, usually without an increase in pulmonary vascular markings, is typical for IP but may not be present if the amount of pericardial fluid is small.
   b. ECG findings are inconsistent and include low-voltage QRS complexes, ST-segment elevation, and T-wave inversion.
   c. Echocardiography is the most sensitive means of detecting pericardial fluid.
   d. The cornerstone of diagnosis of IP is pericardiocentesis. Pericardial fluid should be sent for cell count, glucose, protein, Gram's stain, acid-fast stain, and bacterial, mycobacterial, viral, and fungal cultures. Latex agglutination or CIE of pericardial fluid is often useful.
   e. Blood cultures are positive in 40% to 80% of cases of suppurative pericarditis.
   f. Lumbar puncture to rule out meningitis is generally indicated if *H. influenzae* or *N. meningitidis* pericarditis is present.
   g. A TB skin test should be placed unless bacterial pericarditis is proved.
   h. Viral serologies may be useful if viral pericarditis is suspected.

4. **Therapy:**
   a. Treatment of bacterial pericarditis requires both surgical drainage of pericardial fluid and parenteral antibiotic therapy.
      1) Adequate surgical drainage requires either creation of a pericardial window or anterior pericardiectomy with pericardiostomy tube placement. Percutaneous pericardiostomy tube placement usually does not provide adequate drainage because of the thick, fibrinous nature of the pericardial exudate.
      2) Initial antibiotic therapy should consist of a penicillinase-resistant penicillin plus cefotaxime or ceftriaxone. The antibiotic spectrum can be narrowed after the causative organism is identified. Duration of therapy is generally 2 to 4 weeks.
   b. Tuberculous pericarditis is treated with a three-drug regimen (INH, pyrazinamide, and rifampin) for 9 to 18 months. Corticosteroids are often useful as adjunctive therapy after antituberculous agents have been initiated. Pericardiectomy may be necessary if recurrent tamponade or constrictive pericarditis occurs.
   c. Fungal pericarditis is treated with amphotericin B. Pericardiostomy or pericardiectomy may be necessary in some cases.
   d. Viral pericarditis is treated symptomatically with bedrest and analgesia. Nonsteroidal anti-inflammatory drugs are useful because of their antipyrexic, analgesic, and anti-inflammatory properties. The illness usually resolves in 3 to 4 weeks but may be recurrent.

X. CENTRAL NERVOUS SYSTEM INFECTIONS (Table 6–8):

A. Bacterial Meningitis:

1. **Epidemiology:**
   a. Meningitis is a potentially fatal illness characterized by inflammation of the meninges and caused by a variety of bacteria.

TABLE 6–8.
CSF Findings

	WBC Count (per mm^3)	Predominant Cell Type	Glucose	Protein	Microscopic Examination	Culture
Normal	<5	MNC	>60% serum glucose	<40 mg/dL	–	–
Neonate	<10	PMN, MNC	>50% serum glucose	Term: <60 mg/dL Premature: <130 mg/dL	–	–
Meningitis						
Bacterial	>1,000	PMN	Low	Normal-high	Usually Gram's stain +	Usually +
Aseptic	<1,000	PMN early MNC late	Usually normal	Normal	–	–
Tuberculous	<1,000	MNC	Low	High–very high	Rarely AFB +	Occasionally +
Encephalitis	5–1,000	PMN early MNC late	Normal	Normal–High	–	–
Brain abscess	5–500	Variable	Normal	Normal–High	–	–

AFB = acid-fast bacilli, MNC = mononuclear cells, PMN = polymorphonuclear cells, – = negative, + = positive.

   b. Ninety percent of cases in children occur between ages 1 month and 5 years.
   c. Children between 6 and 12 months are at highest risk for bacterial meningitis.
2. **Etiology:** The etiology of bacterial meningitis varies with age; the most common organisms at various ages are as follows:
   a. Neonates:
      1) Group B streptococcus *(Streptococcus agalactiae).*
      2) *Escherichia coli* and other coliform bacteria.
      3) *Listeria monocytogenes.*
      4) Enterococcus.
      5) *Staphylococcus* and *Candida* (nosocomial).
   b. Infants and preschool children:
      1) Hib
      2) *S. pneumoniae* (pneumococcus)
      3) *N. meningitidis* (meningococcus)
   c. Older children:
      1) *S. pneumoniae*
      2) *N. meningitidis*
3. **Pathogenesis:**
   a. Bacterial meningitis is generally hematogenous in origin (i.e., organisms colonizing the nasopharynx invade the bloodstream and then seed the meninges).
   b. Other routes to the CNS include:
      1) Direct extension from paranasal sinuses or mastoids to the meninges.
      2) Severe head trauma with skull fracture.
      3) Direct inoculation of bacteria into the CSF related to congenital dural defects, neurosurgical procedures, penetrating wounds, or extension from a suppurative parameningeal focus.
   c. CNS injury may be mediated by proinflammatory cytokines triggered by bacterial components.
4. **Clinical manifestations:**
   a. Children and adolescents:
      1) Patients typically have fever, chills, vomiting, irritability, and (if old enough) severe headache.

Occasionally a convulsion may be the first manifestation.

2) As the illness progresses, the patient may develop delirium, obtundation, and coma.
3) The most consistent physical finding in children > 1 year of age is nuchal rigidity, with Brudzinski's and Kernig's signs:
    a) Brudzinski's sign is manifested by flexion of the knees when the neck of a supine patient is rapidly flexed.
    b) Kernig's sign is the presence of marked resistance to extension of the knee when the patient is supine with knees and hips in flexion.
4) Petechial and purpuric lesions are typically associated with meningococcemia, although petechial eruptions may be seen occasionally with Hib or pneumococcal meningitis or sepsis.

b. Signs and symptoms of meningitis are more subtle in infants:
    1) The illness is often characterized by fever, vomiting, convulsions, and a high-pitched cry.
    2) Nuchal rigidity is infrequently present in infants < 18 months.
    3) A tense, bulging fontanelle is often found in young infants.

c. Neonatal meningitis is discussed in Chapter 3 (section II, B2).

5. Differential diagnosis:
    a. Included in the differential diagnosis are aseptic meningitis, tuberculous meningitis, fungal meningitis, brain abscess, brain tumor, intracranial hemorrhage, and lead encephalopathy.
    b. Differentiation depends on the clinical features, careful examination of CSF, and roentgenographic studies. Typical CSF findings are given in Table 6–8.

6. **Diagnosis:**
    a. The diagnosis of bacterial meningitis is based on the clinical picture and examination of the CSF.

b. CSF should be examined for general appearance, red blood cell (RBC) counts, WBC count with differential, glucose and protein concentrations, latex agglutination for bacterial antigens, Gram's stain, and culture.
   1) The WBC count is quite variable but is usually $> 1{,}000/mm^3$ with predominance of PMNs. The WBC count may be normal or near normal very early in the course of illness.
   2) The CSF glucose level is typically less than one half the blood glucose level. The protein concentration is usually moderately increased.
   3) Latex agglutination is used to identity rapidly bacterial antigens in CSF: Hib, *S. pneumoniae, N. meningitidis, E. coli* (K1), and group B streptococcus.
   4) The probability of detecting bacteria on Gram's stain is related to the number of organisms present in the CSF. Usually, organisms are detectable when at least 10^5/mL are present.

7. **Treatment:**
   a. Newborn infants: (Chapter 3)
      1) Initial empiric antibiotic choice for neonatal meningitis is usually ampicillin and ceftriaxone (or cefotaxime).
      2) Ampicillin and an aminoglycoside (gentamicin, amikacin) is an excellent alternative.
      3) Once the antibiotic susceptibilities of the pathogen are available, the most appropriate antibiotic(s) should be selected.
      4) The duration of antibiotic therapy is dependent on the organism involved and the clinical response.
         a) 14 to 21 days of therapy is adequate for most cases of meningitis caused by group B streptococcus or *Listeria*.
         b) 3 weeks of therapy, or at least 2 weeks after sterilization of CSF (whichever is longer), are required for gram-negative enteric meningitis.

b. Infants and children:
   1) Standard therapy for pediatric meningitis has been ampicillin and chloramphenicol. However, expanded spectrum cephalosporins generally have replaced ampicillin and chloramphenicol in the empiric treatment of meningitis in infants and children.
   2) Cefotaxime (200 mg/kg/day) and ceftriaxone (100 mg/kg/day) are both effective against the common pathogens that cause meningitis in this age group.
   3) Once the etiologic agent has been identified, alteration of therapy may be indicated (e.g., to penicillin for *N. meningitidis*).
   4) 7 to 10 days of treatment is satisfactory for most patients with uncomplicated Hib or meningococcal disease; 10 to 14 days is recommended for pneumococcal meningitis.
   5) Fluid restriction to two thirds to three fourths of maintenance is recommended for the first few days.
   6) Dexamethasone is currently under study as adjunctive therapy to antibiotics. The intensity of the inflammatory response may be detrimental to cerebral tissue; corticosteroids may diminish the inflammatory reaction and thus improve the ultimate outcome.

8. **Prevention:** Immunization is the most effective means of prevention of bacterial meningitis in children. Hib, meningococcal, and pneumococcal vaccines are currently available (See Chapter 1.)
9. **Chemoprophylaxis:**
   a. Meningococcal infections:
      1) Household, day care center, and nursery school contacts:
         Rifampin 10 mg/kg (max 600 mg) q12h for 2 days (four doses)
   b. Invasive *Hemophilus* infections:
      1) All household contacts when at least one is ≤48 months:

2) All day care facilitates with children ≤2 years: Rifampin 20 mg/kg (max 600 mg) once daily for 4 days (four doses)
   Rifampin is available in 150- and 300-mg capsules, and a liquid suspension (1% in simple syrup) can be prepared.

10. **Prognosis and sequelae:**
    a. The prognosis of bacterial meningitis is dependent on many factors, including:
       1) Age of the patient.
       2) Duration of illness before effective antibiotic therapy.
       3) Microorganism causing disease.
       4) The number of organisms present in the CSF at the time of diagnosis.
       5) Coexisting disorders that may compromise host response to infection.
    b. Features generally associated with a worse neurologic prognosis include younger age, longer duration of meningitis before treatment, and greater antigenic load at presentation. Beyond the neonatal period, sequelae are most common with *S. pneumoniae* and least common with *N. meningitidis* meningitis.
    c. The mortality rate for bacterial meningitis (beyond the neonatal period) has been reduced to between 1% and 5% with treatment; however, up to 50% of survivors have some sequelae.
    d. Common complications of bacterial meningitis include hearing loss, speech disturbance, mental retardation, motor abnormalities, behavioral problems, seizure disorder, and impaired vision.

B. **Aseptic Meningitis:**

1. **Etiology:**
   a. Aseptic meningitis is a common syndrome associated with a variety of infectious agents and clinical circumstances:
      1) Viral agents: Enteroviruses (poliovirus, coxsackievirus, echovirus), mumps, HSV, varicella-zoster virus, arboviruses, lymphocytic chori-

omeningitis, EBV, rabies, and adenovirus are most common.
   2) Bacteria: Partially treated, tuberculous, cat-scratch fever.
   3) Other infectious agents:
      a) Spirochetes: Lyme disease, syphilis, leptospirosis, rat-bite fever.
      b) Rickettsiae: Typhus, Rocky Mountain spotted fever.
      c) Fungi.
      d) Protozoa and helminths: Toxoplasmosis, malaria, neurocysticercosis, amebiasis.
   4) Tumors: Metastases to meninges, leukemia, carcinomatosis.
   5) Chemical irritation: Contrast media, intrathecal drugs.
   6) Poisons: Lead, arsenic.
   7) Miscellaneous: Sarcoidosis, Kawasaki disease, Behçet's syndrome, Mollaret's meningitis, Vogt-Koyanagi-Harada syndrome.
b. Enteroviruses and mumps virus are the most frequently implicated causative agents. Partially treated bacterial meningitis commonly manifests as an aseptic meningitis-like illness.

2. **Epidemiology:**
   a. The peak incidence for aseptic meningitis is in late summer and early fall, coinciding with the peak incidence for enteroviral infections. However, sporadic illnesses occur throughout the year.
   b. Viral meningitis occurs in children of all ages.
3. **Clinical manifestations:**
   a. Aseptic meningitis is characterized typically by an abrupt onset of headache with fever, signs and symptoms of meningeal irritation, and minimal or no abnormalities in neurologic function.
   b. There may be clinical evidence of other manifestations of the particular viral illness (e.g., a macular or petechial rash of enteroviral infection or the parotid swelling of mumps).
   c. Seizures are uncommon but occur in young children with fever.

4. **Diagnosis:**
   a. The diagnosis of aseptic meningitis requires CSF examination. The CSF characteristically demonstrates pleocytosis, normal to mildly elevated protein concentration, and a normal glucose concentration. Low glucose concentrations are rather common in mumps meningitis.
   b. In the early stages of illness, PMNs are often present in CSF; however, lymphocytes predominate later in the course.
   c. Therefore, when the CSF results are initially equivocal, a second CSF examination 8 to 10 hours later may be of great benefit in differentiating bacterial from viral meningitis. Viral CSF cultures are very often negative in viral meningitis.
5. **Treatment:** Treatment is generally symptomatic and supportive. Once the diagnosis of viral meningitis is secured, antimicrobial therapy is not required.

C. **Encephalitis:**

1. **Etiology:** Encephalitis refers to infection of the brain parenchyma, most frequently caused by a virus. Common causes of acute encephalitis in the United States (and among American travelers abroad) are:
   a. Viruses:
      1) Arboviruses: St. Louis, Eastern equine, Western equine, Venezuelan equine, California, Powassan, Colorado tick fever.
      2) Enteroviruses: Coxsackie A and B viruses, enteric cytopathic human orphan (ECHO) virus.
      3) Others: Herpes simplex types 1 and 2, mumps, varicella-zoster virus, measles, rabies, rubella, EBV, CMV, influenza A and B, lymphocytic choriomeningitis.
   b. Nonviral agents:
      1) Bacteria: Hib, *N. meningitidis, S. pneumoniae,* and other bacterial meningitides often have an encephalitic component.
      2) Spirochetes: Syphilis, leptospirosis, Lyme disease, and other *Borrelia* infections.
      3) Rickettsial infections: RMSF and typhus.

4) Mycoplasmal infections.
5) Fungal agents.
6) Protozoa: *Naegleria* spp., *Acanthamoeba* and toxoplasmosis.
7) Cat-scratch disease.

c. Mumps was the leading cause of meningoencephalitis in the United States before the widespread use of mumps vaccine. Enteroviruses, herpes simplex, and arboviruses are now the leading causes of encephalitis in the United States. Arboviruses are the most important cause of severe encephalitis worldwide.

2. **Epidemiology:** The majority of encephalitis occurs in the summer and fall, the peak season for enteroviral and arboviral infections. However, sporadic cases of encephalitis occur year around.
3. **Pathogenesis:**
   a. For many viruses, primary infection is followed by the virus gaining access to the lymphatic system where viral multiplication occurs, with resultant viremia and spread to the CNS.
   b. Involvement of the CNS may also result from extension of viruses into neuronal and glial cells adjacent to infected capillary endothelial cells, centripetal axonal transport of virus from the olfactory neuroepithelium to the olfactory bulb, or retrograde spread of virus via the peripheral nerves.
   c. Clinical manifestations reflect either direct or indirect effects of an infectious agent on the brain:
      1) Examples in which the virus directly involves tissue cells within the brain include rabies, arbovirus, herpes simplex, and enteroviral encephalitides.
      2) The encephalitic symptoms in rickettsial infections and bacterial meningitides are probably secondary to the vasculitis.
      3) Immunologic reactions are known to play a role in the pathogenesis of encephalitis caused by measles and *M. pneumoniae*.
4. **Clinical manifestations:**
   a. The severity of clinical manifestations varies tremendously.

b. Initial manifestations are usually nonspecific, (i.e., fever, headache, nausea, vomiting, and abdominal pain, which later progress to neurologic abnormalities).

c. Progression of disease may lead to behavioral or personality changes, ataxia, cranial nerve defects, paresis, sensory changes, seizures, stupor, coma, and death.

5. **Diagnosis:**

a. The diagnosis of acute encephalitis is made most frequently on the basis of clinical findings.

b. A careful history is essential to evaluate recent exposure to mosquitoes, ticks, animals, and ill contacts.

c. CSF should be examined to exclude other disorders, as well as to detect specific viral antigens or early antibodies.

1) In viral encephalitis, the CSF is frequently clear.

2) WBC counts range from normal to over a thousand with an initial polymorphonuclear predominance.

3) The protein concentration may be normal or moderately elevated.

4) The glucose concentration is usually normal.

d. Serologic diagnosis may be made with at least a four- fold antibody rise between acute and convalescent titers or specific IgM elevation.

e. If herpes simplex encephalitis (HSE) is being entertained, brain biopsy should be considered. Patients frequently have focal neurologic findings:

1) CT or magnetic resonance image (MRI) scans may show low-density lesions in one or both temporal lobes. Unfortunately, these abnormalities may not develop until several days into the course of the illness.

2) Electroencephalogram (EEG) frequently shows periodic lateralized epileptiform discharges (PLEDS) with HSV encephalitis.

3) Radionuclide scans may demonstrate blood-

brain barrier breakdown in the temporal regions.

6. **Differential diagnosis:** The differential diagnosis of acute encephalitis includes metabolic diseases, Reye syndrome, toxic ingestion, mass lesions, subarachnoid hemorrhage, acute demyelinating disorders, status epilepticus, other CNS infections (e.g., abscess, meningitis), and postinfectious diseases.
7. **Therapy:**
   a. With the exception of acyclovir for HSE, treatment of viral encephalitides is usually nonspecific and supportive.
   b. Therapy is aimed at controlling intracranial pressure (ICP), hyperthermia, and convulsions, as well as maintaining proper water and electrolyte balance.
   c. Acyclovir (30 mg/kg/day divided q8h) is the drug of choice for the treatment of HSE. Therapy should be instituted intravenously as soon as possible.
8. **Prognosis:** The prognosis is guarded in all encephalitides. The prognosis depends to a certain extent on etiology and age:
   a. Young infants usually have a poorer prognosis than older patients.
   b. Many patients with HSE do poorly, even with antiviral therapy.

D. CNS Tuberculosis:

1. **Epidemiology:**
   a. CNS TB has become a relatively rare problem in the United States, occurring in 1 of every 300 primary infections.
   b. It is seen most commonly in children < 6 years and usually appears within 3 to 6 months of an initial infection.
2. **Pathogenesis:**
   a. The tubercle bacillus affects the CNS in various ways, causing TB meningitis, tuberculoma, and tuberculous brain abscess.
   b. TB meningitis arises from the rupture of a caseous focus, which discharges tuberculous bacilli into the subarachnoid space, an area with few host-defense mechanisms.

c. The clinical manifestations of TB meningitis result from the following pathologic processes: proliferative arachnoiditis, vasculitis, and hydrocephalus:
   1) Arachnoiditis is most severe at the base of the brain in the area extending from the pons to the optic nerves. As this process progresses, it may compromise the function of cranial nerves I through VIII in some combination.
   2) Vasculitis with inflammation, constriction, and eventual thrombosis resulting in cerebral infarction may develop in vessels that traverse the basilar exudate. The middle cerebral artery and/or its branches are most frequently involved.
   3) Hydrocephalus develops in the majority of patients with TB meningitis, especially in those who have been symptomatic for more than 2 weeks before therapy. This is most commonly a communicating hydrocephalus because of inflammatory obstruction of the basilar cisterns.

3. **Clinical manifestations:** The course of TB meningitis may be divided into three stages:
   a. The first stage is characterized by fever, listlessness, anorexia, and irritability. Patients in this stage are conscious and rational and may or may not have meningismus.
   b. After 1 to 2 weeks, the disease progresses to a second stage, with signs of increased ICP. These patients are confused or have focal neurologic deficits such as cranial nerve palsies and hemiparesis.
   c. The third stage is characterized by coma, irregular vital signs, and paralysis. Without treatment, death usually occurs within 5 to 8 weeks after onset.
4. **Diagnosis:** The diagnosis of TB meningitis is made by obtaining a history of contact with TB and by the clinical features, as well as by the following:
   a. Tuberculin skin test, the results of which are positive in 50% to 90% of cases.
   b. Chest roentgenogram, which reveals pulmonary changes in 50% to 60% of children.
   c. Most important, characteristic CSF findings:
      1) CSF is usually clear in gross appearance.

2) It typically contains 50 to 500 cells, with PMN leukocytes predominant early and lymphocytes predominant later.
3) The CSF glucose level may be normal very early in the course; however, it falls rapidly during the second and third stages.
4) The protein content may be normal at the time of the first spinal tap, but it rises rapidly to very high concentrations.
5) CT scans are recommended for evaluation of all patients with TB meningitis to detect tuberculomas and hydrocephalus.

5. **Therapy** (See Table A–21):
   a. Therapy should be initiated as soon as the disease is suspected.
   b. The initial choice of therapy should include INH, rifampin, and a third antituberculous drug. Pyrazinamide has become the third agent; because it penetrates into the CSF well, has substantial bactericidal activity even at an acid pH, and is active within macrophages.
   c. In areas of the world where the incidence of primary drug resistance is high, the addition of a fourth antituberculous drug (ethambutol) is advisable.
   d. Antituberculous therapy should be continued for 12 months with INH and rifampin; however, pyrazinamide and/or ethambutol may be discontinued after 2 months in the presence of a good response.
   e. Adjunctive use of corticosteroids probably improves the prognosis, with 2 mg/kg/day of prednisone commonly used for several weeks.
6. **Prognosis:**
   a. A favorable prognosis depends on early institution of treatment, even without confirmation of the diagnosis. The prognosis is related to the clinical stage at the time that therapy is initiated:
      1) Survival in patients treated during the first stage is almost 100% and is 75% in those treated in the second stage.

2) The majority of patients treated during the third stage die or survive with neurologic sequelae.

b. Other poor prognostic factors include hydrocephalus, very young age, and the occurrence of convulsions.

c. The long-term sequelae of TB meningitis include blindness, deafness, paraplegia, and mental retardation.

E. **Fungal Meningitis:**

1. Most CNS fungal infections can be divided into those that occur in normal hosts and those that afflict primarily immunocompromised hosts (infections with specific agents are discussed in Table A–18).
   a. *Coccidioides immitis, Blastomyces dermatitidis,* and the dematiaceous fungi all are fungi that may infect the CNS of normal hosts in the United States.
   b. In contrast, CNS aspergillosis, candidiasis, rhizopus infections, and mucormycosis almost always occur in immunocompromised patients.
   c. Meningitis caused by *Candida* spp. occurs most frequent during infancy but can occur later in life, frequently in nosocomial settings.
   d. Cryptococcal and histoplasmosis infections of the CNS may occur in normal or immunocompromised hosts.
2. The usual clinical manifestation of fungal meningitis is chronic headache and somewhat insidious mental status changes.
3. The CSF characteristically reveals a high opening pressure, lymphocytosis, high protein concentrations, and low glucose concentrations.
4. Amphotericin B is the drug of choice for most CNS fungal infections. Flucytosine may be useful in combination with amphotericin B for treatment of many of these infections. Fluconazole has been demonstrated to be effective for chronic suppressive therapy of cryptococcal meningitis. (See Table A–18.)

F. **Brain Abscess:**

1. **Epidemiology and Etiology:**
   a. Brain abscess is relatively uncommon in children.
   b. Predisposing factors include infection of contiguous

structures (e.g., otitis, mastoiditis, and sinusitis), cyanotic congenital heart disease, trauma to the skull, and meningitis.

c. No primary source of infection can be found in approximately 10% to 25% of patients.
d. Organisms most frequently recovered from brain abscesses are *S. aureus,* viridans streptococci, anaerobic streptococci, Enterobacteriaceae, *Hemophilus* spp., and *Bacteroides* spp.:
   1) Many abscesses contain mixed aerobic and anaerobic flora.
   2) Brain abscesses in neonates are caused more commonly by gram-negative organisms such as *Citrobacter* spp. and *E. coli.*
   3) Hib, *S. pneumoniae, Citrobacter* spp., *E. coli,* and *Salmonella* spp. are usually isolated from brain abscesses associated with meningitis.
   4) In patients with chronic otitis and mastoiditis the most commonly recovered organisms are *Bacteroides* spp., *Proteus* spp., *P. aeruginosa,* and *S. aureus.*
   5) *S. aureus* is the most common pathogen in patients with brain abscess after head trauma.
   6) In patients with cyanotic congenital heart disease, anaerobic or microaerophilic streptococci are the usual pathogens.

2. **Clinical Manifestations:**
   a. Infants may vomit or may have fever and/or seizure activity.
   b. Older children usually have headache and fever, which, if untreated, may progress to vomiting, lethargy, and seizures.
3. **Diagnosis:**
   a. CT or MRI scanning is the diagnostic procedure of choice to confirm the diagnosis of brain abscess.
   b. A lumbar puncture should **not** be performed in a patient with a suspected brain abscess before obtaining a CT scan.
      1) CSF is normal in 10% to 20% of patients with brain abscess.

2) Pleocytosis (5–500 cells/mm^3) with lymphocyte or PMN predominance is usually found.
3) CSF cultures are positive in fewer than 10% of patients.

4. **Treatment:**
   a. Therapy of brain abscess includes parenteral antibiotic therapy with or without surgical excision or needle aspiration.
   b. Medical treatment without surgical intervention should be considered in patients with multiple abscesses or when the abscess is in a location in which surgery may cause damage to vital structures. There have been recent reports of successful outcome in children with brain abscesses treated with antibiotics without surgical intervention.
   c. Surgical therapy consists of drainage by needle aspiration or by total excision:
      1) Aspiration under stereotactic guidance is usually performed in the early stages of disease.
      2) Total excision provides definitive treatment; however, it may not be accomplished if the abscess is very large or located deep within the brain.
   d. Antibiotics should be initiated immediately:
      1) Empiric therapy should consist of a penicillinase-resistant penicillin plus ceftriaxone plus metronidazole.
      2) Antibiotic coverage should be narrowed when Gram's stain and/or culture data are available.
      3) The optimal duration of antimicrobial therapy is not established, but most recommend a minimum of 6 weeks when medical therapy is used alone, 3 to 4 weeks in patients treated by aspiration and antibiotics, and at least 7 to 10 days of antibiotics after surgery in those with excision of an abscess.
   e. Dexamethasone may be helpful in reducing cerebral edema associated with an abscess.

5. **Prognosis and Complications:**
   a. Despite aggressive medical and surgical therapy, the mortality rate continues to be high:
      1) Earlier series reported mortality rates ranging from 27% to 40%.
      2) Since the availability of CT scanning, mortality rates of 5% to 10% have been reported.
   b. 30% to 50% of survivors have some neurologic or developmental sequelae.

G. **Shunt infections:**
1. **Etiology:**
   a. Between 2% and 20% of ventriculoperitoneal shunts are complicated by infection, primarily by coagulase-negative staphylococci, *S. aureus,* and other skin commensals, presumably introduced at the time of surgery.
   b. Gram-negative bacteria such as *E. coli, Klebsiella, Proteus, Enterobacter,* and *P. aeruginosa* cause shunt infections less commonly.
   c. Most shunt infections manifest within 2 months of shunt placement, but they occasionally become apparent even years after surgery.
2. **Clinical manifestations:** Symptoms of shunt infection may be nonspecific; they include fever, vomiting, irritability, lethargy, shunt tract inflammation, and abdominal pain. Evidence of shunt malfunction is often present.
3. **Diagnosis:** Diagnosis is made by examination of ventricular fluid; pleocytosis, diminished glucose levels, and elevated protein concentrations suggest infection. Gram's stain may be positive; however, it is usually negative when infection is caused by coagulase-negative staphylococci. Imaging studies often show evidence of ventricular dilatation related to shunt malfunction.
4. **Therapy:**
   a. Management consists of removal of the infected shunt, with placement of an extraventricular drainage (EVD) system and systemic antimicrobial therapy.

b. Shunt infections caused by staphylococci should be treated with systemic nafcillin or oxacillin (or vancomycin for resistant organisms).
c. Third-generation cephalosporins are the drugs of choice for infection caused by sensitive gram-negative bacilli.
d. Intraventricular antibiotics may be required when IV therapy has not eradicated the infection.
e. Occasionally, the EVD system becomes colonized with bacteria, necessitating replacement of the system.
f. Reinternalization of the shunt should be performed after follow-up cultures are confirmed to be sterile for 7 to 10 days.
g. The value of intraoperative antibiotic prophylaxis is unproved but, if used, should be for very short duration, preferably a single dose.

XI. GENITOURINARY INFECTIONS:

A. Urinary tract infection:

1. **Epidemiology:**
   a. Although the exact incidence of acute urinary tract infection (UTI) is unknown, in one study approximately 3% of girls and 1% of boys had at least one symptomatic UTI by age 11 years.
   b. The male/female ratio for infections in early infancy is between 3:1 and 5:1. The incidence is much higher in uncircumcised compared with circumcised male infants.
   c. After early infancy, girls develop UTI much more often, with male/female ratios of 1:4 for symptomatic infection and 1:25 for asymptomatic infection in school-aged children.
2. **Pathogenesis:**
   a. Most UTIs result from ascending infection from the periurethral area.
   b. In contrast, neonatal UTIs usually occur as a result of bacteremia.
   c. *E. coli,* the most common bacterial agent of acute UTI in children, has surface pili that adhere to spe-

cific glycosphingolipid receptors on uroepithelial cells lining the urinary tract. Susceptibility to UTI (especially to pyelonephritis) may be attributed to the density of the glycosphingolipid receptors on uroepithelial and renal cells.

3. **Etiology:**
   a. *E. coli* is the most frequent etiologic agent of UTI, accounting for 80% to 90% of cases.
   b. Other pathogens include *Klebsiella-Enterobacter* spp., *Proteus* spp., *Enterococcus faecalis,* and coagulase-negative staphylococci.
   c. Adenovirus may cause hemorrhagic cystitis.
   d. Chronic UTIs are frequently related to *Pseudomonas* spp, *Proteus* spp, enterococci, or *Candida* spp.
4. **Clinical manifestations:**
   a. Symptoms related to lower urinary tract inflammation (cystitis) include dysuria, frequency, urgency, enuresis, hematuria, and foul-smelling urine.
   b. Symptoms more typically associated with upper UTI (pyelonephritis) include fever, flank pain, and abdominal distress.
   c. Nonspecific systemic symptoms such as poor feeding, vomiting, diarrhea, irritability, lethargy, and jaundice predominate in early infancy.
5. **Diagnosis:**
   a. The diagnosis of UTI is established by urine cultures. The presence of at least 10^5 organisms/mL of urine of a single genus and species is diagnostic of UTI. However, cultures obtained by suprapubic aspiration (SPA) or by catheterization may contain fewer than 10^5/mL because the bacteria have had insufficient time to multiply before removal of urine from the bladder:
      1) In the incontinent patient, urine for culture should be obtained by catheterization or SPA.
      2) In older children who can void on command, clean-catch specimens are acceptable. A midstream urine sample should be obtained after gentle soap and water cleansing and drying.

b. Microscopic examination of urine is helpful in making a presumptive diagnosis of UTI.
   1) The finding of one or more bacterium per oil immersion field of uncentrifuged urine shows 80% to 95% correlation with bacteriuria of $\geq 10^5$ colony-forming units (CFU)/mL.
   2) Visualization is aided by Gram's stain.
   3) Pyuria, defined as ≥ 5 leukocytes/high-power field (HPF), is less reliable in identifying patients with UTI. Infected individuals may lack pyuria, and, conversely, pyuria can result from noninfectious causes such as chemical inflammation, urethritis, trauma, and contaminated urine specimens.
   4) Leukocyte casts reflect renal tubular inflammation and usually indicate pyelonephritis.
   5) Convenient and inexpensive culture techniques have become available for clinic or office practice. These include filter-strip, dip-slide, and dip-strip techniques.

c. Localization of the site of UTI (i.e., pyelonephritis vs. cystitis) usually is determined by clinical means. Glucoheptonate scan is sometimes useful, especially when clinical manifestations are equivocal. The ESR is generally quite elevated in upper but not lower UTI.

6. **Treatment:**
   a. Except in neonates and young infants or in those who appear very ill and/or very symptomatic, it is preferable to await culture confirmation of UTI before antimicrobial therapy is initiated.
   b. UTI in infants <3 months of age should be managed in the hospital:
      1) Initial therapy should consist of IV ampicillin, 100 mg/kg/day in four doses, and IV gentamicin, 7.5 mg/kg/day in three doses.
      2) Once the identification and sensitivities of the pathogen are known, the antibiotic spectrum should be narrowed appropriately.

3) Parenteral therapy is continued until repeat urine culture is sterile, and the infant has improved clinically and is able to take oral medication. Therapy should be given for a total of 10 days.

c. In older infants and children, the principal determinant of the route and duration of antimicrobial therapy is whether pyelonephritis is likely to be present.

d. Children diagnosed with pyelonephritis should be hospitalized and treated initially with parenteral antibiotics:
   1) Ampicillin and gentamicin, or TMP-SMX are appropriate choices for initial therapy.
   2) Therapy can be changed to oral antibiotics once there is evidence of clinical improvement and urine and blood cultures have become sterile:
      a) TMP/SMX is the drug of choice because of its excellent absorption and tissue penetration and because most urinary pathogens are highly susceptible to this combination of drugs.
      b) Other suitable alternatives are amoxicillin, amoxicillin/clavulanate, or cephalexin.
   3) Children with pyelonephritis should be treated for a minimum of 10 days.
   4) Follow-up urine culture should be obtained after treatment is discontinued.

e. Orally administered sulfonamides, aminopenicillins (e.g., ampicillin) or cephalosporins are satisfactory antibiotic choices in the patient with cystitis. The optimal duration of therapy for lower UTI has not been clearly established:
   1) Antibacterial treatment should be extended 10 days in the patient with clinical evidence of cystitis whose urinary tract has not been evaluated previously.
   2) The patient with cystitis who has normal urinary tract anatomy and a normal voiding pattern requires only a few days of treatment to clear symptoms and eliminate bacteriuria.

3) Follow-up urine culture should be obtained after treatment is discontinued.

7. **Radiologic studies:**
   a. The indications for radiologic studies in children with UTI are the following:
      1) All patients < 2 years.
      2) All boys, regardless of age.
      3) All girls with clinical pyelonephritis or with recurrent UTI.

   b. In the above patients, abnormal urinary tract anatomy, as well as vesicoureteral reflux (VUR), should be ruled out with renal sonography and voiding cystourethrography (VCUG), respectively:
      1) Renal ultrasound can be used to detect urinary tract obstruction or masses and to estimate renal size:
         a) This procedure should be performed as soon as the diagnosis of UTI is established.
         b) In the presence of moderate or severe VUR or if the quality of the sonogram is uncertain, an IV pyelogram (IVP) should be performed.
      2) In contrast, VCUG can be delayed until 4 to 6 weeks after therapy. However, if VCUG is delayed, it may be prudent to administer nitrofurantoin or TMP-SMX in suppressive doses (1–2 mg/kg/day) during the interval between completion of therapy and the procedure.

   c. When necessary, radionuclide scans of the kidneys may be performed to evaluate their functional integrity.

8. **Long-term management:**
   a. VUR is the most common abnormality found in urinary tract evaluation, reported in approximately 30% of children with UTI:
      1) VUR is graded radiographically according to the distance that contrast media refluxes into the ureters.
      2) The majority of grade I and II reflux resolves spontaneously.

3) Grade III and IV reflux are often associated with significant renal damage:
   a) Only 25% of grade III or greater reflux resolves spontaneously.
   b) Ureteral tailoring and/or surgical reimplantation is usually necessary.
4) Children with VUR should be given antibiotic prophylaxis until the child has been free of reflux for at least 1 year and should undergo annual VCUGs until reflux resolves.

b. Recurrent UTIs:
   1) Recurrent UTIs occur in approximately 30% of children after an initial UTI.
   2) The risk of recurrence increases to 75% in children who have had ≥3 UTIs.
   3) Children with ≥3 UTIs within 1 year are candidates for low-dose, daily prophylaxis (e.g., nitrofurantoin or TMP-SMX).
   4) Antibiotics are given for 3 to 6 months, or longer if breakthrough infections occur.

B. Renal and perirenal abscess:

1. **Pathogenesis:**
   a. Intrarenal abscesses are categorized as renal cortical abscesses or renal corticomedullary abscesses.
   b. Renal cortical abscess results as a consequence of a primary focus of infection elsewhere in the body. *S. aureus* is the most common pathogen in cortical abscesses.
   c. The pathogenesis of renal corticomedullary abscess is thought to be a complication of ascending infection associated with VUR, intrarenal reflux, or urinary tract obstruction. Gram-negative bacilli, especially *E. coli,* are most frequently recovered from corticomedullary abscesses.
   d. Perirenal abscess usually results from pyelonephritis or spinal osteomyelitis that ruptures into the retroperitoneal space.
2. **Clinical manifestations:**
   a. Physical examination reveals costovertebral angle tenderness and sometimes a bulging flank mass.

3. **Diagnosis:** Ultrasonography or CT scan.
4. **Treatment:**
    a. Antibiotics, initially consisting of nafcillin and gentamicin, should be given until a specific organism is identified.
    b. Percutaneous drainage should be performed for diagnostic and therapeutic purposes under ultrasound or CT guidance.
    c. Open surgery is necessary when percutaneous drainage is unsuccessful.
    d. Rarely, a patient may have to undergo nephrectomy for uncontrolled infection of a diffusely damaged kidney.
    e. Ultrasonography or CT examination are used to monitor the response to therapy.
    f. The duration of antibiotic treatment depends on the resolution of the abscess. In most cases, antibiotics are continued for at least 10 to 14 days.

C. **Vaginitis:**
1. The major symptoms are vaginal itching, discharge, and dysuria.
2. The most common etiologies of vaginitis are *Candida albicans, Trichomonas vaginalis,* and *Gardnerella vaginalis:*
    a. Vulvovaginal candidiasis is most common in women of reproductive age, especially those taking oral contraceptives, corticosteroids, or antibiotics. It is characterized by:
        1) Itching and dysuria.
        2) Thick white discharge with plaques.
        3) No odor on addition of 10% potassium hydroxide.
        4) pH < 4.5.
        5) Culture positive for yeast.
        6) Treatment is miconazole or clotrimazole intravaginally at bedtime for 3 days.
    b. Trichomoniasis:
        1) *T. vaginalis* infection in prepubertal girls strongly suggests sexual abuse.

2) The diagnosis is apparent with:
   a) Profuse, yellow-green discharge.
   b) Foul odor on addition of 10% KOH.
   c) Motile trichomonads observed on wet preparation.
   d) Vaginal pH: 5.5 to 6.0
3) Treatment is metronidazole 40 mg/kg (maximum 2 g) po once or 15 mg/kg/day (maximum 1 g) divided q8h for 7 days.

c. *Gardnerella* vaginitis:
   1) *Gardnerella* vaginitis, also referred to as bacterial vaginosis, is a polymicrobial infection caused by the interaction of *G. vaginalis* with several anaerobic bacteria.
   2) The diagnosis is made by examination of the vaginal secretions for clue cells (epithelial cells heavily coated with bacteria), fishy odor after the addition of 10% KOH, and a vaginal pH > 4.5.
   3) Although bacterial vaginosis can be acquired sexually, it also causes vaginal discharge in girls without sexual contact.
   4) The treatment of choice is metronidazole (a 7 to 10-day course of 15–20 mg/kg divided q8-12h). Amoxicillin/clavulanate and clindamycin are acceptable alternatives.

D. Pelvic Inflammatory Disease (PID):

1. **Definition:**
   a. PID is the most serious complication of nonviral sexually transmitted diseases (STDs), the result of a vaginal infection that has progressed to involve the fallopian tubes and disseminated to the pelvis.
   b. PID is the single most common cause of infertility in young women.
2. **Etiology:**
   a. *N. gonorrhoeae* and *C. trachomatis* are the most common causes of PID.
   b. Other etiologic agents include *U. urealyticum, E. coli, S. agalactiae,* and anaerobes.

3. **Diagnosis:**
   a. Clinical diagnosis is supported by the presence of lower abdominal pain and tenderness, cervical motion tenderness, and adnexal tenderness. Fever, leukocytosis, elevated ESR, and adnexal mass on abdominal ultrasound further support the diagnosis.
   b. Differential diagnosis includes ectopic pregnancy, endometriosis, ovarian cysts, appendicitis, and mesenteric adenitis.
4. **Treatment:**
   a. Indications for hospitalization for therapy of PID are as follows:
      1) All adolescents (secondary to compliance issues).
      2) Pregnancy.
      3) Presence of an adnexal mass.
      4) Diagnostic uncertainty.
      5) Inability to take oral medications.
   b. Regimens for outpatient treatment of PID include:
      1) One dose of ceftriaxone, 250 mg IM, **plus** tetracycline, 500 mg po q6h for 10 days.
      2) TMP (160 mg) and SMX (800 mg) po q12h for 10 days, **plus** metronidazole, 500 mg po q6h for 10 days.
      3) Or amoxicillin/clavulanate, 500/125 mg po q8h for 10 days, **plus** tetracycline, 500 mg po q6h for 10 days.
   c. Regimens for inpatients with PID include:
      1) Doxycycline, 100 mg IV q12h, **plus** metronidazole, 500 mg IV q6h, **plus** ceftriaxone, 250 mg IM or IV q24h.
      2) Or doxycycline, 100 mg IV q12h, **plus** ceftriaxone, 250 mg IM or IV q24h, or cefoxitin, 2 g IV q6h.
      3) Parenteral therapy should be continued until clinical improvement occurs. The total duration of therapy should be 10 to 14 days.
   d. Patients in whom PID develops after a surgical procedure or while an IUD is worn should be treated with a regimen active against coliform bacilli and

anaerobes, as well as *N. gonorrhoeae* and *C. trachomatis*.

   e. Sexual contacts of women with PID require treatment.

5. Counseling and contraception:
   a. The risk of infertility after a single episode of PID is about 10% . A second episode triples the risk of infertility.
   b. Oral contraceptives decrease both the risk and severity of PID and are therefore indicated for contraception after an episode of PID.

E. **Urethritis:**

1. Urethritis is uncommon in prepubertal children and is most common in sexually active males. Sexual abuse must be considered when the diagnosis of urethritis is confirmed in sexually immature children.
2. Symptoms include dysuria, genital itching, and discharge.
3. Urethritis is usually caused by *N. gonorrhoeae* or *C. trachomatis*.
4. Treatment of gonorrhea in the prepubertal child consists of a single dose of:
   a. Aqueous procaine penicillin G, 100,000 units/kg IM, and probenecid, 25 mg/kg.
   b. Or amoxicillin, 50 mg/kg, and probenecid.
   c. Or ceftriaxone, 5 mg/kg IM.
   d. Or cefuroxime, 25 mg/kg IM.
   e. Spectinomycin, 40 mg/kg IM.
   f. Regimens c, d or e are used in penicillin-allergic patients or in patients thought to be infected with penicillinase-producing *N. gonorrhoeae*.
   g. In addition, because 25% to 35% of children with gonococcal infection are coinfected with *C. trachomatis,* they should also be treated with erythromycin (10 mg/kg/dose q6h for 7 days) or tetracycline if > 8 years old.
5. The following regimens should be used in the treatment of uncomplicated anogenital gonorrhea in adolescents and adults:
   a. Amoxicillin, 3.0 g po.

   b. Aqueous procaine penicillin G, 4.8 million units IM.
   c. Ceftriaxone, 250 mg IM.
   d. Or spectinomycin, 2.0 g IM.
   e. These patients also need to be treated for nongonococcal urethritis.
6. Nongonococcal or nonspecific urethritis (NSU) is more prevalent than gonococcal urethritis. Approximately 60% of NSU cases are caused by *C. trachomatis* or *U. urealyticum*. Others are caused by *T. vaginalis, C. albicans,* or viruses:
   a. The typical urethral discharge in NSU is clear and watery.
   b. The diagnosis of NSU is made presumptively based on symptoms and a negative gonococcal culture.
   c. Tetracycline or doxycycline is the drug of choice because both *Chlamydia* and *Ureaplasma* are susceptible. Erythromycin is an alternative. Treatment should be continued for 10 to 14 days.

F. **Balanitis:**

1. Balanitis is inflammation of the glans penis and is usually associated with a redundant foreskin and poor penile hygiene.
2. Most cases can be treated with frequent diaper changes, improved penile hygiene, sitz baths, and use of a mild soap.
3. Circumcision may be required if the previous measures are unsuccessful and if phimosis is present.
4. Antibiotics are usually unnecessary.

G. **Epididymitis:**

1. Acute epididymitis is uncommon in prepubertal boys; however, it is important in the differential diagnosis of patients with acute scrotal swelling, which includes torsion of the spermatic cord, testicular trauma, orchitis, acute hydrocele, and hernia.
2. Diagnosis is aided by radionuclide scan and scrotal sonogram. A urethral specimen for smear, Gram's stain of the urine, and urine culture should be obtained.
3. The most common cause of epididymitis in young men are the organisms that cause urethritis (i.e., *C. tra-*

chomatis and *N. gonorrhoeae*). In prepubertal children, coliform organisms are sometimes recovered; however, no etiologic agent is identified in most cases of prepubertal epididymitis.

4. The treatment of epididymitis depends on the specific etiology:
   a. In the prepubertal child with minimal systemic symptoms, an oral cephalosporin or TMP-SMX should be given. Patients with obvious systemic involvement should receive IV gentamicin 6 mg/kg/day in three divided doses.
   b. Treatment in pubertal or postpubertal patients with epididymitis consists of tetracycline, 500 mg qid, or amoxicillin, 500 mg tid, and erythromycin , 500 mg qid, for 10 days.

H. Orchitis:

1. Acute infection of the testes is rare in boys.
2. Orchitis develops as a result of extension of inflammation from the epididymis, from hematogenous origin, or through lymphatic spread. It may be pyogenic, viral, or traumatic.
3. Bacterial orchitis:
   a. The most common causes of bacterial orchitis are *E. coli, K. pneumoniae,* streptococci, staphylococci, and *P. aeruginosa*.
   b. Needle aspiration may be necessary for diagnosis; scrotal sonography may facilitate diagnosis and aspiration.
   c. Antibiotics should be started on the basis of the Gram stain until culture and sensitivity are available. In the absence of a positive Gram's stain, cephalexin may be given empirically until culture susceptibility data are known.
4. Mumps orchitis:
   a. Mumps orchitis occurs in approximately 20% of boys who develop parotitis; however, it usually occurs only in those who are postpubertal.
   b. Onset typically occurs 4 to 6 days after parotitis, and it may occur even without parotid involvement.
   c. Orchitis is unilateral in 70% of cases.

d. Treatment consists of bed rest, scrotal support, and use of analgesics.
e. Although some degree of testicular atrophy occurs in 50% of postpubertal mumps orchitis, sterility is an uncommon sequela of unilateral mumps.

5. After treatment, evaluation to detect an underlying congenital urologic anomaly is recommended.

I. Condyloma Acuminata (Genital Warts):

1. Genital warts are caused by human papillomavirus (HPV). HPV are implicated as the etiologic agents of cervical, vulvar, and anal cancer.
2. In adults, genital papillomas are transmitted by sexual intercourse. Genital papillomas in children usually relate to sexual abuse by an infected adult. It is not known if children can acquire genital warts by other modes of contact.
3. Vulvar warts are treated with liquid nitrogen.
4. Cervical warts:
   a. Cervical warts should be closely evaluated colposcopically and monitored by a gynecologist.
   b. They often require excisional biopsy for accurate diagnosis and may be treated by laser cautery.
   c. A woman or adolescent with genital warts should be observed carefully for several years to detect early cervical dysplasia and neoplasia.

J. Chancroid:

1. Chancroid is caused by *Hemophilus ducreyi,* a small gram-negative rod.
2. It typically manifests as a small genital papule that becomes pustular and ulcerative within 2 to 3 days and is associated with painful inguinal adenopathy in 50% of cases.
3. Diagnosis of chancroid is made by culture or by monoclonal antibody stains.
4. The treatment of choice for chancroid is a single IM dose of ceftriaxone, 5 mg/kg (maximum 250 mg). Alternative drugs include TMP-SMX, erythromycin, and amoxicillin/clavulanate, each for 5 to 7 days.
5. Patients with chancroid should be evaluated for other STDs and children for sexual abuse. Sexual consorts of

persons with chancroid should be treated presumptively for chancroid and examined for other STDs.

K. Lymphogranuloma Venereum:

1. Lymphogranuloma venereum (LGV) is a sexually transmitted disease caused by *C. trachomatis*.
2. The primary lesion of LGV occurs at the inoculation site as a papule, vesicle, or small ulcer.
3. Tender and often suppurative lymphadenitis follows, with its anatomic location depending on the lymphatic drainage from the primary site.
4. Diagnosis depends on isolation of *C. trachomatis* from a fluctuant lymph node or by demonstration of chlamydial elementary bodies on direct fluorescent antibody staining. Confirmatory serologic tests are as follows:
   a. Complement fixation titer against chlamydial genus-specific antigen ≥1:64.
   b. Or microimmunofluorescence titer against *C. trachomatis* ≥1:256.
5. Treatment of choice is tetracycline, 10 mg/kg/dose q6h, or doxycycline, 2 mg/kg/dose q12h, for 14 to 21 days. Alternative treatment for patients < 7 years or those unable to take tetracycline is sulfisoxazole, 50 mg/kg/dose bid for 2 weeks.

XII. GASTROINTESTINAL INFECTIONS:

A. Peritonitis:

1. **Epidemiology and etiology:**
   a. Peritonitis is inflammation of the serous lining of the peritoneal cavity caused by infection or chemical irritation.
   b. Peritonitis is referred to as **primary** when infection reaches the peritoneum via the bloodstream or lymphatics or **secondary** when it occurs as a result of disease within the abdominal cavity:
      1) Most cases of primary peritonitis occur in children with ascites related to nephrotic syndrome or cirrhosis. Some are idiopathic.
      2) The majority of peritonitis in children is secondary to perforation of intra-abdominal viscera with spillage of fecal material into the perito-

neal cavity, extension from an intraabdominal abscess, or as a result of an indwelling catheter in patients with continuous ambulatory peritoneal dialysis (CAPD). The most common predisposing conditions include appendicitis, necrotizing enterocolitis, biliary tract disease, pseudomembranous colitis, amebic colitis, and trauma. Other underlying processes include intussusception, volvulus, ruptured Meckel's diverticulum, inflammatory bowel disease, and incarcerated hernia.

c. The organisms most commonly involved in primary bacterial peritonitis are *S. pneumoniae* and *S. pyogenes,* followed by *S. aureus, E. coli,* and other enteric organisms.
d. Secondary bacterial peritonitis is typically polymicrobial, reflecting fecal flora:
    1) Numerically, anaerobes predominate, especially *Bacteroides fragilis,* which is frequently positive for β-lactamase. Other anaerobes include anaerobic cocci, streptococci, and clostridia.
    2) The major aerobes include *E. coli, Klebsiella* spp., and *Pseudomonas* spp.
    3) Enterococci are found frequently; however, their role in the pathogenesis of intra-abdominal infection remains unclear.
    4) Although *Entamoeba histolytica* and *Clostridium difficile* are less common etiologic agents, they should be considered when the etiology of an intestinal perforation is not apparent.

2. **Clinical presentation:**
    a. Clinical findings include anorexia, nausea, vomiting, fever, and abdominal tenderness and guarding.
    b. Laboratory abnormalities usually include an elevated WBC count with a left shift. Other findings may include coagulation abnormalities and pyuria from irritation of the bladder by an adjacent abscess.
    c. Localized abscesses are most accurately identified by CT; ultrasound may be useful as well.

3. **Treatment:**
   a. Treatment consists of surgery when indicated (e.g., drainage of a localized abscess or resection of necrotic bowel) and antibiotic therapy.
   b. Primary peritonitis therapy can be guided initially by Gram's stain of peritoneal fluid and modified on the basis of culture results.
   c. When peritonitis occurs after intestinal perforation, antibiotic coverage against β-lactamase-producing strains of *B. fragilis* and aerobic gram-negative rods, including *P. aeruginosa,* should be provided:
      1) Clindamycin and an aminoglycoside are an acceptable combination.
      2) Metronidazole is preferred over clindamycin for treatment of clindamycin-resistant strains of *B. fragilis*.
      3) Ceftazidime is an alternative to an aminoglycoside, especially in patients with renal dysfunction.
   d. When peritonitis occurs in a patient undergoing CAPD, antibiotic (e.g., cephapirin [cefadyl] or vancomycin) may be added directly to the dialysate. Antibiotic should be selected on the basis of the organism isolated from the peritoneal fluid.
   e. Duration of therapy is determined by the extent of infection, adequacy of surgical procedure, and clinical response:
      1) A 7 to 10-day course of antibiotic therapy should be adequate for uncomplicated peritonitis after intestinal perforation.
      2) A more prolonged course of antimicrobial therapy is required for the patient with multiple abscess formation.
4. **Complications:** The most frequent infectious complications in these patients are wound infections postoperatively and development of subphrenic or pelvic abscess. Intestinal obstruction secondary to the development of adhesions may occur as a late complication after surgery.

B. Infectious Gastroenteritis:

1. Introduction:
   a. *Epidemiology:* Acute infectious gastroenteritis is one of the most common infectious syndromes of humans. It is a major cause of morbidity and mortality among infants and young children, especially in developing areas of the world, primarily because of dehydration. Worldwide, approximately 5 million deaths occur annually from diarrhea.
   b. *Etiology:* The causative agent is most often a bacterium or a virus. See Table 6–9.
2. Bacterial gastroenteritis:
   a. *Pathogenesis:*
      1) Bacteria usually cause gastroenteritis in one of two ways:
         a) Growth within the GI tract where the bacteria either invade the tissue or secrete exotoxins.
         b) Secretion of a preformed exotoxin that is then ingested by the host.
      2) Bacterial pathogens that colonize and multiply within the GI tract include *Salmonella, Shigella,* some *E. coli,* and *V. cholerae.*
      3) Illnesses caused by ingestion of preformed exotoxin include botulism and staphylococcal and clostridial food poisoning.
      4) The term **dysentery** refers to abdominal cramping, tenesmus, and pus and blood in the stool.

TABLE 6–9.
Etiology of Gastroenteritis

Viruses	Bacteria	Protozoa
Rotaviruses 1–3	*Salmonella*	*Giardia lamblia*
Norwalk-like agents	*Shigella*	*Entamoeba histolytica*
Enteric adenoviruses	*E. coli*	*Cryptosporidium*
Calicivirus	*Vibrio cholerae*	
	Other vibrios	
	Campylobacter fetus	
	Yersinia enterocolitica	

These symptoms are associated with bacterial invasion of the intestinal wall, usually of the colon. The mucosal invasion is visible as ulcerations and results in blood and pus in the stool. Shigellae are the prototype of invasive organisms causing dysentery.

5) The more common **diarrhea syndrome** refers to profuse watery isotonic diarrhea reflecting dysfunction of the small intestine. *V. cholerae* is the prototype organism that causes profuse efflux of fluid because of the effects of its enterotoxin on intestinal cells. No mucosal invasion occurs in cholera.
6) Table 6–10 lists the characteristics of common bacterial infections.

b. **Clinical manifestations** (Table 6–11)

c. *Diagnosis:*

1) The age of the patient, geographic setting, and clinical manifestations provide clues to identifying the etiologic agent.

TABLE 6–10.
Characteristics of Gastroenteritis

Organism	Diarrhea	Dysentery	Enterotoxin	Site
Salmonella typhi	0	±	0	Small bowel
Salmonella enteritidis	±	+	+	Small bowel
Shigella dysenteriae	+	+	+	Small bowel
Shigella flexneri	±	+	+	Large bowel
Shigella sonnei	±	+	+	Large bowel
V. cholerae	+	0	+	Small bowel
E. coli				
Enterotoxigenic	+	0	+	Small or large bowel
Enteroinvasive	0	+	0	Small or large bowel
Enteropathogenic	+	±	0	Small or large bowel
Enterohemorrhagic	+	+	+	Small or large bowel
C. fetus	+	+	+	Large bowel
Y. enterocolitica	±	+	+	Large bowel

TABLE 6–11.
Clinical Manifestations

Organism	Epidemiologic Considerations	Usual Manifestations
Salmonella spp.	Travel, exposure to carrier, food exposure	Watery diarrhea or dysentery with fever; bacteremia or focal infection may occur
Shigella spp.	Exposure to an infected person	Watery diarrhea or severe dysentery with fever; may be accompanied by meningismus and convulsions
E. coli		
Enterotoxigenic	Travel	Watery diarrhea in travelers to developing countries and in infants
Enteropathogenic	Exposure to an infected person, outbreaks in nurseries	Acute and chronic diarrhea in infants
Enteroinvasive	Food exposure	Dysentery with fever, rapid onset
Enterohemorrhagic	Food exposure, exposure to an infected person	Nausea, vomiting, severe abdominal cramps; grossly bloody diarrhea, associated with hemolytic-uremic syndrome
V. cholerae	Travel, food, or water exposure	Sudden onset of profuse, painless, watery diarrhea; dehydration and shock are common sequelae
C. fetus	Animal or food exposure	Watery diarrhea or dysentery
Y. enterocolitica	Animal or food exposure	Watery diarrhea or dysentery; may be accompanied by arthritis and erythema nodosum

2) Laboratory data (Table 6–12):
   a) Stool examination demonstrating leukocytes and blood is indicative of an invasive process.
   b) Routine stool cultures can detect *Salmonella, Shigella, Campylobacter,* and *Yersinia enterocolitica*. Because *V. cholerae* is a rare pathogen in the United States, the laboratory should be alerted if it is a suspected pathogen.
   c) Laboratory confirmation of disease caused by *E. coli* is not generally available.
   d) The peripheral blood smear often reveals more band forms than segmented neutrophils in *Shigella* infection.

d. *Therapy:*
   1) Fluid replacement is necessary either orally or intravenously.

TABLE 6–12.
Fecal Leukocytes in Gastroenteritis*

Infectious Agent	Fecal Leukocytes
Rotavirus	No
Other viral agent	No
Giardia	No
Cryptosporidium	No
Vibrio cholerae	No
Toxigenic *E. coli*	No
Food poisoning	No
Typhoid fever	Yes, 95% MNC
Other salmonellosis	Yes, 75% PMN
Shigella	Yes, 80% PMN
Invasive *E. coli*	Yes, 80% PMN
Campylobacter	Yes, PMN
Yersinia	Yes

*Modified from Harris et al: *Ann Intern Med* 1972; 76:697. MNC = mononuclear cells, PMN = polymorphonuclear cells.

2) Electrolytes should be measured in moderate to severe dehydration and corrected when necessary.
3) Motility inhibitors, e.g., diphenoxylate hydrochloride (Lomotil), are not recommended in children because they do not alter the course of illness and may actually prolong symptoms.
4) Empiric antibiotic therapy should be started in the severely ill hospitalized patient with suspected bacterial gastroenteritis and/or bacteremia. TMP-SMX is a logical choice because it is effective against *Shigella* and *Salmonella* (including ampicillin-resistant strains).
5) Table 6–13 lists the most appropriate antimicrobial agents and dosage for specific pathogens.

3. Traveler's diarrhea:
   a. **Etiology:**
      1) Traveler's diarrhea, also referred to as **turista** or **Montezuma's revenge,** is the most common illness encountered by persons from the United States and Northern Europe who travel to Latin America, Asia, or Africa.
      2) Enterotoxigenic *E. coli* is the most commonly identified pathogen. However, a variety of bacteria, viruses, and parasites have been implicated, including *Shigella, Salmonella, Campylobacter,* rotavirus and *Giardia lamblia*.
   b. **Clinical manifestations:**
      1) The clinical illness is variable, depending in part on the causative agent.
      2) Typically, travelers experience watery diarrhea, cramps, and nausea within several weeks of arrival to the foreign country.
      3) Less frequently, patients may have bloody diarrhea, vomiting, and fever.
   c. **Treatment:**
      1) Although several agents, including bismuth subsalicylate, TMP-SMX, and doxycycline, appear to prevent traveler's diarrhea, prophylactic antibiotics are not generally recommended.

TABLE 6–13.
Antimicrobial Agents and Dosage for Specific Pathogens

Pathogen	Antimicrobial Agent	Dosage
Salmonella		
Gastroenteritis	None (unless patient < 3 mo or compromised host)	
Bacteremia	Ampicillin	200 mg/kg/day IV q6h for 2 wk
	or	
	chloramphenicol	75 mg/kg/day IV or po q6h for 2 wk
	TMP-SMX	TMP-10 mg/kg/day q12h for 2 wk
S. typhi (typhoid fever)	Amoxicillin, chloramphenicol, or TMP-SMX	Dosages as above for 14–21 days
Shigella	TMP-SMX (25% resistant in Latin America)	Dosages as above for 5 days
	or	
	ampicillin (20%–40% resistant)	50–75 mg/kg/day po q6h for 5 days
E. coli		
Enterotoxigenic	None or TMP-SMX	
Enteropathogenic	None or TMP-SMX or neomycin	Dosages as above for 5 days
Enteroinvasive	TMP-SMX	
Enterohemorrhagic	TMP-SMX	
V. cholerae	TMP-SMX	Dosage as above for 2 days
	or	
	tetracycline (> 7 or 8 y old)	25–50 mg/kg/day q6h for 2 days
C. fetus	None or erythromycin	40 mg/kg/day po q6h for 5–7 days
Y. enterocolitica	None or TMP-SMX	Dosage as above for 5 days.

2) TMP-SMX (10 mg/kg/day of TMP q12h for 5 days) is an effective therapeutic agent if acute diarrhea develops.
3) Water, uncooked food, and unpasteurized milk should be avoided.

4. Viral enteropathogens:
   a. Rotavirus:
      1) Rotavirus is one of the most important enteric pathogens worldwide, especially in infants.
      2) In the winter months, it is responsible for 50% to 60% of diarrheal illnesses in infants and young children.
      3) Diarrhea, vomiting, and fever are the most prominent clinical features.
      4) Reinfection may occur because there are several serotypes.
      5) Diagnosis is made by rapid enzyme immunoassays or latex agglutination tests to detect rotavirus in stools.
      6) Treatment is symptomatic.
      7) Oral antirotavirus antibodies are under study for prevention of rotavirus illness among high-risk groups (e.g., infants in day-care centers).
   b. Norwalk virus:
      1) These agents are frequently responsible for community outbreaks of gastroenteritis.
      2) Illness caused by Norwalklike viruses typically produces an explosive, self-limited disease lasting 24 to 48 hours.
      3) Diagnosis is made by immune electron microscopy or by serology. Commercial assays are not available.
      4) There is no specific treatment or immunization available at this time.
   c. Enteric adenovirus (specific serotypes):
      1) Adenovirus diarrhea is typically mild and self-limited.
      2) Symptoms include watery stools, vomiting, and low-grade fever.
      3) Infants are especially susceptible to these agents.
      4) Treatment is supportive.
5. Parasitic enteropathogens:
   a. The most frequent causes of parasitic diarrhea in persons living in the United States are *G. lamblia* (usually chronic, with malabsorption), *E. histolytica*

TABLE 6–14.
Therapy of Protozoal Enteropathogens

Pathogens	Therapy	Dosage
G. lamblia	Quinacrine	6 mg/kg/day po tid × 7 days
	metronidazole or	15 mg/kg/day po tid × 7–10 days
	furazolidone	9 mg/kg/day po tid × 10 days
E. histolytica		
Asymptomatic excretor	Iodoquinol or paromomycin	30 mg/kg/day po tid × 20 days
Intestinal amebiasis	Metronidazole	30–50 mg/kg/ day po tid × 10 days
	Plus iodoquinol	30 mg/kg/day po tid × 20 days
Cryptosporidium	None effective	

(usually acute, bloody), and *Cryptosporidium* (chronic, seen in AIDS patients). *Cryptosporidium* also causes acute self-limited diarrhea in day-care children.

b. Therapy for these pathogens are as follows (Table 6–14):

C. **Viral Hepatitis:**

1. Introduction: Although hepatitis occurs with many infections (e.g., EBV, CMV, toxoplasmosis, rubella, and malaria), the liver is not the primary target organ in these conditions. This section discusses liver disease caused by hepatitis A virus (HAV), hepatitis B virus (HBV), hepatitis D virus (HDV), hepatitis C virus (HCV), and hepatitis E virus (HEV).
2. HAV (infectious hepatitis):
   a. **Epidemiology:**
      1) HAV is highly contagious; the dominant mode of transmission is fecal-oral. HAV occurs worldwide.
      2) In developing countries, most infections occur early in life as subclinical or anicteric illnesses,

resulting in early acquisition of immunity. In developed areas, early infection is more common in lower socioeconomic groups.

3) Risk factors for HAV in the United States include contact with a person with known hepatitis, male homosexuality, foreign travel, and contact with a child attending a daycare center.

b. **Virology:**
   1) HAV is a picornavirus (the group comprising the enteroviruses and rhinoviruses) with only a single-known serotype.
   2) The HAV genome is single-stranded RNA with 7,478 nucleotides.

c. **Pathogenesis:**
   1) After ingestion of HAV, replication occurs in the liver, with production of viral RNA polymerase and protease and synthesis of viral RNA and proteins.
   2) The precise mechanisms of liver damage are unknown, but data suggest that injury is immunologically mediated:
      a) Lymphocytic infiltration occurs.
      b) Cytokines are released.
      c) CD8+ suppressor T-lymphocytes isolated from liver in acute hepatitis A are specifically cytotoxic for HAV-infected cells.

d. **Clinical manifestations:**
   1) Asymptomatic, subclinical HAV infection is common, particularly in children.
   2) When present, symptoms include nausea, vomiting, fever, abdominal discomfort, headache, and myalgias, developing 15 to 50 days after exposure (median 30 days).
   3) Tender hepatomegaly and icterus may be noted on examination.
   4) Symptoms subside after 3 to 7 days in most HAV-infected patients, especially children. However, in some, an icteric phase occurs, with elevated serum bilirubin levels. Elevated serum liver transaminase levels correlate with the degree of hepatocyte damage.

5) Infrequently, fulminant hepatitis A develops, with a high fatality rate.
6) There is no chronic form of HAV hepatitis.

e. **Diagnosis:**

1) HAV infection is diagnosed by detection of serum IgM-anti-HAV, which is almost always positive at clinical presentation and persists for several months.
2) Serum IgG-anti-HAV appears during convalescence and persists usually for life, conferring immunity to HAV infection.

f. **Management:**

1) Passive immunization: Pooled human immune serum globulin (ISG) protects against HAV.
   a) ISG in proper dosage (0.02 mL/kg) is up to 87% effective for household contacts if given within 2 weeks of exposure.
   b) ISG may prevent infection completely or may ameliorate severity of infection.
   c) ISG is recommended in the following situations:
      i) Household and sexual contacts of individuals with HAV.
      ii) Contacts in institutions for the retarded and those related to day-care centers.
      iii) For travelers going to countries where HAV is endemic.
2) Active immunization: Development of an effective and safe HAV vaccine is the goal of current research.
3) Prevention:
   a) Handwashing effectively prevents person-to-person spread of HAV.
   b) Careful disposal of excreta and avoidance of contamination of the water supply reduce the risk of fecal-oral transmission of HAV.

3. HBV (serum hepatitis):

a. **Epidemiology:**

1) Transmission of HBV occurs primarily by parenteral, sexual, or vertical (mother-infant) routes.

2) Individuals at high risk for HBV include IV drug abusers, male homosexuals, those who are sexually promiscuous, health care workers, hemophiliacs, and transfusion recipients.
3) Certain geographic areas associated with high rates of chronic HBV infection include Southeast Asia, sub-Saharan Africa, Oceania, and the Mediterranean region.
4) The World Health Organization estimated in 1990 that 1 billion individuals have been infected with HBV; > 200 million worldwide are currently infected; and 1 to 2 million deaths each year are attributed to HBV.
5) HBV is clearly oncogenic, associated with 80% of primary hepatocellular carcinoma (hepatoma).

b. **Virology:**
1) HBV belongs in the Hepadna class of viruses.
2) The intact virion, or the Dane particle, is comprised of an outer layer of hepatitis B surface antigen (HBsAg) and a core comprised of hepatitis B core antigen (HBcAg), hepatitis B e antigen (HBeAg), DNA polymerase, and a circular, mostly double-stranded DNA genome.

c. **Pathogenesis:**
1) The pathogenesis of HBV infection involves the host response to HBV.
2) Hepatocyte necrosis is most likely the result of T-cell cytotoxicity directed against HBV and/or hepatocyte membrane antigens:
   a) Individuals with impaired T-cell function (e.g., HIV infection, neonates, malignancy) are therefore more likely to have a relatively mild acute illness, followed by smoldering, persistent chronic HBV infection.
   b) In contrast, those with normal T-cell function tend to have more severe acute illness; however, they are more likely to terminate the infection, with clearance of HBsAg from liver and serum and development of anti-HBs, a sign of resolution.

d. **Clinical manifestations:**
   1) The incubation period between infection and symptoms is 45 to 180 days (median 120 days).
   2) Clinical manifestations of acute HBV are similar to acute HAV but with a more insidious onset and a propensity to become chronic. Icterus is more common.
   3) Individuals infected with HBV may have asymptomatic disease, symptomatic self-limited disease, or fulminant disease.
   4) Extrahepatic manifestations include:
      a) A serum sickness–like syndrome with rash, fever, and polyarthritis.
      b) Chronic membranous glomerulonephritis and nephrosis.
      c) A papulovesicular rash on the face, buttocks, and extremities (Gianotti-Crosti syndrome).
   5) The icteric phase of acute HBV lasts 2 to 6 weeks.
   6) Physical examination frequently reveals hepatomegaly, often with splenomegaly, and icterus.
   7) Unlike HAV, many HBV-infected individuals become chronically infected, frequently for life. This is particularly true of neonates. HBsAg, anti-HBc, HBeAg or anti-HBe, DNA polymerase, and HBV DNA persist in serum of these patients.
   8) Chronic HBV may take one of three forms:
      a) Chronic HBsAg carriage: These individuals are asymptomatic with minimal or no liver disease.
      b) Chronic persistent HBV: Mild portal triaditis is present with only mildly elevated serum transminase levels. Resolution occurs within 1 year without development of cirrhosis.
      c) Chronic active HBV: This is the serious form of chronic HBV, with more elevated transaminase levels and T-cell inflammation, which traverses beyond the portal triad across the limiting plate and into the lobules.

Fibrosis and cirrhosis may develop, leading to portal hypertension. These patients are at particularly great risk for hepatoma. Interferon-α therapy appears promising in these patients, but pediatric experience is lacking.

e. **Diagnosis:**
   1) The diagnosis of HBV is made serologically. (Table 6–15).
   2) Serum HBsAg appears late in the incubation period and persists during the clinical stage of acute HBV:
      a) HBsAg is measured by radioimmunoassay (RIA) or enzyme-linked immunosorbent assay (ELISA).

TABLE 6–15.
Hepatitis B Serologic Markers

HBsAg hepatitis B surface antigen (Australia antigen): Appears in serum late in incubation period and persists through most of acute clinical illness and throughout chronic infection or chronic carriage; disappearance from serum usually means termination of HBV infection. HBV vaccine is comprised of pure HBsAg.

Anti-HBs antibody to HBsAg: Appears in serum during convalescence after HBsAg has become undetectable; indicates recovery (or response to HBV vaccine), persists for many years, and is *protective* against reinfection.

HBcAg hepatitis B core antigen: Does *not* appear in serum but is found in hepatocytes, correlating with viral replication.

Anti-HBc antibody to HBcAg: Appears in serum late in incubation period, and declines to low levels with convalescence. May persist at low levels for many years in those who have recovered.

IgM anti-HBc igM antibody to HBcAg: Appears in serum (except in young infants) early and persists only a short time, strongly suggesting recent acute HBV infection.

HBeAg hepatitis B e antigen: Appears in serum late in incubation period, correlating with DNA polymerase activity and active viral replication, increased infectivity, and increased severity of liver disease. May be quite transient or persist for many decades.

Anti-HBe antibody to HBeAg: Appears in serum shortly after HBeAg becomes nondetectable and correlates with lower infectivity, less viral replication, and decreased severity of liver disease.

b) HBsAg is present in body fluids, including serum, saliva, breast milk, and semen.

3) The disappearance of HBsAg almost always indicates termination of HBV infection.
4) HBeAg is associated with DNA polymerase activity, and it serves as a marker of significant chronic liver disease and increased infectivity.
5) Serum DNA polymerase and HBV DNA indicate active HBV replication. Therefore, their disappearance correlates with termination of HBV infection.
6) Anti-HBc appears late in the incubation period and diminishes to low levels during convalescence. It may persist at this low level for years. Anti-HBc may be the only HBV marker during the interval between the disappearance of HBsAg and the appearance of anti-HBs. This is the "core window."
7) Anti-HBs appears later in convalescence, often considerably after HBsAg has disappeared, and signifies termination of HBV infection and protection against reinfection.

f. **Management:**

1) Passive immunization: Hepatitis B immune globulin (HBIG) is used in the following circumstances:
   a) After an inadvertent needle stick from an HBsAg-positive individual.
   b) After ingestion of HBsAg-positive material.
   c) After contamination of an open skin wound or an eye splash with HBsAg-positive material.
   d) For sexual contacts of patients with acute HBV within 14 days of exposure.
   e) Household contacts < 1 year of age of patients with acute HBV.
   f) Infants born to HBsAg-positive mothers.
2) Active immunization: Safe and effective HBV vaccine containing recombinant HBsAg synthesized by yeast is now available:

a) Three doses (at 0, 1, and 6 months) result in anti-HBs in approximately 95% of recipients.
b) HBV vaccine is indicated for the following high-risk individuals:
    i) Health professionals.
    ii) Hemodialysis patients.
    iii) Residents and staff of chronic care institutions.
    iv) IV drug abusers.
    v) Prostitutes.
    vi) Household or sexual contacts of HBV carriers.
    vii) High-risk populations (e.g., Alaskan Eskimos or immigrants from Southeast Asia, Haiti, and sub-Saharan Africa).
    viii) Homosexually active men.
    ix) International travelers (>6 months in an endemic area).
    x) Recipients of certain blood products.
    xi) All neonates (even those not at high risk). See Chapter 1.
c) HBV vaccine in combination with HBIG is indicated in the following circumstances:
    i) After needle-stick or splash exposures with HBsAg-positive material.
    ii) In neonates born to HBV-infected mothers.
    iii) To sexual contacts of patients with acute hepatitis B.
    iv) Household contacts of persons with acute HBV infection.

3) Interferon-α appears to be beneficial in reducing the disease activity in chronic HBV infections.

4. HDV:
    a. HDV is a defective RNA virus that can infect only HBsAg-positive individuals and can replicate only in the presence of HBV.
    b. HDV may occur simultaneously with acute HBV, may be an acute infection superimposed on chronic HBV, or may be a chronic infection superimposed on chronic HBV infection.

c. Coinfection with HDV and HBV leads to more fulminant acute hepatitis than infection with HBV alone.
d. Modes of transmission of HDV are identical to HBV.
e. With HDV infection, δ-antigen and HDV RNA are present in the liver, and anti-δ-antibody is demonstrable in serum.
f. Studies evaluating interferon-α for treatment of chronic HDV are in progress.

5. Non-A, Non-B (NANB) viral hepatitis:
   a. NANB is now responsible for 80% to 90% of posttransfusion hepatitis and 25% to 50% of spontaneous hepatitis.
   b. Almost 150,000 cases of NANB hepatitis occur annually in the United States, with 15,000 progressing to chronic active hepatitis and/or cirrhosis.
   c. Two distinct modes of transmission for NANB suggests that at least two viral agents are responsible:
      1) One form, which is transmitted primarily parenterally and causes posttransfusion hepatitis (HCV).
      2) A water-borne form with fecal-oral transmission that causes epidemics in developing countries (HEV).
   d. In recent years, many cases of NANB hepatitis have been shown to represent HCV infection:
      1) Seroconversion to HCV may occur as long as 6 to 12 months after infection and 4 to 10 months after onset of hepatitis.
      2) About 50% of those who acquire posttransfusion HCV develop chronic hepatitis.
      3) Interferon-α may be effective in treatment of chronic hepatitis C.
   e. HEV is a form of NANB hepatitis characterized by fecal-oral transmission and shorter incubation period (usually 2 – 9 weeks).
      1) HEV typically occurs in developing countries in outbreaks most often associated with fecal contamination of the water supply.
      2) An antigen associated with E-NANB hepatitis

has been identified in hepatocytes of experimentally infected primates.

3) Pregnant women are at risk for particularly severe illness. Chronic liver disease is not known to result from HEV.

D. Pyogenic liver abscess:

1. **Epidemiology and etiology:**
   a. Pyogenic liver abscesses occur infrequently in normal children.
   b. Patients who are immunocompromised, especially those with chronic granulomatous disease (CGD) or neutropenic leukemia, are at greater risk for developing liver abscess.
   c. The most common source of liver abscess in children is bacteremia with hematogenous spread to the liver.
   d. Bacteria also can establish infection in the liver by the following routes:
      1) Direct extension from contiguous structures (e.g., biliary tract infection).
      2) Via the portal system (e.g., secondary to umbilical vein catheterization or omphalitis).
      3) After trauma to the liver as a result of bacterial proliferation within resultant collections of blood and bile.
   e. *S. aureus* is the most common isolate in children, especially from solitary liver abscess in CGD. Gram-negative enteric bacilli and anaerobes are frequently isolated when multiple abscesses are present. Multiple small fungal abscesses, particularly caused by *C. albicans,* are frequently seen in leukemia.
2. **Clinical manifestations:**
   a. Fever, nausea, vomiting, anorexia, malaise, and abdominal pain are the most prominent symptoms.
   b. Hepatomegaly is present in the majority of patients. Right pleural effusion may be present.
3. **Diagnosis:**
   a. Because of its nonspecific manifestation, one must have a high index of suspicion to diagnose liver abscess. Liver function test results are often normal.
   b. CT provides the most accurate information concerning the size, location, and number of abscesses.

4. **Treatment:**
   a. Surgical drainage and antibiotics are the basic treatment for hepatic abscesses.
   b. A penicillinase-resistant penicillin plus an aminoglycoside or a third-generation cephalosporin should be started empirically in a patient with suspected liver abscess until Gram's stain and/or culture data are obtained.
   c. Anaerobic coverage is indicated for multiple abscesses or if putrid drainage is obtained. Clindamycin, chloramphenicol, and metronidazole are effective against most anaerobes; penicillin is usually adequate for gram-positive anaerobes.
   d. The optimal duration of antimicrobial therapy is not established, but most recommend a minimum of 6 weeks, with the first 2 to 4 weeks consisting of parenteral antibiotics. For multiple abscesses (i.e., less amenable to complete surgical drainage), a longer course of antibiotic therapy is recommended.
   e. Drainage of liver abscess may be accomplished by abdominal exploration or by percutaneous drainage under CT guidance.
5. **Complications:**
   a. Complications of hepatic abscesses include peritonitis, pleural and pulmonary inflammation, subphrenic and subhepatic abscesses, and hemobilia.
   b. Mortality rates depend on underlying pathologic conditions.

E. **Cholangitis:**

1. **Epidemiology and Etiology:**
   a. Cholangitis is defined as inflammation of the bile ducts.
   b. It occurs most frequently in children who have undergone a surgical procedure involving the biliary tree, sometimes with an intestinal conduit (i.e., patients who have undergone the Kasai procedure or after orthotopic liver transplanation).
   c. Cholangitis in children results less often from biliary tract obstruction of other etiologies, including gallstones in the common bile duct, cysts, tumors, and infections.

   d. Gram-negative enteric bacilli, especially *E. coli* and *Klebsiella* spp, are the most common pathogens. Other intestinal organisms, as well as *Pseudomonas* spp, are also seen. The role of anaerobes in the pathogenesis of cholangitis is unclear.

2. **Clinical manifestations:** Fever, obstructive jaundice, and right upper quadrant abdominal pain. However, patients with intestinal-biliary conduits often have only fever and leukocytosis.
3. **Treatment:**
   a. Empiric therapy should consist of cefoperazone and an aminoglycoside. Cefoperazone is recommended because it achieves high biliary concentrations.
   b. If prolonged fever occurs, the addition of metronidazole for *B. fragilis* coverage should be considered.
   c. Cholangitis should be treated with IV antibiotics for a minimum of 10 days.
   d. Surgical intervention to relieve biliary tract obstruction and stasis (removal of gallstones, tumors, cysts, etc.) should be performed as soon as the patient is clinically stable and is receiving antibiotics.
4. **Prognosis:** Recurrences are common in patients with intestinal conduits whose biliary obstruction is not correctable surgically. Prophylactic oral TMP-SMX (5 mg/kg/day as TMP) is often used for 1 to 2 years after surgery.

F. Pseudomembranous Colitis

1. **Etiology:**
   a. Pseudomembranous colitis (PMC) usually occurs as a result of antibiotic therapy.
   b. The specific cause of PMC is a toxin produced by *C. difficile*.
   c. It is presumed that in some individuals an antibiotic upsets the balance of intestinal microflora, resulting in proliferation of *C. difficile* with production of toxin.
   d. Although most antibiotics can cause this syndrome, it is most often associated with clindamycin, a penicillin, or a cephalosporin.
2. **Clinical manifestations:**
   a. The illness typically occurs between the fourth and ninth days of antibiotic therapy; however, onset of

illness can be as late as several weeks after completion of antibiotics.

b. Diarrhea, with or without blood, low-grade fever, abdominal pain, nausea, and vomiting are manifestations of PMC.

3. **Diagnosis:** The diagnosis of PMC is made on the basis of the clinical setting, demonstration of *C. difficile* and its toxin in the feces, and by characteristic changes of yellow or white plaques of fibrinous exudate on colonoscopy (when performed).
4. **Therapy:**
   a. The most important therapeutic measure in PMC is the discontinuation of the offending antibiotic.
   b. Specific therapeutic agents should be considered in the severely ill patient or in those patients with persistent or worsening symptoms.
      1) Vancomycin (50 mg/kg/day po q6h for 7 days) is the treatment of choice.
      2) Metronidazole (30 mg/kg/day po or IV q6h) is an alternate form of therapy and is much less expensive than oral vancomycin.
      3) Cholestyramine may be helpful in conjunction with vancomycin or metronidazole, perhaps by binding *C. difficile* toxin, thereby preventing its adsorption.

XIII. SKIN AND SOFT TISSUE INFECTIONS:

A. Normal and Pathogenic Skin Flora:

1. Anaerobic and facultative diphtheroids *(Propionibacterium, Corynebacterium),* coagulase-negative staphylococci, and micrococci constitute the majority of normal bacterial skin flora. These organisms are usually benign but may be pathogenic in certain circumstances.
2. *S. aureus,* streptococci, enteric organisms, and *Candida* may intermittently colonize the skin and may be pathogenic. *S. aureus* and group A streptococci account for most common skin and soft tissue infections.

B. Impetigo:

1. **Epidemiology, etiology, and pathogenesis:**
   a. Impetigo is chiefly a disease of children and is most common in warm, humid climates. It may be epi-

demic among families or groups in close physical contact (schools, athletic teams). Bullous impetigo is much less common than classical impetigo and may occur among neonates in nursery epidemics.

b. Group A streptococci and *S. aureus* are the chief causative agents of impetigo. Bullous impetigo is exclusively staphylococcal in origin.

c. Impetigo results from bacterial invasion of disrupted skin (insect bites, minor trauma). The characteristic lesions of bullous impetigo are caused by an epidermolytic toxin produced by the infecting staphylococci.

2. **Clinical findings:**
   a. The classic lesions of impetigo begin as erythematous papules in traumatized areas. They quickly evolve into honey-colored crusted plaques with surrounding erythema up to 2 cm in diameter. The infection is typically indolent and may heal spontaneously.
   b. Bullous impetigo is characterized by flaccid superficial bullae 1 to 2 cm in diameter arising from normal skin. When the bullae rupture, a thin, clear coating forms over the denuded area. The bullae may be confused with thermal burns or with other bullous dermatoses. Diagnosis is made by demonstrating the infecting organisms on Gram's stain or culture. Skin biopsy is rarely necessary.
   c. Impetigo caused by certain strains of group A streptococci may lead to acute poststreptococcal glomerulonephritis (APSGN), usually manifested by edema, hematuria, proteinuria, and hypertension, occurring a few weeks after the primary infection. APSGN occurs in $<1\%$ of cases of impetigo.
3. **Prevention and therapy:**
   a. Good personal hygiene and prompt attention to minor skin wounds are the cornerstones of prevention.
   b. Either an oral antibiotic or topical mupirocin ointment is the preferred therapy for impetigo. Antiseptic washes are not of value.
   c. Both classical and bullous impetigo may be treated

with oral erythromycin, clindamycin, or amoxicillin-clavulanate, usually for 10 days.

d. Mupirocin is a relatively new topical antimicrobial that is at least as effective as oral antibiotics for treatment of impetigo of limited extent. It is usually applied for 7 to 10 days.

e. Antibiotic therapy does not alter the incidence of APSGN. Rheumatic fever does not develop after streptococcal impetigo.

C. **Acne:**

1. **Etiology and pathogenesis:**
   a. The pathogenesis of acne is a multifaceted, complex process that takes place in sebaceous follicles. This summary focuses on the infectious aspects of lesion formation.
   b. The main steps involved in formation of the characteristic lesions of acne are as follows:
      1) Microcomedone formation, resulting from failure to slough epidermal cells lining the follicular canal, with subsequent keratin plug formation.
      2) Open comedo formation, resulting from dilation of the follicular orifice above the microcomedone; or closed comedo formation, resulting from impaction of sebum and sloughed epidermal cells behind a follicular orifice that has failed to dilate.
      3) Formation of inflammatory lesions (papules, pustules, cysts) resulting largely from action of *P. acnes* on the impacted sebaceous follicle.
   c. The organism involved in acne pathogenesis is *Propionibacterium acnes*. It plays a role in inflammatory lesion formation.
   d. *P. acnes* is a normal skin inhabitant found in higher concentration in the sebaceous follicle. The organism may proliferate in response to increased sebum production. *P. acnes* produces chemotactic factors that attract neutrophils into the follicle. The neutrophils ingest the bacteria and release hydrolytic enzymes that cause follicular damage. Rupture of the follicle into the dermis results in a local foreign body reac-

tion with further inflammation. The classical and alternate complement pathways may also be activated by *P. acnes,* resulting in further perpetuation of the inflammatory response.

2. **Clinical findings:**
   a. Acne usually occurs on the face, back, and chest in pubertal or postpubertal individuals.
   b. The earliest clinically apparent lesions of acne are the open comedone (blackhead) and the closed comedone (whitehead). These lesions frequently progress to papules and pustules, with nodule or cyst formation occurring in more severe cases.
3. **Therapy:**
   a. Therapy of acne involves primarily antimicrobials that decrease the population of *P. acnes* and agents that decrease microcomedone formation. However, eradication of *P. acnes* from the skin does not result in cure, emphasizing the multifaceted nature of the disease.
   b. Topical benzoyl peroxide is a cornerstone of acne therapy. It decreases the concentration of *P. acnes* in the sebaceous follicle by oxidizing bacterial proteins. It may also have mild comedolytic effects.
   c. Topical erythromycin and clindamycin, usually in liquid solutions, are also active against *P. acnes* and are clearly efficacious. An oral antibiotic, usually tetracycline, may be used in more severe cases of acne.
   d. Tretinoin is a topical medication that is comedolytic and also prevents microcomedone formation. It is a useful first-line drug, along with benzoyl peroxide and topical antibiotics.
   e. Accutane (13- *cis* -retinoic acid) is very effective for therapy of severe nodulocystic acne recalcitrant to other forms of treatment. However, it may have pronounced side effects, including mucous membrane inflammation, hypertriglyceridemia, and pseudotumor cerebri, and should be prescribed only by a physician experienced with its use. It is also a teratogen and should never be used by pregnant women. It has multiple effects, including a decrease in sebum production, comedolysis, and antibacterial effects.

D. **Cellulitis (nonfacial):**

1. **Etiology and pathogenesis:**
   a. Cellulitis is caused by coagulase-positive staphylococci and group A β-hemolytic streptococci. Hib may occasionally cause nonfacial cellulitis in young children.
   b. Cellulitis is an infection of primarily the subcutaneous and dermal tissues. Erysipelas, caused by group A streptococci, is more superficial, involving mainly the dermis.
   c. Infection typically occurs in an area of prior trauma, usually on the extremities.
2. **Clinical findings:**
   a. Cellulitis manifests as an area of warmth, erythema, edema, and tenderness with indistinct borders. Erysipelas, a more superficial process, has well-demarcated borders with skin induration. Bullae may occur in areas involved by erysipelas or cellulitis.
   b. Cellulitis may extend to involve deeper tissues and can be associated with septic arthritis and osteomyelitis.
3. **Therapy:**
   a. Nonfacial cellulitis of limited extent unaccompanied by signs of systemic illness may be treated with an oral antibiotic such as dicloxacillin or erythromycin, which is active against streptococci and staphylococci.
   b. Extensive cellulitis, or cellulitis accompanied by signs of toxicity, should be treated with a parenteral antistaphylococcal antibiotic such as nafcillin or cephalothin. Oral therapy can be instituted to finish a 10-day course when substantial clinical improvement is seen.

E. **Facial (Buccal) Cellulitis:**

1. **Epidemiology, etiology, and pathogenesis:**
   a. Two distinct classes of facial cellulitis:
      1) Buccal cellulitis is an uncommon but distinctive infection occurring in children 6 months to 3 to 5 years of age. No portal of entry for infection is apparent on examination.

2) Facial cellulitis secondary to local trauma or dental infection tends to occur in older patients.

b. **Etiology:**

1) Buccal cellulitis is nearly always caused by Hib, with occasional cases caused by *S. pneumoniae*.
2) Causative organisms in facial cellulitis depend on the portal of entry. Anaerobes are often isolated in cases of cellulitis secondary to a dental abscess, whereas *S. aureus* may be found in cases secondary to local skin trauma.

c. **Pathogenesis:**

1) The pathogenesis of buccal cellulitis is somewhat controversial but probably involves direct seeding of the buccal mucosa from the bloodstream. Lymphatic extension from ipsilateral otitis media is another postulated mechanism.
2) Facial cellulitis secondary to trauma or dental infection is a result of direct extension of the primary infection.

2. **Clinical findings:**

a. Buccal cellulitis manifests with rapid onset of fever and unilateral cheek swelling and discoloration, usually evolving in less than 24 hours. Patients are usually quite ill appearing. The cheek discoloration is usually poorly demarcated and ranges from salmon pink to violaceous. A violaceous hue is consistent with but not diagnostic of Hib infection. A portal of entry is not evident on examination. For unknown reasons, the right cheek is involved more often than the left.

b. Examination of patients with secondary forms of facial cellulitis reveals a portal of entry for infection (skin trauma, dental abscess).

c. Meningitis has been reported to occur in 5% to 10% of patients with buccal cellulitis, sometimes without clinical evidence of meningeal irritation.

3. **Laboratory evaluation:**

a. Leukocytosis is usually present.

b. Blood cultures are positive in 40% to 60% of cases of buccal cellulitis but are rarely positive in other forms of facial cellulitis.

c. Culture of a leading edge aspirate is positive in 25% to 50% of cases of buccal cellulitis. Facial wounds or dental abscesses associated with cellulitis should be cultured.
d. Urine CIE or latex agglutination test for bacterial antigen detection may be helpful when cultures are negative.
e. Because of the association of subclinical meningitis with buccal cellulitis, lumbar puncture should be strongly considered in these patients as part of the initial evaluation.

4. **Therapy:**
   a. Patients with buccal cellulitis without a portal of entry for infection should be considered bacteremic and initially treated with maximal doses of ceftriaxone or cefuroxime; therapy can be tailored after culture results become available. Parenteral therapy should be continued until the patient is afebrile and the cellulitis is substantially resolved. The patient should receive oral antibiotics to finish a 10-day course of therapy. Positive blood or CSF cultures mandate a full course of parenteral antibiotics.
   b. Patients with facial cellulitis clearly secondary to local skin trauma may be treated with a penicillinase-resistant penicillin such as nafcillin. Those with dental infection–associated cellulitis should receive parenteral penicillin. Oral therapy may be instituted when the patient is afebrile and substantial improvement has been noted.

F. **Myositis:**

1. **Etiology, epidemiology, and pathogenesis:**
   a. Myositis is defined as a primary infection or inflammation of muscle tissue.
   b. Bacteria, parasites *(Trichinella spiralis),* and viruses are recognized causes of myositis.
      1) The most common form of bacterial myositis is tropical pyomyositis, caused chiefly by *S. aureus*.
      2) Group A streptococci and occasionally staphylococci cause a less common but more virulent infection, termed **acute bacterial myositis.**

3) Influenza virus and Coxsackie B virus are the main causes of viral myositis.
4) The tissue nematode *T. spiralis* causes a distinctive form of myositis (trichinosis).

c. **Epidemiology:**

1) Tropical pyomyositis occurs chiefly in tropical regions but has been reported in various areas of the United States, especially Texas. It is more common in males.
2) Acute bacterial myositis is a disease mainly of adults and is usually associated with prior physical exertion or minor trauma.
3) Influenza infection may rarely be associated with a self-limited myositis, which occurs as other symptoms of infection subside. True postinfluenza myositis must be distinguished from the myalgias that commonly accompany influenza infection.
4) Coxsackie B viruses may cause a self-limited myositis of the chest and abdominal muscles, resulting in the symptom complex of pleurodynia, or "devil's grip." The disease occurs predominantly in those < 20 years of age.
5) Trichinosis occurs in persons ingesting undercooked meat, usually pork, which contains viable encysted larvae. Its incidence has been declining in recent decades.

d. **Pathogenesis:**

1) Tropical pyomyositis probably results from a primary transient staphylococcal bacteremia that seeds previously traumatized muscle, resulting in one or more discrete muscle abscesses.
2) The pathogenesis of acute bacterial myositis is probably similar to that of tropical pyomyositis. However, acute bacterial myositis is characterized by diffuse infection of one or more muscle groups without discrete abscess formation. The differences between the two diseases may be related to organism virulence and the extent of prior muscle trauma.

3) Viral myositis may result from primary muscle infection or a secondary immune-mediated process. Viruses have not been isolated from muscle tissue obtained from individuals with suspected viral myositis.
4) Trichinosis results from ingestion of infectious larvae, which then multiply in the intestine, enter the bloodstream, and invade muscle tissues. The larvae form encapsulated cysts after the fifth week of infection. The cysts calcify after several months.

2. **Clinical and laboratory findings:**
   a. Tropical pyomyositis typically manifests with low-grade fever, pain in the involved muscle(s), and sometimes swelling of the affected limb. The muscles of the thighs and trunk are most frequently involved. Abscesses in the psoas and other trunk muscles may manifest with abdominal pain and can be confused with visceral abscesses. Muscle enzyme levels are usually normal. Ultrasonography may be useful in demonstrating muscle abscesses that may be deep-seated and difficult to palpate.
   b. Acute bacterial myositis typically manifests with the abrupt onset of high fever, diffuse tenderness of the involved muscles, and, in severe cases, septic shock. Blood cultures are frequently positive and muscle enzyme levels are markedly elevated.
   c. Postinfluenza myositis is usually localized to the calf and manifests with severe lower leg pain lasting 1 to 3 days. Leukopenia and elevated muscle enzymes may be present.
   d. Coxsackie B virus myositis manifests with fever and sharp pains in the chest and abdomen secondary to muscle inflammation in those areas. The virus may be isolated from the throat or stool of infected individuals.
   e. Trichinosis is characterized by fever, generalized muscle pain, eyelid and facial edema, and eosinophilia on the peripheral blood smear. The extraocular muscles, masseters, diaphragm, and neck and back

muscles are most frequently involved. Myocarditis is a serious potential complication. Various serologic methods for detection of antibodies to *Trichinella* exist, but none is perfect, and diagnostic confirmation by muscle biopsy is recommended.

3. **Treatment:**
   a. Tropical pyomyositis requires surgical drainage of muscle abscesses, together with parenteral administration of an antistaphylococcal agent until substantial clinical improvement occurs. Oral antibiotics can then be continued to finish a 2-week course of therapy.
   b. Acute bacterial myositis requires aggressive therapy with high doses of a parenteral penicillinase-resistant agent, usually for 3 to 4 weeks. Antibiotic coverage may be narrowed when the causative organism is isolated.
   c. Viral myositis is self-limited and requires only supportive therapy with analgesics.
   d. Trichinosis is treated with mebendazole or thiabendazole (see Chapter 10 and Table A–20). Corticosteroids may be useful in decreasing inflammation.

XIV. BONE AND JOINT INFECTIONS:

A. Septic Arthritis:

1. **Etiology:**
   a. Hib is the most common etiologic agent of suppurative arthritis in children 6 months to 5 years of age.
   b. *S. aureus* is recovered from patients of all ages and overall is the second most common cause of septic arthritis in children.
   c. *S. pneumoniae*, group A streptococcus, and *N. gonorrhoeae* also cause septic arthritis throughout childhood.
   d. Group B streptococcus, *S. aureus*, and Enterobacteriaceae are the most common agents in the neonate.
2. **Pathogenesis:**
   a. Organisms reach joints by:
      1) Hematogenous spread.
      2) Extension from contiguous infected areas (e.g., osteomyelitis).

3) Direct puncture wounds. The synovium is extremely vascular and contains no limiting basement membrane, thereby enabling easy seeding from blood.

3. **Clinical manifestations:**
   a. The majority of children have acute onset of fever, severe joint pain and swelling, and refusal to bear weight or to use the extremity. Examination reveals warmth, tenderness, varying degrees of effusion, and limited range of motion. The joint is typically held in the position of least pain (usually flexion).
   b. Septic arthritis in the neonate is usually subtle; however, there is usually evidence of limited motion on careful examination. Osteomyelitis often precedes septic arthritis in the neonate, with rupture into the joint space.
   c. Joint involvement is usually monoarticular, but involvement of more than one joint does not exclude septic arthritis. The knees are most frequently affected, followed by hips, elbows, shoulders, and ankles.
4. **Diagnosis:**
   a. Joint aspiration should be carried out immediately and synovial fluid sent for culture, Gram's stain, cell count and differential, and glucose and protein concentrations. Culture yield can be increased by diluting the fluid, as, for example, by inoculating a drop into a blood culture bottle.
   b. Synovial fluid WBC counts $>100,000$ cells/mm^3 and glucose < 20 mg/dL are seen almost exclusively in septic arthritis (Table 6–16). WBC counts between 2,000 and 100,000/mm^3 can be seen in many conditions, including septic arthritis.
   c. Blood cultures should be obtained, because they are positive in 40% to 50% of cases.
   d. Radiographic findings are not particularly helpful early in the disease process.
5. **Differential diagnosis:**
   a. The differential diagnosis includes systemic lupus erythematosus (SLE), juvenile rheumatoid arthritis

TABLE 6–16.
Synovial Fluid

		Arthritis		
	Normal	Septic	Nonseptic Inflammatory	Reactive
Color	Pale yellow	Yellow-green	Yellow	Clear, slightly turbid
Clarity	Clear	Cloudy	Cloudy	Variable
Viscosity	High	Low	Low	Variable
WBC/mm^3	<200	≥70,000	3,000–50,000	5,000–30,000
Neutrophils %	<25	>90	70	Variable
Mucin clot	Good	Poor	Poor	Fair to good
Glucose (% blood)	80–100	<60	<80	<80

(JRA), rheumatic fever, viral arthritis, osteomyelitis with a sympathetic effusion, toxic synovitis, and leukemia.

6. **Treatment:**
   a. Antibiotic therapy:
      1) Gram's stain of synovial fluid should guide initial antibiotic therapy. When Gram's stain is negative, therapy should be directed toward the most common pathogens in that particular age group.
      2) Cefuroxime (100–150 mg/kg/day IV in three divided doses) is effective against the most common causes of septic arthritis in normal children between 2 months and 10 years of age.
      3) For normal children > 10 years of age, IV nafcillin or oxacillin provides adequate initial coverage.
      4) If *S. aureus* is recovered, oxacillin or nafcillin (150–200 mg/kg/day in four divided doses) is continued. First-generation cephalosporins and clindamycin are alternatives for penicillin-allergic patients.
      5) In the neonate, nafcillin or oxacillin **and** an aminoglycoside or a third-generation cephalosporin provide adequate initial antibiotic coverage.

6) Duration of therapy varies with the situation:
   a) Hib infections may be treated with 2 weeks of parenteral therapy.
   b) Arthritis caused by *S. aureus* or Enterobacteriaceae should be treated for 3 weeks.
   c) Septic arthritis caused by *N. gonorrhoeae* can often be treated with only 7 days of antibiotic therapy.

b. Surgical therapy:
   1) The infected joint should be drained by needle aspiration or by surgical incision and drainage. Needle aspiration is usually adequate except for the hip joint.
   2) Surgical incision and drainage of the hip is considered mandatory because suppurative arthritis of the hip can compromise the blood supply to the femoral head.

B. Osteomyelitis:

1. Epidemiology, etiology, and pathogenesis:
   a. Osteomyelitis is most frequently bacterial; however, it may also be caused by fungi and perhaps by viruses. Its annual incidence is approximately 1 in 5,000 children $<$ 13 years. Male/female ratio is 2.5:1.
   b. Microorganisms are introduced into the bone by one of three ways: (1) Most often by hematogenous infection secondary to bacteremia. (2) By local spread from a contiguous area of infection (e.g., cellulitis). (3) By direct inoculation, usually after trauma or surgery.
2. Hematogenous osteomyelitis:
   a. **Pathogenesis:**
      1) The infection begins in the metaphysis of a long bone adjacent to the epiphyseal growth plate. The metaphyseal blood supply consists of a high capillary network without lining phagocytes and with sluggish blood flow; therefore, bacteria can easily lodge on the venous side of the capillary loop where circulation is most sluggish. Venous occlusion with thrombus then prevents the phago-

cytes from reaching the bacteria and allows the organisms to proliferate. The proliferation of bacteria then leads to bone necrosis.

2) The lower extremities are most often affected. The sites of involvement in decreasing order of frequency are femur, tibia, humerus, fibula, radius, calcaneous, ilium , and ulna.

b. **Etiology:**

1) *S. aureus* is the primary pathogen, accounting for 80% of cases. Other common agents include group A streptococci, Hib, tuberculosis, Enterobacteriaceae, *S. pneumoniae, Candida* spp., and anaerobes. Sickle cell patients with osteomyelitis frequently have *Salmonella* as the causative agent.

2) Unusual causes include actinomycosis, coccidiomycosis, aspergillosis, and brucellosis.

3) Specific agents are associated with certain clinical circumstances:

Circumstance	Agent
Human bite	Anaerobes
Dog or cat bite	*Pasteurella multocida*
Nail puncture wound	*P. aeruginosa*
IV drug use	*Pseudomonas* spp.
Sickle cell disease	*Salmonella* spp.
Diabetes mellitus	Fungi
Neonates	Group B streptococci, staphylococci, enterobacteriaceae
Hemodialysis patients	*S. epidermidis*

c. **Clinical manifestations:**

1) The neonate may or may not have systemic symptoms, (e.g., appearing septic or with pseudoparalysis). Physical examination may reveal massive local swelling because neonates have thin bony cortex, allowing the infection to dissect into the surrounding tissues.

2) Older infants and children have more specific symptoms; well-localized pain with point tenderness is usually present. Often the child refuses to use the affected extremity. Fever and malaise are usually present.

d. Laboratory data:
   1) Leukocytosis with predominance of polymorphonuclear cells is seen; mild normochromic, normocytic anemia is common. The ESR is almost always elevated.
   2) Definitive diagnosis is made by isolation of bacteria from bone. Blood cultures are positive in about 50% of patients.
   3) Radiographic changes: (a) Soft tissue swelling in the metaphyseal region within 3 days after onset of symptoms. (b) Swelling of the muscles and obscured translucent fat lines about 3 to 7 days after onset of symptoms. (c) The typical changes of bone destruction and new periosteal bone formation that are apparent 10 to 21 days after the onset of symptoms.
   4) Radionuclide imaging is a very valuable adjunct to the diagnosis of osteomyelitis:
      a) The major advantage of radionuclide scanning with short half-life isotopes such as technetium 99 is its high overall accuracy, exceeding 90%, and its ability to show bone involvement before x-ray changes.
      b) Technetium bone scans are often nondiagnostic in neonates and infants < 6 months.
      c) Gallium 67 scan may be of value when technetium scan is nondiagnostic.

e. **Differential diagnosis:**
   1) The differential diagnosis includes septicemia, cellulitis, septic arthritis, toxic synovitis, leukemia, Ewing's sarcoma, rheumatologic disorders, thrombophlebitis, and bone infarction secondary to sickle cell disease.

f. **Treatment:**
   1) Acute bacterial osteomyelitis should always be treated with parenteral antibiotics.

2) Until the pathogen is identified, empiric therapy should be directed toward *S. aureus,* group A streptococci, and Hib (in infants and toddlers).
3) Therefore, initial (empiric) antibiotic choices may consist of a penicillinase-resistant semisynthetic penicillin or a first-generation cephalosporin in the older child and cefuroxime in infants and toddlers.
4) Antibiotics should be modified based on culture results.
5) The minimum duration of therapy for acute osteomyelitis is 3 weeks of parenteral antibiotics.
6) Surgical drainage and debridement may hasten recovery, especially if the diagnosis is delayed and abscess has already formed.
7) Indications for surgery:
   a) The need to obtain adequate specimens for culture.
   b) A suppurative collection, especially in the subperiosteal space or other tissue planes, that should be drained.
   c) *Pseudomonas* osteochondritis after a puncture wound of the foot.
   d) Failure of clinical response within 48 to 72 hours of initiating parenteral antibiotic therapy.

g. **Prognosis:** The prognosis for children with hematogenous osteomyelitis is generally good, especially if the diagnosis is made rapidly and the treatment is adequate. Aggressive therapy should prevent evolution to chronic osteomyelitis.

3. Nonhematogenous osteomyelitis:
   a. Contiguous osteomyelitis:
      1) An infected contiguous focus leading to osteomyelitis is much less common in children than in adults.
      2) Most cases of osteomyelitis acquired in this manner are nosocomial (e.g., decubitus) or secondary to an infected burn.
      3) More than one half of cases are caused by multi-

ple organisms. *S. aureus* and streptococci are most common; anaerobes and gram-negative enterics are also frequently encountered.

b. Puncture wound osteomyelitis most frequently involves the foot or patella:
   1) Osteomyelitis of the foot, more commonly termed osteochondritis, is most frequently caused by *P. aeruginosa,* although staphylococci and streptococci are sometimes isolated:
      a) Symptoms and signs typically consist of localized pain, swelling, and erythema over the puncture wound entrance. Constitutional symptoms are uncommon, with little or no fever.
      b) Treatment consists of surgical debridement and antipseudomonal therapy (e.g., ticarcillin and gentamicin) for 1 to 3 weeks.
   2) Osteomyelitis of the patella:
      a) This is most frequently seen in childhood before the patellar vessels have atrophied, but overall it is rare.
      b) Constitutional symptoms are uncommon; extension of the leg results in pain over the anterior aspect of the patella.
      c) The most common etiologic agent is *S. aureus*.
      d) The diagnosis is made by isolating the organism from the patella; x-ray film does not reveal periosteal elevation; however, rarefaction and sclerosis may be seen.
      e) The treatment is the same as that for other forms of osteomyelitis.

4. Spinal osteomyelitis:
   a. Discitis (not true osteomyelitis):
      1) Signs and symptoms include backache, limp, refusal to walk, hip pain, tenderness to palpation, limitation of movement, and low-grade fever.
      2) *S. aureus* is sometimes recovered; less common isolates include coagulase-negative staphylococci, pneumococci, and gram-negative enterics. The

role of these organisms is unclear. Similar manifestations may occur with noninfectious disc necrosis.

3) Discitis occurs most frequently in children less than 5 years of age and almost exclusively in the lumbar region.
4) X-ray studies may reveal disc space narrowing 2 to 4 weeks after the onset of symptoms, followed by destruction of margins of vertebral bodies adjacent to the disc space.
5) Treatment should be started with an antistaphylococcal agent; oral antibiotics are frequently used after an initial period of parenteral therapy. Prolonged therapy (4–6 months) may be necessary.
6) Prognosis is good for young children; however, spontaneous spinal fusion is common in older children.

b. Vertebral osteomyelitis:
   1) Because of the sluggish blood flow through the vertebral veins, vertebral bodies are predisposed to infection.
   2) Signs and symptoms include dull back pain, pain on exertion, fever, and exquisite tenderness to percussion.
   3) X-rays reveal progressive destruction of the vertebral body (usually anteriorly), followed by changes in adjacent vertebrae with new bone formation. Paraspinal abscess can form.
   4) *S. aureus* is the most common etiologic agent, followed by gram-negative enterics, especially those associated with UTI. *P. aeruginosa* may be isolated, especially in IV drug abusers. *M. tuberculosis* may also cause vertebral osteomyelitis (Pott's disease).
   5) The best method of establishing the diagnosis is bone biopsy culture.
   6) Because > 80% is caused by *S. aureus,* initial treatment should be directed at this organism. The average duration of therapy is 2 months.

7) Immobilization is usually required, either with bed rest or a body cast.
8) Surgical drainage should also be considered.

5. Chronic osteomyelitis:
   a. **Clinical manifestation:**
      1) Local findings include pain, soft tissue swelling, and draining sinus tracts.
      2) Acute systemic signs are not usually present; children are usually afebrile, have normal WBC count and differential, and may have a normal ESR. Many demonstrate elevated ESRs.
      3) Roentgenographic findings include sclerosis, lytic lesions, and adjacent soft tissue swelling.
   b. **Etiology:**
      1) Because the range of infecting organisms is much wider than with acute osteomyelitis, special effort should be made to isolate a pathogen. However, recovering a causative agent can be difficult even with invasive measures.
      2) Chronic osteomyelitis is usually the sequel of acute osteomyelitis, a traumatic injury, or the placement of foreign bodies.
   c. The differential diagnoses of diseases causing radiologically similar lytic or sclerotic bone lesions include tuberculosis, congenital syphilis, sarcoidosis, cat-scratch disease, eosinophilic granuloma, osteoid osteoma, and other tumors.
   d. **Treatment and prognosis:**
      1) Surgical debridement with removal of infected sequestra (devitalized pieces of bone) usually is necessary.
      2) The recommended duration of antimicrobial therapy is $\geq$ 6 months:
         a) Parenteral drug therapy should be maintained for the first 6 weeks.
         b) The remaining therapy may be continued with oral antibiotics on an outpatient basis if patient compliance and adequate drug levels can be achieved.

3) Even with appropriate therapy, some patients with chronic osteomyelitis may continue to have relapses.

XV. MISCELLANEOUS INFECTIONS:

A. Kawasaki Disease:

1. **Definition and epidemiology:**
   a. An acute febrile illness of unknown etiology that affects predominantly young infants. It is typically characterized by at least 5 days of fever (temperature 38.9°C–40°C) and at least four of five criteria:
      1) Polymorphous exanthemous rash that can be urticarial, maculopapular, erythema multiforme-like, etc.
      2) Bulbar conjunctival injection, usually without exudate and with sparing of the limbus.
      3) Inflammatory changes of the lips and oral mucosa, with swelling, erythema, and fissuring.
      4) Swelling and redness of the hands and feet, with subsequent desquamation beginning in the periungual region.
      5) Cervical adenopathy (≥1.5 cm in diameter), usually unilateral.
   b. Incomplete or atypical cases occur, posing diagnostic dilemmas.
   c. Approximately 20% to 25% of patients develop coronary artery aneurysms if untreated, and these account for the long-term morbidity and mortality of Kawasaki disease.
   d. Epidemiologic features:
      1) Median age is 2 years; 80% of cases occur in patients aged ≤ 5 years.
      2) Males predominate (1.5:1).
      3) Attack rates are highest in children of Japanese or Korean ethnicity, but in areas with relatively small Asian populations, most cases occur in the general population of children.
      4) Cases tend to occur in clusters every 2 to 4 years, but person-person transmission is not apparent.

2. **Clinical features:**
   a. Major features are listed above.
   b. Additional symptoms and signs:
      1) Arthralgia or arthritis, particularly in girls > 3 years old.
      2) Irritability.
      3) Acute cardiac features include myocarditis, small pericardial effusions, and tachycardia.
      4) Hydrops of the gallbladder, with occasional obstructive jaundice; mild hepatitis is common.
3. **Diagnostic considerations:**
   a. No specific diagnostic test exists.
   b. Laboratory features include mild leukocytosis, marked elevation of ESR, mild anemia, mild-moderate hypoalbuminemia, mild CSF lymphocytic pleocytosis, and sterile pyuria; thrombocytosis develops during convalescence.
   c. Illnesses with similarities that often need to be excluded include streptococcal infection, drug reactions, measles, and toxic shock syndrome.
   d. Patients with an incomplete clinical picture but with supportive laboratory findings (e.g., very elevated ESR) may warrant therapy to prevent coronary disease.
   e. Serial echocardiograms are critical for assessing status of coronary arteries.
4. **Treatment:**
   a. **Acute stage** (≤ 10 days of onset of fever):
      1) IV γ-globulin, 2 g/kg over 10 to 12 hours as a single dose.
      2) Aspirin, 80 to 100 mg/kg/day in four divided doses until the 14th day of illness, then 3 to 5 mg/kg/day as a single dose.
   b. **Convalescent stage:**
      1) Aspirin, 3 to 5 mg/kg/day as a single dose until 4 weeks after onset.
      2) Patients with coronary abnormalities: Aspirin 3 to 5 mg/kg/day, with or without dipyridamole (Persantine), 5 mg/kg/day divided tid.

c. **Chronic stage:**
   1) Patients with mild persistent coronary abnormalities should continue low-dose aspirin as listed earlier.
   2) Patients with moderate persistent coronary abnormalities:
      a) Low-dose aspirin as listed earlier.
      b) Plus dipyridamole as listed earlier.
   3) Patients with severe coronary abnormalities (stenoses, thromboses):
      a) Low-dose aspirin as listed earlier.
      b) Plus warfarin sodium (Coumadin).

B. Cat-Scratch Disease CSD:

1. **Definition:** CSD is a self-limited illness characterized by regional lymphadenopathy after an animal scratch, usually from a cat or kitten.
2. **Epidemiology:**
   a. CSD occurs worldwide, probably more often in semitropical areas.
   b. In temperate zones, incidence of CSD is higher during fall and winter.
   c. About 80% of cases occurs in individuals <21 years of age.
3. **Etiology:**
   a. The cause of CSD is a small gram-negative bacillus (*Afipia felis*) that is more abundant in early nodal involvement. Frequently, excised lymph nodes do not demonstrate organisms, suggesting this is a **postinfectious** condition.
   b. Illness follows a scratch or a lick from a kitten or cat in > 90% of patients.
   c. Cats that transmit CSD are not ill; the majority are immature.
   d. An inoculation site can be found in >50% of patients.
4. **Pathology:**
   a. Pathology of lymph nodes in CSD is not specific but can strongly suggest the diagnosis.
   b. Lymph nodes initially enlarge with reticulum cell hyperplasia, then with granulomas, and ultimately microabscess formation.

c. Pathologic findings may be confused with tularemia, lymphogranuloma venereum, brucellosis, toxoplasmosis, tuberculosis, or sarcoidosis.
d. Clusters of bacilli may be demonstrated by the Warthin-Starry silver impregnation stain.

5. **Clinical manifestations:**
   a. 3 to 5 days after contact with a cat, a skin papule forms, which progresses through a vesicular and crusting stage.
   b. Lymphadenopathy develops about 2 weeks after the scratch:
      1) The enlarged node(s) are invariably tender initially.
      2) Multiple sites are involved in approximately one third of patients.
      3) Node size usually varies from 1 to 6 cm.
      4) The most frequently affected sites (in descending order) are axillary, cervical, submandibular, inguinal, preauricular, and epitrochlear.
      5) Enlarged nodes may persist for several months and as long as 24 months.
      6) Suppuration of nodes occurs in less than one fourth of cases.
   c. Initially, fever, malaise, headache, anorexia, and sore throat may be present.
   d. Despite significant lymphadenopathy, patients usually do not appear very ill.
   e. Atypical manifestations include:
      1) Oculoglandular syndrome of Parinaud (conjunctivitis and preauricular lymphadenopathy).
      2) Erythema nodosum.
      3) Osteolytic lesions.
      4) Atypical pneumonia.
      5) Thrombocytopenic purpura.
      6) Severe chronic systemic disease (hepatosplenomegaly, fever, adenopathy).
      7) Neurologic complications:
         a) Encephalopathy, meningitis, myelitis, radiculitis, or cerebral arteritis develops in approximately 1%.

b) Encephalopathy appears suddenly, with convulsions often the first manifestation, usually 1 to 6 weeks after onset of CSD. Patients may become combative, lethargic, or comatose. Treatment is mainly supportive, and recovery is usually rapid and complete.

6. **Differential diagnosis:**
   a. Bacterial adenitis: *S. aureus,* group A streptococcus, anaerobes.
   b. Other infections: Atypical mycobacteria, TB, lymphogranuloma venereum, infectious mononucleosis, tularemia, and toxoplasmosis.
   c. Noninfectious: Hodgkin's disease, cystic malformations, non-Hodgkin's lymphoma, histiocytosis, sarcoidosis, Kawasaki disease.
7. **Diagnosis:**
   a. Diagnosis of CSD is based on clinical criteria:
      1) Single (usually) or regional lymphadenopathy.
      2) Cat contact.
      3) Identifiable inoculation site.
      4) A positive skin test result with cat-scratch antigen (if necessary).
   b. Hanger-Rose (cat-scratch) skin test is available in some centers. Skin test material is prepared from aspirated suppurative material:
      1) 0.1 mL of test antigen is injected intradermally.
      2) A positive reaction consists of $\geq$ 5-mm induration surrounded by erythema $>$ 10 mm in diameter at 48 to 72 hours.
      3) Testing should be deferred to at least 1 week after onset of adenopathy to avoid false negative results.
      4) In one series, 99% of patients meeting clinical criteria for CSD had positive results.
      5) Thousands of patients have had skin tests administered with no reported serious untoward effects.
8. **Treatment:**
   a. Antimicrobials appear to have little affect on the course of CSD. Rifampin, ciprofloxacin, TMP-SMX, and gentamicin have been used in immunocompromised patients.

   b. Suppurative nodes may be treated by needle aspiration.
   c. Surgical excision is unnecessary except when needed for diagnosis.
9. **Prognosis:**
   a. Most patients have a benign course.
   b. CSD with complications such as encephalopathy or osteolytic lesions may have a more prolonged course; however, long-term prognosis remains good.
   c. Reinfection is extremely rare.

C. Toxic Shock Syndrome

1. **Epidemiology:**
   a. Toxic shock syndrome (TSS) first was described in 1978 in children; however, the disease became widely recognized in 1980 when TSS was reported in menstruating women using tampons. More recently streptococcal TSS due to group A streptococci has been identified.
   b. Patients considered at high risk include menstruating women using tampons or other inserted vaginal devices and those with focal *S. aureus* infection.
   c. No evidence of person-to-person transmission exists for staphylococcal TSS.
   d. The median incubation period is 2 days.
2. **Clinical manifestations:**
   a. TSS is an acute febrile illness with mucocutaneous manifestations and multisystem involvement. It often is accompanied by vomiting and diarrhea at onset of illness.
   b. Temperature usually is higher than 38.9°C.
   c. The rash is usually sunburn-like initially, with desquamation of the skin of the palms and soles occurring 7 to 10 days later. Diffuse rash is usually not present in patients with streptococcal TSS.
   d. Hypotension and shock with multiorgan dysfunction can occur.
3. **Etiology:** The etiologic agent in most patients is a TSS toxin-1 (TSST-1)–producing strain of *S. aureus*. Streptococcal TSS has been associated primarily with streptococcal pyrogenic exotoxin A (SPE-A) producing strains of *S. pyogenes*.

4. **Diagnosis:**
   a. The diagnosis of TSS is based on a strict case definition (See Table 6–17).
   b. The isolation of TSST-1–producing *S. aureus* or of SPE-A–producing *S. pyogenes* is supportive evidence.
   c. Differential diagnosis includes measles, Kawasaki disease, Rocky Mountain spotted fever, streptococcal scarlet fever, leptospirosis, and Stevens-Johnson syndrome.
5. **Therapy:**
   a. Aggressive intravenous fluid replacement and vasopressor agents may be necessary.
   b. The most important component of therapy is elimination of the source of presumed staphylococcal or

TABLE 6–17.
Criteria for Toxic Shock Syndrome

Fever >38.9°C (102°F)
Rash:
1. Diffuse macular erythroderma
2. Desquamation after 1–2 weeks, especially on palms and soles

Hypotension:
1. Systolic <90 mm Hg in adults or <5th percentile in children <16 years
2. Orthostatic drop >15 mm Hg in diastolic blood pressure from lying to sitting; orthostatic syncope or dizziness

Multisystem involvement (>3):
1. *GI:* Vomiting or diarrhea at onset
2. *Muscular:* Severe myalgias or CPK more than twice upper normal limit
3. *Mucosae:* Vaginal, oropharyngeal, or conjunctival hyperemia
4. *Renal:* BUN or creatinine more than twice upper normal limits or urine sediment with >5 WBC per high-power field (without infection)
5. *Hepatic:* Total bilirubin, or alanine or aspartate transaminase values more than twice upper limit of normal
6. *Hematologic:* Platelets <100,000/mm^3
7. *CNS:* Disorientation or altered consciousness without focality when fever and hypotension are absent

Normal laboratory results (if tests performed):
1. Rocky Mountain spotted fever, leptospirosis, measles titer
2. Blood (may be positive for *S. aureus*), throat, CSF cultures

streptococcal infection or colonization and toxin production. This may involve removal of any foreign body (e.g., tampons, wound packing), drainage of an abscess, or debridement and irrigation of a wound. Streptococcal TSS frequently is associated with severe cellulitis or fasciitis.

c. Anti-staphylococcal antibiotics are recommended to eradicate the focus of TSST-1–producing *S. aureus,* although they probably do not affect the outcome of the acute illness. Anti-streptococcal therapy is important in treatment of streptococcal TSS.

D. Other Infections:

TABLE 6–18.
Infections Potentially Transmitted in Day Care Centers*

Mode of Transmission	Viruses	Bacteria	Parasites
Respiratory	Adenovirus	*H. influenzae* type b	
	Herpes simplex	Nontypable *H. influenzae*	
	Influenza A and B	*N. meningitidis*	
	Measles	Pertussis	
	Parainfluenza	*S. pyogenes*	
	Parvovirus B19	Tuberculosis	
	Respiratory syncytial virus		
	Rhinoviruses		
	Varicella		
Fecal-Oral	Enteroviruses	*Campylobacter*	*Cryptosporidium*
	Hepatitis A	*C. difficile*	*E. histolytica*
	Rotavirus	*Salmonella*	*E. vermicularis*
	Calicivirus	*Shigella*	*G. lamblia*
Skin Contact	Herpes simplex	*S. pyogenes*	Scabies
		S. aureus	Pediculosis
Blood, urine, saliva contact	Cytomegalovirus		Tinea capitis
	Herpes simplex		Tinea corporis
	Hepatitis B		

*Modified from *Redbook.* Elk Grove Village, Ill, 1991, American Academy of Pediatrics.

TABLE 6–19.
Important Infectious Diseases in Refugee Children and Foreign-Born Adoptees

Bacterial	Viral	Helminthic	Protozoal	Arthropoda
Campylobacter	Cytomegalovirus	Ascariasis	Amebiasis	Scabies
Salmonella	Hepatitis A	Hookworm	Giardiasis	Lice
Shigella	Hepatitis B	Liver flukes	Malaria	
Syphilis	Human immunodeficiency virus	Lung flukes		
Tuberculosis		Schistosomiasis		
Typhoid	Poliomyelitis	Tapeworm		
		Trichuriasis		

BACTERIAL PATHOGENS 7

I. COMMON BACTERIAL PATHOGENS:

A. Bacteroides:

1. **Microbiology:**
   a. Anaerobic gram-negative bacilli.
   b. Multiple species, especially *Bacteroides fragilis, Bacteroides oralis,* and *Bacteroides melanogenicus.*
2. **Normal sites:**
   a. *B. fragilis:* gut (90% of gut flora are anaerobes, especially *Bacteroides*).
   b. *B. oralis, B. melanogenicus:* Oral cavity.
3. **Infections:**
   a. *B. fragilis:*
      1) Intra-abdominal, including appendiceal, subphrenic, hepatic, or subhepatic abscess.
      2) Sepsis secondary to intra-abdominal process or focus.
      3) Brain abscess.
      4) Sepsis in compromised host.
   b. *B. oralis, B. melanogenicus:* Adenitis, peritonsillar abscess, Ludwig's angina, sinusitis.
4. **Therapy:**
   a. Drainage of abscess (foul-smelling pus).
   b. Antibiotic treatment: Chloramphenicol, clindamycin metronidazole, or cefoxitin.
   c. Consider hyperbaric oxygen in very serious infections.

B. Bordetella pertussis:

1. **Microbiology:**
   a. Strictly aerobic tiny gram-negative coccobacilli resembling *Hemophilus influenzae.*
   b. Grows slowly on Bordet-Gengou agar containing fresh blood, yielding small colonies after 3 to 7 days.
2. **Normal sites:** None.

3. **Infections:** Pertussis (whooping cough) is a protracted respiratory tract infection characterized by an early catarrhal phase with rhinorrhea and a later paroxysmal phase in which moderate to severe episodes of coughing paroxysms followed by a characteristic whooping inspiratory sound occur.
4. **Diagnosis:**
   a. *B. pertussis* can be cultured from nasopharyngeal secretions but only during the catarrhal phase.
   b. Organisms can be identified by fluorescent antibody staining of slides swabbed with nasopharyngeal secretions during the paroxysmal phase.
5. **Therapy:**
   a. Erythromycin (estolate preferably), 50 mg/kg/day po divided q6h for 10 days, has little or no effect on the disease but prevents transmission to others.
   b. Household and other close contacts may benefit from prophylaxis with erythromycin.

C. Campylobacter (including Helicobacter):

1. **Microbiology:** Curved spiral gram-negative microaerophilic bacilli. Four important species: *Campylobacter jejuni, Campylobacter fetus, Campylobacter coli, Campylobacter pylori* (renamed *Helicobacter pylori*).
2. **Epidemiology:**
   a. Commonly found in animals (birds, fowl, cattle, cats, dogs).
   b. *C. jejuni:* Spring and summer prevalence. Asymptomatic gastrointestinal (GI) carriage is rare in developed world (except day care centers), but common in Third World. Human fecal-oral transmission is rare (except day care centers).
3. **Infections:**
   a. *C. jejuni:* Common agent of acute gastroenteritis; rarely extraintestinal foci; occasional cause of reactive postinfectious arthritis or Reiter's syndrome.
   b. *C. coli:* Less common agent of gastroenteritis.
   c. *C. fetus:* Septicemia (relapsing) in immuncompromised hosts and occasionally in neonates (including meningitis).

d. *H. pylori:* Associated with gastritis and peptic ulcer disease.

4. **Diagnosis:**
   a. *Enteritis:* Frequently associated with blood, fecal leukocytes; 1% aqueous basic fuchsin stain of stool smear enables rapid diagnosis.
   b. *Gastritis or peptic ulcer:* Histologic examination of biopsy or culture of aspirates or biopsy specimens.
5. **Therapy:**
   a. *Enteritis:* Supportive; antibiotics usually unnecessary; antibiotics of possible value are erythromycin stearate, tetracyclines, ciprofloxacin, and clindamycin.
   b. *Sepsis:* Erythromycin, gentamicin, chloramphenicol, or quinolones.
   c. *Gastritis:* Bismuth subcitrate, amoxicillin (unproved), ciprofloxacin.

D. CHOLERA (Vibrio cholerae):

1. **Microbiology:**
   a. Comma-shaped, motile, gram-negative bacilli (pathogens are serogroup 01).
   b. *V. cholerae* non-01: Nonpathogenic.
   c. Other pathogens (rarely): *Vibrio vulnificus, Vibrio mimicus, Vibrio parahaemolyticus.*
2. **Epidemiology:**
   a. Waterborne transmission (fecal-oral).
   b. Humans are the only documented host.
   c. Seen in Asia, Africa, Mediterranean, and Gulf of Mexico coast.
   d. Non–*V. cholerae*: Sea water exposure.
3. **Infections:**
   a. *V. cholerae:* Severe toxin-mediated secretory diarrhea, without blood, mucus, or leukocytes (rice-water stools).
   b. Non–*V. cholerae:* Wound infections in healthy hosts and primary sepsis with occasional extraintestinal foci in compromised hosts.
4. **Diagnosis:**
   a. Geographic history.
   b. Dark field microscopy of stool: Rapidly motile comma-shaped bacilli.
   c. Culture on specific bile salt–containing media.

5. **Therapy:**
   a. Vigorous rehydration.
   b. *V. cholerae:* Tetracycline for those > 7 or 8 years old or trimethoprim-sulfamethoxazole (TMP-SMX) or ciprofloxacin.
   c. *V. vulnificus:* Tetracycline and aminoglycoside for those > 7 or 8 years or chloramphenicol.
   d. *V. parahaemolyticus:* Tetracycline for those > 7 or 8 years or ciprofloxacin.

E. Enterococcus

1. **Microbiology:**
   a. Formerly classified as group D streptococci, now a separate genus.
   b. Most are α-hemolytic or nonhemolytic gram-positive cocci, but some are β-hemolytic; they grow in 6.5% NaCl unlike other streptococci.
   c. Species include *Enterococcus faecalis* and *Enterococcus faecium*.
2. **Normal Sites:** GI tract.
3. **Infections:**
   a. Occasional neonatal infections (sepsis, etc.).
   b. Urinary tract infections (UTIs).
   c. Endocarditis (rarely in children).
   d. Intra-abdominal infections.
4. **Diagnosis:** Isolation from normally sterile site (blood, peritoneum, urine).
5. **Treatment:**
   a. UTIs usually can be treated with ampicillin.
   b. All other infections require synergy between penicillin or ampicillin and an aminoglycoside (usually best with gentamicin) for cure.
   c. Vancomycin should replace ampicillin for resistant strains or in penicillin-allergic patients.

F. Escherichia coli:

1. **Microbiology:**
   a. Aerobic gram-negative enteric bacilli.
   b. Many different serotypes based on K (capsular) and O (lipopolysaccharide) antigens. Some serotypes (termed enteropathogenic) produce diarrhea by one of several distinct mechanisms.

2. **Normal sites:** GI tract.
3. **Infections:**
   a. *Neonatal infections,* including sepsis and meningitis, particularly serotypes with K1 capsular antigen.
   b. *UTIs,* particularly with *E. coli* that are piliated (possess fimbriae, long filamentous organelles).
   c. *Gastroenteritis* caused by *E. coli* strains that are enteroadherent, enterotoxigenic, enteroinvasive, enteropathogenic, or enterohemorrhagic.
4. **Diagnosis:**
   a. *E. coli* is easily cultured from normally sterile sites, e.g., urine, blood, cerebrospinal fluid (CSF), when infection is present.
   b. Readily available methods for identifying enteropathogenic strains of *E. coli* in stool are not available.
5. **Therapy:** Generally susceptible to standard antibiotics (e.g., cephalosporins, ampicillin, and extended spectrum penicillins, aminoglycosides).

G. Hemophilus influenzae:

1. **Microbiology:**
   a. Aerobic (facultatively anaerobic) gram-negative coccobacilli.
   b. Absolute requirement for the oxidized form of nicotinamide adenine dinucleotide (NAD^+).
   c. Unencapsulated (nontypable) or encapsulated (types a–f) organisms differ in clinical significance. Type b is by far most important.
2. **Normal sites:**
   a. Nontypable organisms: Respiratory tract.
   b. Type b organisms: Upper respiratory tract ($\leq$ 5% normal children).
3. **Infections:**
   a. Nontypable *H. influenzae:* Otitis media, sinusitis, conjunctivitis, possibly lower respiratory tract infections.
   b. *H. influenzae* type b: Hematogenous infections, including meningitis, epiglottitis, septic arthritis, pericarditis, pneumonitis, buccal or facial cellulitis, and periorbital cellulitis; rarely, others.
   c. Antibody to type b capsule is protective by opsonic activity.

4. **Diagnosis:**
   a. *H. influenzae* is cultivated on chocolate agar (i.e. sheep blood agar that has been heated to lyse red blood cells [RBCs] to release NAD^+).
   b. Antigen detection assays (latex agglutination, counter-immunoelectrophoresis [CIE]) enable rapid detection of capsular polysaccharide (especially type b) in urine, CSF, etc).
5. **Therapy:**
   a. Antibiotic treatment: Ampicillin, chloramphenicol, ceftriaxone , cefuroxime (not for meningitis).

H. Mycobacterium:

1. **Microbiology:**
   a. Very slow-growing strictly aerobic acid-fast bacilli; acid fastness indicates resistance to decolorization once stain has been taken up by the lipid-rich cell wall.
   b. *Mycobacterium tuberculosis (TB):* The most important species; infects only humans naturally; requires complex medium (e.g., Lowenstein-Jensen).
   c. Other (atypical) mycobacteria:
      1) Photochromogens: *Mycobacterium kansasii, Mycobacterium marinum* —become pigmented only after exposure to light.
      2) Scotochromogens: *Mycobacterium scrofulaceum, Mycobacterium szulgai* —are pigmented with or without exposure to light.
      3) Nonchromogens: *Mycobacterium avium-intracellulare* (MAI) complex—nonpigmented.
      4) Rapid growers: *Mycobacterium fortuitum, Mycobacterium chelonei* —free-living, rapid growing (3–7 days) organisms.
   d. *Mycobacterium leprae:* Not cultivable in vitro.
   e. *Mycobacterium bovis:* Similar to *M. tuberculosis.*
2. **Epidemiology:**
   a. *M. tuberculosis:* Person-person transmission, primarily via droplets.
   b. Atypical mycobacteria: Environmental reservoirs rather than person-person transmission.
   c. *M. leprae:* Major reservoir is infected humans; low infectivity requiring prolonged close exposure.

d. *M. bovis:* now rare; cattle pathogen, with transmission to humans by milk from infected herds.

3. **Infections:**
   a. *M. tuberculosis:* Typical tuberculosis involving lungs, CNS, kidneys, and (rarely) other organs.
   b. Atypical mycobacteria:
      1) Photochromogens: *M. kansasii* —pulmonary disease that mimics TB; *M. marinum* —a fish pathogen that causes ulcerating granulomatous skin lesions after an abrasion.
      2) Scotochromogens: *M. scrofulaceum* —common cause of granulomatous cervical adenitis in children (also caused by MAI, *M. fortuitum*).
      3) Nonchromogens: MAI causes chronic cavitary pulmonary infections, disseminated infections in acquired immunodeficiency syndrome (AIDS) with positive blood cultures, chronic cervical adenitis in children.
      4) Rapid growers: Rare infections.
   c. *M. leprae:* Leprosy.
   d. *M. bovis:* Gastrointestinal (GI), bone infections.
4. **Diagnosis:**
   a. *M. tuberculosis:* Tuberculin skin test positivity; positive acid-fast smears and/or cultures from sputum, bronchial secretions, lymph node aspirates, etc.
   b. Atypical mycobacteria: Positive acid-fast smears and/or cultures.
   c. *M. leprae:* Acid-fast stains of infected tissue (nasal mucosa, earlobes, skin).
   d. *M. bovis:* Positive culture from infected tissue.
5. **Therapy:**
   a. *M. tuberculosis* (see Table A–21).
   b. Atypical mycobacteria:
      1) *M kansasii:* Prolonged antituberculous drugs, including rifampin.
      2) *M. scrofulaceum:* Surgical excision, limited role for antituberculous drugs.
      3) MAI: No effective therapy for disseminated disease.

4) *M. fortuitum:* Resistant to antituberculous agents; surgical excision; amikacin, cefoxitin, and probenecid may be useful.

c. *M. leprae:*

1) Tuberculoid leprosy: Dapsone, 1 mg/kg daily, and rifampin, 10 mg/kg once monthly.

2) Lepromatous or borderline leprosy: Dapsone, 1 mg/kg daily, and clofazime, 1 mg/kg daily, and rifampin, 10 mg/kg once monthly for at least 2 years.

d. *M. bovis:* Same therapy as for *M. tuberculosis* infection.

I. Neisseria gonorrhoeae (Gonococcus):

1. **Microbiology:**
   a. Aerobic gram-negative cocci that occur in pairs (diplococci) with adjacent sides flattened.
   b. Usually catalase and cytochrome oxidase positive. Growth is enhanced in the presence of carbon dioxide.
2. **Normal sites:** None.
3. **Infections:**
   a. *Ophthalmia neonatorum:* Severe neonatal conjunctivitis acquired during passage through infected birth canal.
   b. *Neonatal sepsis* or *septic arthritis*.
   c. *Vaginitis, urethritis* in children: Often associated with sexual abuse.
   d. *Salpingitis, pelvic inflammatory disease*.
   e. *Pharyngitis* (rare): Often associated with sexual abuse.
4. **Diagnosis:** Usually cultured on chocolate blood agar, if specimen is from a normally sterile site, or on Thayer-Martin medium (contains nystatin, vancomycin, colistin to suppress other flora) if specimen is from contaminated area (e.g., rectum, cervix).
5. **Therapy:** Antibiotic therapy with penicillin and probenecid, amoxicillin and probenecid, spectinomycin for infections with penicillinase-producing organisms, or ceftriaxone.

J. Neisseria meningitidis (Meningococcus):

1. **Microbiology:**
   a. Aerobic gram-negative cocci that occur in pairs (diplococci) with adjacent sides flattened.

   b. Usually catalase and cytochrome oxidase positive. Growth is enhanced in presence of CO_2.
   c. Nine serogroups on basis of polysaccharide capsule, the most important being A, B, C, W-135, and Y.
2. **Normal sites:** Nasopharyngeal carriage without disease occurs relatively commonly.
3. **Infections:**
   a. *Meningococcemia,* a frequently catastrophic illness with a high mortality rate, characterized by hemorrhagic manifestations and shock.
   b. *Meningitis,* relatively mild if not associated with clinical evidence of meningococcemia; hematogenous pathogenesis.
   c. Occasionally causes pneumonia, other purulent infections.
4. **Diagnosis:**
   a. CSF Gram's stain may be diagnostic.
   b. Organisms grow rapidly on blood or chocolate agar.
   c. Rapid antigen detection assays (latex agglutination, CIE) can demonstrate capsular antigen in CSF, urine, and other fluids.
5. **Treatment:**
   a. Intravenous (IV) penicillin; alternatives include ceftriaxone, chloramphenicol.
   b. Rifampin prophylaxis (10 mg/kg to maximum 600 mg orally q12h for four doses over 2 days).
   c. The value of corticosteroids in meningococcemia has not been established. Monoclonal antibody preparations are under evaluation as adjunctive therapy.

K. Pseudomonas:

1. **Microbiology**
   a. Aerobic motile gram-negative bacilli that grow in almost any environment.
   b. *Pseudomonas aeruginosa* is the most important species and is the most consistently antibiotic-resistant of the common medically important bacteria. Resistance is largely related to the structure of outer membrane porins.
   c. Approximately ten other *Pseudomonas* species cause infection, especially *Pseudomonas cepacia, Xantho-*

monas maltophilia, and *Pseudomonas pseudomallei.*

2. **Normal sites:** *P. aeruginosa;* GI, occasionally throat. All pseudomonads are found in water, soil, and vegetation.
3. **Infections:**
   a. *P. aeruginosa:* Invasive infections in immunocompromised hosts and burn patients, and pulmonary infections in cystic fibrosis; osteomyelitis after puncture wounds.
   b. *P. pseudomallei:* Melioidosis in tropical areas.
   c. *P. cepacia, P. maltophilia,* and other non-*aeruginosa* species cause opportunistic infections almost exclusively.
4. **Diagnosis:**
   a. Culture from a normally sterile site (blood, CSF, etc.).
   b. Cultures of *P. aeruginosa* or non-*aeruginosa* pseudomonads from endotracheal tubes and other nonsterile sites generally reflect colonization rather than infection.
5. **Therapy:**
   a. *P. aeruginosa* infections require an expanded spectrum penicillin (e.g., piperacillin, ticarcillin) with an aminoglycoside or ceftazidime.
   b. Non-*aeruginosa* organisms are often sensitive to other antibiotics such as TMP-SMX or chloramphenicol.

L. Salmonella:

1. **Microbiology:**
   a. Aerobic gram-negative enteric bacilli, nonlactose-fermenters.
   b. Three homogenous species (*Salmonella typhi, Salmonella paratyphi* A, and *Salmonella cholerasuis*) and one very heterogeneous group containing >1,500 serotypes distinguished by O (somatic) and H (flagellar) antigens.
2. **Epidemiology:**
   a. *S. typhi* only infects humans; all other salmonellae are found in animals, especially domestic cattle and poultry.
   b. Infection most commonly spreads from contaminated food or water.
   c. Some individuals excrete *Salmonella* in stool chronically, occasionally with a gallbladder focus (usually in adults).

3. **Infections:**
   a. *Gastroenteritis:* Most common, self-limited.
   b. *Enteric fever:* Particularly with *S. typhi, S. cholerasuis, S. paratyphi* A, and occasional other serotypes; patients manifest bacteremia and enteritis.
   c. Occasional pyogenic infections: Osteomyelitis, etc.
4. **Diagnosis:**
   a. Culture from a normally sterile site; positive blood culture in enteric fever.
   b. Positive stool culture with gastroenteritis and enteric fever.
5. **Therapy:**
   a. *Gastroenteritis:* Antibiotics are given only to the very young (< 3 months) or immunocompromised hosts; fluid replacement.
   b. *Enteric fever* (bacteremia) or pyogenic infections: Ampicillin, TMP-SMX, chloramphenicol, or ceftriaxone.

M. Shigella:

1. **Microbiology:**
   a. Aerobic nonmotile lactose-nonfermenting gram-negative enteric bacilli.
   b. Four species: *Shigella dysenteriae* (group A), *Shigella flexneri* (group B), *Shigella boydii* (group C), and *Shigella sonnei* (group D). Groups A to C are subdivided into > 30 serotypes.
2. **Epidemiology:**
   a. Not normal flora; very rarely found in asymptomatic individuals unless they are convalescing from recent illness.
   b. Strictly a human pathogen, not found in animals.
   c. Transmission by contaminated fingers, food, or water.
   d. Highly communicable; < 100 organisms required to initiate infection.
3. **Infections:**
   a. *Gastroenteritis,* mediated both by toxin production (Shiga toxin) and invasiveness (plasmid mediated). Bacteremia is rare except with infections caused by *S. dysenteriae* type 1 (Shiga's bacillus).

4. **Diagnosis:**
   a. Stool culture yields non-lactose-fermenting organisms with biochemical characteristics of *Shigella* and reaction with antisera to group A, B, C, or D.
   b. Blood and pus in stool supports the diagnosis.
5. **Therapy:**
   a. Supportive management, including fluids.
   b. TMP-SMX, tetracycline, or quinolones (not in children); ampicillin resistance has been increasing.

N. Staphylococcus:

1. **Microbiology:**
   a. Aerobic (and facultatively anaerobic) gram-positive cocci that tend to grow in grapelike clusters.
   b. Divided into coagulase-positive (*Staphylococcus aureus*) and coagulase-negative (*Staphylococcus epidermidis, Staphylococcus saprophyticus,* and nine other species).
2. **Normal sites:** *S. aureus* and coagulase-negative staphylococci frequently colonize anterior nares and skin of healthy individuals.
3. **Infections:**
   a. Coagulase-negative staphylococci: UTIs, opportunistic infections in compromised hosts, infections of prosthetic devices or tubing (e.g., cardiac valves, CSF shunts).
   b. *S. aureus:* Purulent infections, often in healthy individuals (e.g., osteomyelitis, pneumonia, arthritis); postoperative infections, skin infections.
   c. Toxin-mediated disorders: Toxic shock syndrome results from infection or colonization by a toxin-producing strain of *S. aureus*.
4. **Diagnosis:**
   a. Culture of *S. aureus* from a normally sterile site (e.g., bone, blood) generally represents infection.
   b. Culture of coagulase-negative staphylococci from normally sterile sites frequently represent contamination unless confirmed by repeat cultures.
5. **Therapy:**
   a. Penicillinase-resistant penicillins (nafcillin, oxacillin, methicillin), first- or second-generation cephalosporins,

and clindamycin are effective agents unless methicillin resistance is present.

b. Methicillin-resistant *S. aureus* are particular problems, requiring treatment with vancomycin. A large proportion of coagulase-negative staphylococci also require vancomycin because of methicillin resistance.

c. In particularly severe infections, rifampin or an aminoglycoside such as gentamicin is added for a synergistic effect.

d. Surgical drainage of an abscess or removal of a foreign body is frequently necessary.

O. Streptococcus (see Enterococcus):

1. **Microbiology:**

a. Aerobic (and facultatively anaerobic) gram-positive cocci that grow in chains.

b. Divided on the basis of hemolysis on blood agar into α-streptococci (viridans), β-streptococci, and nonhemolytic (γ) streptococci.

c. α-Streptococci include *Streptococcus sanguis, Streptococcus salivarius, Streptococcus mutans,* and many others; these differ from *Streptococcus pneumoniae* by lack of bile solubility and lack of optochin sensitivity.

d. β-Streptococci are subdivided by serologic reactivity of cell wall carbohydrate into group A (*Streptococcus pyogenes*), group B (*Streptococcus agalactiae*), group C (four species), nonenterococcal group D, etc.

2. **Normal sites:**

a. α streptococci are found in the oral cavity and respiratory tract.

b. β streptococci: Group A may colonize skin and may colonize pharynx; group B colonizes the vagina and throat; group C, G, and F colonize the pharynx occasionally; group D colonizes the GI tract.

3. **Infections:**

a. α-Streptococci: Dental caries, endocarditis.

b. β-Streptococci:

1) Group A: Pharyngitis, adenitis, impetigo, scarlet fever, miscellaneous pyogenic infections; postinfectious acute glomerulonephritis, acute rheumatic fever.

2) Group B: Puerperal and neonatal infections.
3) Groups C, G, and F: Occasional pharyngitis, other pyogenic infections.

4. **Diagnosis:**
   a. Isolation from a normally sterile site.
   b. Group A streptococci on throat culture (or positive rapid antigen detection test result).
   c. Interpretation of other β-hemolytic streptococci recovered from throat cultures is difficult because these can be normal flora.
5. **Therapy:**
   a. Streptococci (not enterococci) are penicillin-sensitive organisms.
   b. Alternate agents include other penicillins, erythromycin, clindamycin, and cephalosporins.

P. Streptococcus pneumoniae (Pneumococcus):

1. **Microbiology:**
   a. Aerobic gram-positive oval cocci that usually occur in pairs with their axes end to end.
   b. Multiple (> 80) serotypes determined by capsular polysaccharides; immunity is type-specific.
   c. Most strains remain highly penicillin sensitive, but relatively resistant and multiply resistant strains are known.
2. **Normal sites:** Upper respiratory tract.
3. **Infections:**
   a. Bacteremia, often without a focus of infection, especially in highly febrile children 6 months to 3 years of age.
   b. Meningitis, pneumonitis, septic arthritis, and other focal purulent hematogenous infections are relatively common.
   c. Otitis media and sinusitis occur frequently.
4. **Diagnosis:**
   a. Organisms are readily grown on standard medium, producing α-hemolysis on blood agar.
   b. Antigen detection assays (latex agglutination, CIE) using polyvalent antisera to multiple pneumococcal capsular types enable rapid demonstration of antigen in CSF, urine, etc.

5. **Therapy:** β-Lactam antibiotics (penicillins and cephalosporins); alternatives include clindamycin and erythromycin.

II. UNCOMMON BACTERIAL PATHOGENS:

A. Acinetobacter:

1. **Microbiology:**
   a. Aerobic gram-negative coccobacillus (nonfermentive, nonmotile) that can resemble *Neisseria* or *Hemophilus* on Gram's stain.
   b. Previously classified as *Herellea, Moraxella, Mima, Alcaligenes, Achromobacter,* and *Bacterium.*
   c. Single species: *Acinetobacter calcoaceticus,* with two important biotypes *Acinetobacter calcoaceticus* var. *anitratus* (formerly *Herellea vaginicola*) and var. *lwoffi* (formerly *Mima polymorpha*).
2. **Epidemiology:**
   a. Ubiquitous in soil, water, and sewage.
   b. Frequently colonize skin and other sites, only in hospitalized patients.
3. **Infections:** Nosocomial infections, including catheter-related bacteremia, ventilator-associated pneumonitis, and catheter-related bladder infection.
4. **Therapy:**
   a. Removal of implicated foreign bodies.
   b. Antibiotic treatment: TMP-SMX, aminoglycoside with expanded-spectrum penicillin, imipenem.

B. Actinomycosis (Actinomyces israelii):

1. **Microbiology:**
   a. Filamentous, branching elongated gram-positive rods that grow slowly (4–10 days) and only in anaerobic or microaerophilic circumstances.
   b. Colonies form yellow-orange "sulfur granules" in vivo comprised of densely intertwined branching filaments.
   c. Most human infections are caused by *A. israelii.*
2. **Epidemiology:**
   a. Normal inhabitants of the GI tract from the oropharynx to the colon.
   b. Confined normally to the mucosal surface.
   c. Person-person transmission does not occur.

3. **Infections:**
   a. Infection develops only if *Actinomyces* penetrates the mucosal barrier to areas of tissue with sufficiently low oxygen tension to enable replication.
   b. Infections typically invade locally without respect to anatomic boundaries or tissue planes. Lesions are comprised of polymorphonuclear neutrophils (PMN)–filled sinus tracts that may drain spontaneously. Chronic indolent infections are the rule.
   c. The most common form of actinomycosis is "lumpy jaw," cervicofacial actinomycosis, usually related to poor dental hygiene or oral trauma. Patients manifest indolent submandibular swelling and obscuring of the angle of the mandible.
   d. Thoracic and/or abdominal actinomycosis is rare in children.
4. **Diagnosis:**
   a. Diagnosis is suspected on clinical grounds.
   b. Confirmation requires culture and/or histologic demonstration of *Actinomyces*. Culture can be difficult because of small gram-negative rods (Actinobacillus) that are commonly present as well. Culture of sulfur granules provides the highest yield.
5. **Therapy:**
   a. Prolonged high-dose penicillin G is treatment of choice. Response to treatment may not be apparent for at least 4 to 6 weeks.
   b. Alternate antibiotics include erythromycin, clindamycin, and tetracycline.

C. **Anthrax:**
   1. **Microbiology:** *Bacillus anthracis* is an aerobic, nonmotile spore-forming gram-positive rod.
   2. **Epidemiology:** Domestic herbivorous animals (horses, sheep, cattle, swine, goats) are infected by ingestion of spores that contaminate soil, establishing an animal-soil-animal cycle. Humans are infected by direct contact with contaminated animal products (e.g., goatskins, West Asian cashmere). Workers involved in industrial processing of imported animal products are now vaccinated.
   3. **Infections:** Now very rare in the United States, with the

majority being **cutaneous** anthrax, with a papule at the site of initial inoculation leading to a vesicle and then to a characteristic black eschar surrounded by secondary vesicles and edema. Patients are acutely ill and 5% are bacteremic. **Inhalation** and **GI anthrax** are very rare in children.

4. **Diagnosis:** Direct smear and culture of vesicular fluid from skin lesion. Blood culture. Serologic responses can be seen by 3 weeks after onset.
5. **Therapy:** Penicillin (300,000–400,000 units/kg/day) IV for 14 days for systemic anthrax and for cutaneous anthrax if patient is toxic, if lesions are on head or neck, or if extensive edema is present. Oral penicillin has been used for mild cutaneous anthrax.

D. Brucellosis:

1. **Microbiology:**
   a. Nonmotile obligate aerobic gram-negative coccobacilli or short rods arranged singly or less commonly in short chains. They are non-spore-forming and lack capsules.
   b. Species infective for humans, with usual hosts: *Brucella suis* (swine), *Brucella abortus* (cattle), *Brucella melitensis* (goats and sheep), and *Brucella canis* (dogs).
2. **Epidemiology:** *Brucella* organisms are harbored by domestic animals in many areas of the world. Spread to humans occurs mainly from ingesting unpasteurized milk or milk products (cheeses), from direct contact with infected animals (farm or abattoir workers), or from inhalation of contaminated aerosols.
3. **Infections:** Childhood infections are commonly associated with high spiking fevers for ≥ 1 month, hepatosplenomegaly, generalized adenopathy, myalgia, arthralgia, weight loss, hepatitis, and leukopenia with left shift, anemia. More unusual manifestations include meningitis, encephalitis, spondylitis, osteomyelitis. Many childhood infections are apparently self-limited.
4. **Diagnosis:** Recovery of organism from blood, bone marrow, or other site or demonstration of a rise in antibody titer (usually agglutination titer).
5. **Therapy:**
   a. For children < 7 or 8 years: oral trimethoprim-sulfamethoxazole (10/50 mg/kg/day) for 3 weeks, with in-

tramuscular (IM) gentamicin (5 mg/kg/day) for the first 5 days.

b. For those > 7 or 8 years: oral doxycycline (5 mg/kg/day) or oxytetracycline (30 mg/kg/day) for 3 weeks, with IM gentamicin (5 mg/kg/day divided in two doses) for the first 5 days.

E. Clostridium:

1. **Microbiology:**
   a. Gram-positive spore-forming anaerobes, some of which produce potent exotoxins.
   b. Important organisms regarding human disease:
      1) Gas gangrene group, especially *Clostridium perfringens.*
      2) *Clostridium tetani,* the cause of tetanus.
      3) *Clostridium botulinum,* the cause of botulism.
      4) *Clostridium difficile,* the cause of pseudomembranous colitis.
2. **Epidemiology:** Found in lower GI tract and in soil (particularly in soil contaminated by animal feces); spores allow prolonged survival in hostile environments.
3. **Infections**
   a. *C. perfringens:* Produces **gas gangrene** after dirt-contaminated wounds, **anaerobic cellulitis, clostridial endometritis,** and **clostridial food poisoning** after ingestion of large numbers of enterotoxin-producing organisms.
   b. *C. tetani:* **Tetanus** ("lockjaw") from spore-contaminated wounds, including **neonatal tetanus** after umbilical cord contamination in developing countries.
   c. *C. botulinum:* **Botulism** from ingestion of preformed toxin-containing foods (frequently home-canned foods) or contaminated wounds (**wound botulism**); **infant botulism** from absorption of toxin produced in the infant intestine after ingestion of spores.
   d. *C. difficile:* **Pseudomembranous colitis,** or antibiotic-associated colitis, a toxin-mediated colitis after antibiotic therapy that has led to overgrowth of *C. difficile.*
4. **Diagnosis:**
   a. *C. perfringens* infections: Usually clinical diagnosis.
   b. Tetanus: Clinical diagnosis

c. Botulism: Clinical diagnosis; also demonstration of botulinum toxin in blood, intestinal contents, or remaining food.

d. Pseudomembranous colitis: Endoscopic appearance of colon, isolation of *C. difficile* from stool, and detection of *C. difficile* toxin in stool of symptomatic patient.

5. **Therapy:**
   a. Gas gangrene: Excision of devitalized tissue, massive doses of penicillin, hyperbaric oxygen.
   b. Tetanus: Supportive measures, removal of site of entry if possible, human tetanus immune globulin to neutralize unbound toxin, penicillin.
   c. Botulism: Supportive measures and horse botulinum antitoxin to neutralize unbound toxin.
   d. Infant botulism: Supportive measures, **no** antibiotic or antitoxin.
   e. Pseudomembranous colitis: Withdrawal of inciting antibiotic agent; oral metronidazole or vancomycin.

F. Corynebacterium:

1. **Microbiology:**
   a. *Corynebacterium diphtheriae:* Aerobic and facultatively anaerobic gram-positive pleomorphic bacilli that are non-spore-forming and arrange themselves to form "Chinese Letters"; usually nonhemolytic; produces a powerful exotoxin (diphtheria toxin).
   b. **Diphtheroids:** Mostly nonpathogenic commensals; group JK causes opportunistic infections.
2. **Epidemiology:**
   a. *C. diphtheriae:* Transmitted by droplets from person to person; some patients become carriers and serve as source of spread of infection.
   b. Diphtheroids: nonpathogenic normal flora of pharynx, nasopharynx, urethra, and skin.
3. **Infections:**
   a. *C. diphtheriae:* Diphtheria, which is a superficial pharyngeal infection with gray-white membrane formation, elaboration of a toxin that is absorbed, circulates, and binds to myocardium and cranial and peripheral nerves to produce myocardial dysfunction and nerve palsies.
   b. Diphtheroids: Usually contaminants but occasionally cause infections of foreign bodies.

c. Group JK: Important cause of opportunistic infections in compromised hosts.

4. **Diagnosis:**
   a. Diphtheria: A clinical diagnosis, confirmed by culture of toxin-producing *C. diphtheriae* on tellurite media.
   b. Diphtheroid infection, including JK: Repeated culture from a normally sterile site.
5. **Therapy:**
   a. Diphtheria: Equine diphtheria antitoxin, penicillin, supportive measures.
   b. Diphtheroid infections: Usually penicillin-susceptible; JK organisms, however, are usually sensitive only to vancomycin.

G. Legionella:

1. **Microbiology:**
   a. Aerobic pleomorphic gram-negative bacilli that require a complex-enriched media for growth.
   b. More than 20 species are described, with *Legionella pneumophila* the most important; *L. pneumophila* includes at least 12 serotypes.
2. **Epidemiology:** Organisms contaminate cooling towers, air-conditioning systems, and shower heads; person-person transmission is not documented.
3. **Infections:** Two forms of illness, both rare in children:
   a. **Legionnaire's disease:** Severe pneumonitis, with a substantial mortality rate.
   b. **Pontiac fever:** A nonpneumonic febrile illness that is self-limited and non-life-threatening.
4. **Diagnosis:**
   a. Direct immunofluorescence demonstration of organisms in lung or tracheal aspirate specimen.
   b. Culture of organisms on buffered charcoal yeast extract medium but not on standard medium.
   c. Serologic demonstration of a rising serum indirect immunofluorescence antibody titer.
5. **Treatment:** Erythromycin is the drug of choice; alternatives include tetracycline, quinolones, and rifampin.

H. Leptospirosis (Leptospira interrogans):

1. **Microbiology:** Spirochete with at least 180 serotypes identified.

2. **Epidemiology:**
   a. Rodents are the most important reservoir; however, almost all mammals, including dogs, can serve as reservoirs of leptospirosis.
   b. Humans acquire leptospirosis after contact with blood, urine, tissues, or organs of infected animals. Therefore, this is a zoonosis.
   c. Leptospirosis is most frequent in summer and early fall.
   d. Disease is associated with farming, sewers, abattoirs, and contact with pet dogs.
3. **Infection:**
   a. Leptospirosis is usually a biphasic illness. The initial, or septicemic, phase usually lasts 4 to 7 days and is characterized by fever, headache, myalgia, nausea, vomiting, and abdominal pain. Conjunctivitis, pharyngitis, lymphadenopathy, hepatosplenomegaly, icterus, macular exanthem, and proteinuria may be seen. During this phase, organisms multiply in monocytes.
   b. The second, or immune, phase begins 1 to 3 days after cessation of symptoms and lasts 4 to 30 days. This phase is characterized by fever, rash, headache, uveitis, and meningitis. Leptospiruria is present.
   c. About 10% of patients develop a severe form of disease (Weil's disease, or ictohemorrhagic fever), characterized by prolonged fever, jaundice, hemorrhage, azotemia, and vascular collapse.
4. **Diagnosis:**
   a. Leptospires may be cultured from blood during the initial phase or from urine during the second phase.
   b. A fourfold or greater rise in microscopic agglutination titer may be seen.
   c. Rapid diagnosis may be made by determining specific IgM using the enzyme-linked immunosorbent assay (ELISA) method.
5. **Therapy:** Generally, leptospirosis is a self-limited disease with a favorable prognosis. To be effective, treatment with penicillin or tetracycline must be initiated early in the course of disease. Duration of therapy should be 7 to 10 days.

I. Listeria:

1. **Microbiology:**
    1) *Listeria monocytogenes* is a gram-positive rod that resembles corynebacteria. Narrow rim of β-hemolysis surrounds colony on blood agar.
    2) Characteristic tumbling motility in fluid media.
2. **Epidemiology:**
    1) Foodborne transmission is important, with coleslaw and Mexican cheese implicated recently.
    2) Widespread in nature, with frequent colonization or infection of animals and transient human colonization.
3. **Infections:**
    1) Neonatal sepsis and/or meningitis, related to colonization of the birth canal.
    2) Granulomatosis infantiseptica: Stillborn with intrauterine disseminated abscesses and/or granulomata.
    3) Puerperal sepsis.
    4) Occasional infections in acquired immunodeficiency syndrome (AIDS) or other compromised hosts or in the very elderly.
4. **Diagnosis:** Culture from a normally sterile site (usually blood or CSF).
5. **Therapy:** Penicillin, ampicillin, erythromycin, and chloramphenicol are effective agents.

J. Nocardiosis *(Nocardia asteroides* and *Nocardia brasiliensis)*:

1. **Microbiology:**
    a. Gram-positive branching rods that, unlike *Actinomyces,* are strict aerobes and weakly acid-fast positive. They have a beaded appearance with Gram's staining.
    b. Growth occurs aerobically in 2 days on blood agar, with colonies having a dry chalky appearance.
2. **Epidemiology:**
    a. Frequently found in soil and in other environmental sources.
    b. Not considered normal flora.
3. **Infections:**
    a. Skin and subcutaneous infection: Most typically a pustule associated with fever and lymphadenitis follows a

traumatic lesion (e.g., thorn prick) with or without soil contamination. *N. brasiliensis* is the usual pathogen.

b. Pulmonary nocardiosis: Typically inhalation of *N. asteroides* from dust or soil leads to a confluent pneumonia that may progress to multiple abscesses and/or pleural extension. About one half of these infections occur in hosts with impaired T-cell function. Dissemination, particularly to the brain, can occur.

4. **Diagnosis:**
   a. Diagnosis is easier than in actinomycosis because organisms are more uniformly distributed. Weak acid fastness is useful to distinguish from *Mycobacterium* and from *Actinomyces*.
   b. Culture is relatively easy if the laboratory is notified to seek *Nocardia*.
5. **Therapy:**
   a. The treatment of choice is a combination of systemic sulfonamides and surgical drainage.
   b. Other possible agents include ampicillin, ceftriaxone, aminoglycosides, and trimethoprim-sulfamethoxazole. Antituberculous agents are ineffective.

K. *Pasteurella multocida*:

1. **Microbiology:** Small gram-negative coccobacillus that grows on blood agar.
2. **Epidemiology:** Transmitted to humans by a dog or cat bite (the most common cause of infected dog or cat bite).
3. **Infections:** Infected animal bite. Rarely a more invasive infection.
4. **Diagnosis:** Easily cultured from the infected bite.
5. **Therapy:** Highly susceptible to penicillin. Alternatives include tetracycline and ceftriaxone but not first- or second-generation cephalosporins.

L. Plague *(Yersinia pestis)*:

1. **Microbiology:**
   a. Pleomorphic, nonmotile, gram-negative bacilli.
   b. Strains of *Y. pestis* vary in virulence.
2. **Epidemiology:**
   a. Plague is transmitted to humans by the bite of an infected flea, through direct contact with an infected animal (through skinning and/or evisceration), or by inha-

lation of infected droplets from a patient with pneumonic plague.

b. Domestic animals may be responsible for some cases of human plague, but rodents are the most important reservoir. This is a zoonosis.
c. In the United States, cases occur most often in southwestern states.
d. An average of 18 cases were reported annually in the United States in the 1980s.

3. **Infections:**
    a. The portal of entry of *Y. pestis* largely determines which form the disease will take.
    b. Most common site of entry is the skin; the organism enters the skin and moves by lymphatics to regional lymph nodes. It may localize here or disseminate via the bloodstream to involve the liver, spleen, lungs, kidneys, and meninges.
    c. A mass of large, tender, and fixed nodes, known as a "bubo," is visible in bubonic plague. Most commonly involved are groin, axilla, and neck nodes.
    d. When the portal of entry is the lung (pneumonic plague), the disease is particularly fulminant. Severe pneumonitis and septicemia occur. The patient usually dies unless early treatment is begun.
    e. Onset of illness is abrupt, with fever, shaking chills, malaise, and headache.
    f. Neurologic manifestations such as delirium, stupor, and disorder of speech are common.
    g. Other manifestations may include acute tubular necrosis, elevated liver enzymes, and disseminated intravascular coagulopathy.
    h. Severity of disease largely reflects the degree of endotoxemia.
4. **Diagnosis:** Definitive diagnosis is made by culture of *Y. pestis* from infected tissue or body fluid (most often bubo aspirate or blood culture).
5. **Therapy:**
    a. Therapy should be begun as soon as plague is suspected.
    b. Streptomycin is the drug of choice for acutely ill patients.

c. Mild cases can be treated with chloramphenicol or tetracycline. TMP-SMX may be useful.

d. Chloramphenicol should be given if meningitis develops.

M. Rat Bite Fever:

1. **Microbiology:** Two different etiologic agents.
   a. *Spirillum minus:* Gram-negative spiral organism with two to three regular spirals and polar flagella; animal inoculation is required for isolation of organism.
   b. *Streptobacillus moniliformis:* Gram-negative pleomorphic microaerophilic rod; requires enriched media for growth.
2. **Epidemiology:**
   a. Both organisms represent flora of rodent mouth, particularly rats and mice.
   b. Infection is seen primarily in urban children and laboratory workers.
3. **Disease:**
   a. **Rat bite fever:** Acute fever, rash, and adenitis.
      1) *S. minus* infection: Long incubation period of 14 to 18 days, development of eschar or ulcer at inoculation site, relapsing fever, myalgias, macular plaque-like rash, regional adenitis, may remit and relapse over several months; the classic illness is termed **sodoku.**
      2) *S. moniliformis* infection: Short incubation period of 1 to 3 days, chills, headache, vomiting, blotchy rash, arthritis; may have a biphasic course.
   b. **Haverhill fever:** A similar *S. moniliformis* infection that is the result of ingestion of raw milk contaminated with *S. moniliformis*.
4. **Diagnosis:**
   a. *S. minus* infection: Demonstration of organism in blood, wound exudate, or adenitis; false positive test result for syphilis.
   b. *S. moniliformis:* Recovery of organism from blood, joint fluid, or infected bite wound; false positive serologic test result for syphilis.
5. **Therapy:**
   a. *S. minus:* Highly sensitive to penicillin; tetracycline or aminoglycosides are alternatives.

b. *S. moniliformis:* Sensitive to penicillin but less so than *S. minus;* recommend 1.2 million units of procaine penicillin daily or 2 g of oral penicillin V daily (adult doses) for 7 to 10 days.

N. Tularemia *(Francisella tularensis)*:

1. **Microbiology:** Aerobic, fastidious, nonmotile gram-negative coccobacilli.
2. **Epidemiology:**
   a. Transmissible to humans by bites of infected ticks, deer flies, fleas, mites, as well as by contact with infected animals, especially rabbits, sheep, squirrels, and deer. Rabbits are the most important reservoir. This is, therefore, a zoonosis.
   b. Most infections occur during warm months.
   c. Tularemia has been reported throughout the United States; most frequently occurs in the southcentral states (Arkansas, Missouri, Oklahoma, Texas, and Louisiana).
   d. Incidence is < 200 cases/year in the United States.
3. **Infections:**
   a. Organisms enter the body via skin, conjunctivae, oropharynx, or the respiratory tract.
   b. Symptoms consist of fever, chills, vomiting, headache, and generalized aches. Skin rash may appear.
   c. Six clinical patterns of disease are described: ulceroglandular, glandular, typhoidal, oculoglandular, oropharyngeal, and pneumonic.
   d. Ulceroglandular syndrome accounts for approximately 75% of cases. It is characterized by a painful, swollen papule at the site of entry. About 2 days after the appearance of general symptoms, tender enlarged lymph nodes, most often axillary or inguinal, develop. The papule ruptures and develops into an ulcer with raised margins that can persist > 1 month. The skin over these areas may be inflamed. Generalized lymphadenopathy, as well as hepatosplenomegaly, may be present.
4. **Diagnosis:**
   a. History of possible exposure (wild animal exposure, family members).
   b. Fourfold rise in serum agglutination titers.

c. False positive titers may occur with *Brucella* infections.
d. The organism may be cultured from blood, skin, ulcers, or lymph nodes; however, the risk of aerosol inhalation by laboratory personnel is high.

5. **Therapy:**
   a. Parenteral streptomycin or gentamicin for 7 to 10 days.
   b. Clinical improvement occurs within several days of onset of antibiotic therapy.
   c. Oral tetracycline or chloramphenicol are effective; however, because of high relapse rates, these bacteriostatic drugs should be continued for at least 2 weeks.

O. Yersinia:

1. **Microbiology:**
   a. Gram-negative non-lactose-fermenting coccobacilli with bipolar staining.
   b. Three important species of *Yersinia:*
      1) *Yersinia pestis* (see Section L).
      2) *Yersinia pseudotuberculosis* (formerly *Pasturella*): Seven antigenic groups based on somatic O antigens.
      3) *Yersinia enterocolitica:* 34 serogroups based on O antigens.
2. **Epidemiology:**
   a. *Y. pseudotuberculosis:* GI portal of entry, with many species of wild animals, as well as humans, serving as reservoirs; winter predominance.
   b. *Y. enterocolitica:* Water, food, and animals are primary reservoirs, with primary GI portal of entry; late fall and winter seasonality.
3. **Infections:**
   a. *Y. pseudotuberculosis:* Fever and abdominal pain that mimics acute appendicitis, representing **acute mesenteric lymphadenitis;** causes pseudotuberculosis in animals.
   b. *Y. enterocolitica:* A usually self-limited **enterocolitis** in children, with fever, abdominal pain, and diarrhea, sometimes with **polyarthritis; acute mesenteric lymphadenitis** as listed earlier can occur.
4. **Diagnosis:**
   a. *Y. pseudotuberculosis:* Rarely isolated on stool culture;

occasionally cultured from lymph node or blood; antibody titers can enable serologic diagnosis.

b. *Y. enterocolitica:* Isolation from stool is more frequent, particularly if "cold enhancement" is employed; serologic diagnosis is possible, with highest titers in those with arthritic manifestations.

5. **Therapy:**
   a. *Y. pseudotuberculosis:* Role of antibiotic therapy is unclear; organism is usually sensitive to ampicillin, cephalosporins, aminoglycosides, tetracyclines, and chloramphenicol.
   b. *Y. enterocolitica:* Role of antibiotic therapy is unclear; usually sensitive to aminoglycosides, TMP-SMX, ceftriaxone, and quinolones.

VIRAL PATHOGENS 8

I. ADENOVIRUSES

A. Microbiology:

1. Double-stranded DNA viruses.
2. Almost 100 different serotypes known.

B. Epidemiology:

1. Spread occurs via respiratory or fecal-oral route.
2. Infections can occur any time of the year, but are most frequent during the late winter and early spring months.
3. Outbreaks of adenovirus conjunctivitis caused by inadequately chlorinated swimming pools have been reported.

C. Infections:

1. Many clinical syndromes are associated with adenovirus infection, including upper respiratory tract infection (URI), pharyngitis, conjunctivitis, pneumonia, croup, bronchiolitis, hemorrhagic cystitis, and acute gastroenteritis.
2. Infection with adenoviruses often is subclinical.

D. Diagnosis:

1. Viruses can be isolated by cell culture.
2. Diagnosis also may be made by serologic testing of acute and convalescent sera.

E. **Therapy:** There is no vaccine or specific therapy for adenovirus infection at this time.

II. ARBOVIRUSES (Table 8–1)

III. ENTEROVIRUSES:

A. Microbiology:

1. Group of small RNA viruses in the picornavirus family.
2. They include poliovirus 1 to 3, Coxsackie viruses, echoviruses, and those simply designated enteroviruses.

TABLE 8–1.
Selected Arboviruses of Significance in Humans

Genus (Family)	Vector	Usual Disease Expression	Geographic Distribution	Age Affected	Morbidity
Alphavirus (Togaviridae)					
Western equine encephalitis	Mosquito	Encephalitis	North America	Very young, very old	Low
Eastern equine encephalitis	Mosquito	Encephalitis	North America	All	High
Flavivirus (Flaviviridae)					
St. Louis encephalitis	Mosquito	Encephalitis	North America	Elderly	Rare
Dengue	Mosquito	Febrile illness or hemorrhagic fever	All tropical zones	All	Rare, if patient survives
Yellow fever	Mosquito	Hemorrhagic fever	Africa, South America, Carribean	All	Rare, if patient survives
Bunyavirus (Bunyaviridae)					
California encephalitis	Mosquito	Encephalitis	North America	Children	Low

B. Epidemiology:

1. Enteroviruses are found worldwide.
2. Humans are the major hosts.
3. Epidemics usually occur during the summer and fall months.
4. Spread of infection is usually through direct or indirect fecal-oral transmission.
5. Incubation periods vary; however, short intervals (2–10 days) are typical.

C. Infections:

1. **Polioviruses:**
   a. Most infections are subclinical or mild.
   b. The disease may manifest as a nonspecific febrile illness, aseptic meningitis, or paralytic poliomyelitis.
   c. The extent of involvement in paralytic poliomyelitis is very variable.
   d. Vaccination against polio has resulted in a dramatic decline in paralytic cases (see Chapter 1, section I).
2. **Coxsackie viruses, echoviruses, and other enteroviruses:**
   a. Most infections are subclinical.
   b. Clinical syndromes associated with these viruses include aseptic meningitis and encephalitis, poliomyelitis-like disease, exanthems and enanthems, pericarditis and myocarditis, conjunctivitis, and generalized disease of the newborn.

D. Diagnosis: Diagnosis can be made by virus isolation from throat, body fluids, stool, or tissues and further supported by a fourfold rise in neutralizing antibody titer between paired acute and convalescent serum samples.

E. Therapy: No specific therapy is available.

IV. HERPESVIRUSES:

Herpesviruses are large, double-stranded DNA viruses. Within this group, many cause human infections, including two herpes simplex viruses (HSVs), cytomegalovirus (CMV), varicella-zoster virus (VZV), Epstein-Barr virus (EBV), and human herpesvirus type 6. Herpesviruses are ubiquitous, and diseases caused by these viruses vary from asymptomatic infections to fatal illnesses. Primary infection with these viruses results in an overt clinical illness, which is typically followed by a period of latency. The virus, which is present in the cell, may be reactivated, which then results in recurrent infection.

A. **Herpes Simplex Virus:**

1. **Microbiology:**
   a. There are two distinct antigenic types: HSV-1 and HSV-2.
   b. Many strains of each virus exist.
2. **Epidemiology:**
   a. HSV are found worldwide.
   b. The mode of spread is by direct contact with infected secretions.
   c. In the United States, HSV-1 antibody is found in approximately 50% of middle class populations and in almost 90% of lower socioeconomic groups.
   d. HSV-2 antibody is isolated from approximately 20% to 35% of sexually active adults.
3. **Infection:**
   a. Clinical manifestations of HSV-1 infection include the following:
      1) Gingivostomatitis: This is often the primary infection, and it appears most frequently in toddlers. Ulcerative lesions may be found on the buccal mucosa, tongue, gums, and pharynx. These may be associated with fever and irritability.
      2) Recurrent cold sores; Reactivation usually results in cold sores, which recur over the lips, anterior buccal mucosa, or perioral area of the face.
      3) Herpetic whitlow: This is an infection of the finger or fingernail area, which results from the inoculation of secretions infected with HSV-1 through a break in the skin. Lesions are painful and vesicular; they are often misdiagnosed as staphylococcal infection.
      4) Corneal infection: HSV-1 infection of the eye with resultant corneal scarring is one of the most common causes of blindness. Aggressive local antiviral therapy (acyclovir, vidarabine) is indicated.

5) Encephalitis: Approximately 1 in 100,000 persons infected with HSV-1 develop HSV encephalitis. Typically, focal neurologic signs are present, and the temporal lobe (or lobes) is most frequently affected. Untreated, the mortality rate is high.

b. HSV-2 infections:

1) Genital herpes: The majority (approximately 70%) of genital herpes is caused by HSV-2. Primary genital herpes is associated with systemic symptoms; subsequent episodes are usually less severe.

2) Neonatal herpes: Usually results from contact with infected maternal secretions during the time of delivery. Because they are relatively immunocompromised, HSV infection in the neonate is associated with high morbidity and mortality. Manifestations of neonatal HSV infections include:

a) Disseminated disease with widespread organ involvement.

b) CNS disease.

c) Infections localized to the skin, eyes, and mouth.

4. **Diagnosis:** Diagnosis is usually made on clinical grounds and supported by demonstration of HSV in infected secretions or lesions by culture or immunoassay. Serologic studies can also be used to document recent infection (presence of IgM antibody; fourfold rise in IgG titer) or past infection.

5. **Therapy (see Table A–22):**

a. Acyclovir is an inhibitor of HSV DNA polymerase.

b. It is an effective and commonly used drug for HSV infections. Foscarnet is also effective against HSV, including those strains resistant to acyclovir.

B. Cytomegalovirus:

1. Microbiology:

a. CMV contains the largest genome of the herpesviruses.

b. Strains isolated from different persons reveal genomic and phenotypic heterogeneity.

2. Epidemiology:
   a. More than 80% of adults have antibody to CMV, reflecting previous infection.
   b. CMV infection is frequently acquired during the first 5 years of life or during young adulthood.
   c. During the period of latent infection, CMV resides primarily in leukocytes.
   d. Infection is acquired through contact with infected secretions.
3. Infections:
   a. Diseases commonly associated with CMV infection include congenital CMV, heterophile-negative mononuclesis, and infections in immunosuppressed patients (i.e., interstitial pneumonia, posttransplant syndrome, chorioretinitis, encephalitis, esophagitis and duodenitis).
   b. Most infections are asymptomatic.
   c. Congenital CMV infection may manifest as jaundice, hepatosplenomegaly, pneumonia, thrombocytopenia, microcephaly, intracerebral calcifications, chorioretinitis, and sensorineural deafness (see Chapter 3).
4. Diagnosis:
   a. Diagnosis of CMV infection requires isolating the virus or demonstrating a rise in antibody titer. Large, inclusion-bearing cells in the urine sediment may be seen in patients with widespread CMV infection.
5. Therapy:
   a. Ganciclovir has been shown to reduce the severity of retinitis, esophagitis, and colitis associated with CMV. Ganciclovir and immune globulin used concurrently probably decreases mortality due to CMV pneumonia in bone-marrow transplant patients.
   b. Foscarnet has been used successfully in treatment of patients unable to tolerate ganciclovir or those infected with ganciclovir-resistant CMV.

C. Epstein-Barr Virus:

1. Microbiology:
   a. EBV is similar to other herpesviruses; however, there are fewer genomic strain differences.
   b. EBV selectively infects β-lymphocytes.

2. Epidemiology:
   a. EBV is acquired by contact with infected secretions.
   b. Humans are the only source of EBV.
   c. There is no seasonal predilection to EBV infection.
   d. The period of communicability is unknown.
3. Infections:
   a. Infectious mononucleosis is the most common manifestation of EBV:
      1) It is characterized by fever, exudative pharyngitis, lymphadenopathy, splenomegaly, and atypical lymphocytosis.
      2) Complications include airway obstruction, pneumonia, aseptic meningitis, encephalitis, Guillain-Barré syndrome, and thrombocytopenia.
      3) In patients with congenital or acquired cellular immune deficiencies, B-cell lymphomas or fatal disseminated infection may occur.
      4) "Chronic" infectious mononucleosis has been reported; however, this remains a topic of controversy.
   b. EBV is associated with several malignancies, including Burkitt's lymphoma, anaplastic nasopharyngeal carcinoma (commonly seen in Southeast Asia), and certain B-cell lymphomas.
4. Diagnosis:
   a. Diagnosis depends on the clinical manifestations and serologic testing.
   b. Heterophil antibody (Monospot test) is most commonly used; however, it is unreliable in children <4 years; results are frequently negative despite EBV infection.
   c. EBV-specific antibodies can be measured:
      1) IgM to viral capsid antigen (VCA) appears early in illness and disappears within 1 to 2 months. Therefore, it is an indicator of recent primary infection (Table 8–2).
      2) IgG to VCA appears early in illness and persists for life.
      3) Antibody against early antigen (EA) appears several weeks after onset of illness and persists for 3

TABLE 8–2.
Serologic Markers of Epstein-Barr Virus

	No previous Infection	Acute Infection	Recent Infection	Past Infection
Anti-VCA-IgG	–	+	+	+
Anti-VCA-IgM	–	+	±	–
Anti-EA (diffuse)	–	±	±	–
Anti-EBNA	–	–	±	+

EA = early antigen, EBNA = Epstein-Barr nuclear antigen, VCA = viral capsid antigen; – indicates <1:10 for VCA or EA tests, <1:2 for EBNA.

to 6 months. Therefore, its presence indicates recent infection.

4) Antibody against EBV nuclear antigen (EBNA) can be demonstrated within weeks to months after the onset of illness and persists for life.

5. Therapy:
   a. No specific therapy is available.
   b. Although corticosteroids have been reported to alleviate some of the symptoms associated with infectious mononucleosis, we do not recommend their use in routine cases.

D. Varicella-Zoster Virus:

1. Microbiology:
   a. VZV is morphologically very similar to HSV.
   b. Only one serotype is known.
2. Epidemiology:
   a. VZV is highly contagious, and most people contract the primary infection (chickenpox) before adulthood.
   b. The major mode of transmission is respiratory.
   c. The incubation period is 10 to 23 days.
   d. Immunity is generally lifelong.
3. Infections:
   a. Chickenpox (primary VZV infection) is characterized by a generalized, pruritic, vesicular rash.
   b. Chickenpox lesions begin on the head and spread to the neck, trunk, and extremities.
   c. There may be mucous membrane involvement.

d. Reactivation of latent VZV results in herpes zoster, which is usually a unilateral vesicular eruption in a dermatomal distribution.
e. Complications of varicella include encephalitis, pneumonia, hepatitis, coagulopathy and bacterial superinfection, particularly with group A streptococcus. Complications occur more frequently in immunocompromised patients.

4. Diagnosis:
   a. Diagnosis is usually made clinically.
   b. The presence of a herpesvirus can be demonstrated by a Tzanck smear that demonstrates inclusions.
   c. Infection can be confirmed by acute and convalescent titers of VZV antibody.
5. Therapy
   a. Intravenous acyclovir should be given to immunocompromised patients with varicella or herpes zoster.
   b. Oral acyclovir given to healthy children with varicella within 24 hours of onset of rash results in decrease in the number and duration of skin lesions. This should be considered in adolescents and adults with varicella.
   c. Varicella-zoster immune globulin (VZIG) should be given, within 96 hours of exposure, to susceptible patients who are at high risk for severe or complicated varicella. The following persons should receive VZIG after significant exposure:
      1) Immunocompromised, susceptible children who have had household exposure, shared a hospital room, or played indoors for at least 1 hour with children with contagious VZV.
      2) Normal susceptible adults, especially pregnant women.
      3) Newborn infant of a mother who had onset of chicken pox within 5 days before or 48 hours after delivery.
      4) Hospitalized premature infant (>28 weeks gestation) whose mother has not had chicken pox.
      5) All hospitalized premature infants <28 weeks gestation or weighing <1,000 gm.

V. INFLUENZA VIRUSES:

A. Microbiology:

1. Members of the orthomyxovirus group, which are enveloped, single-stranded RNA viruses.
2. Three major serotypes: A, B, and C.
3. Influenza A and B contain glycoproteins, hemagglutinin, and neuraminidase.

B. Epidemiology:

1. Humans are the major hosts.
2. The most common mode of transmission is by direct droplet spread.
3. Infections occur most frequently during midwinter months.
4. Major outbreaks of influenza A occur at 2- to 3-year intervals.

C. Infections:

1. Incubation period is an average of 2 days.
2. Onset is usually abrupt, with development of fever, headache, and myalgia.
3. Nonproductive cough frequently develops.
4. Patient usually improves within 1 week.
5. Occasionally patients develop pneumonia, which may be lethal.
6. Other uncommon manifestations of influenza include myositis, myocarditis, and central nervous system (CNS) abnormalities.
7. Reye's syndrome has been associated with influenza.
8. The most common complication of influenza virus infection is bacterial superinfection, usually with *Streptococcus pneumoniae, Hemophilus influenzae,* and *Staphylococcus aureus*.

D. Diagnosis: May be established by virus isolation (e.g., from nasopharyngeal and throat swabs), direct immunofluorescent detection of viral antigen from respiratory tract epithelial cells, or by demonstrating a fourfold or greater increase in antibody titers between acute and convalescent specimens.

E. Prevention: Killed viral vaccine prepared from strains closest to the antigenic subtypes causing infections are available. Vaccination is recommended for the elderly, individuals of any age at high risk (e.g., with chronic lung or heart disease, immunodeficiency), and those in high-risk occupations (e.g., medical personnel). Amantadine is effective in preventing illness when started before exposure to influenza A.

F. **Therapy:** Treatment is mostly symptomatic. Amantadine therapy may have modest benefit when begun within 48 hours after the onset of illness.

VI. MEASLES:

A. **Microbiology:**

1. Measles virus is a single-stranded RNA virus in the paramyxovirus family.
2. Only a single serotype is known to cause human infection.

B. **Epidemiology:** Measles is usually a childhood disease. It typically spares infants < 6 months because of maternal antibodies. The infectivity rate is very high, and most of those infected become ill. The disease is communicable from 3 to 5 days before the onset of rash to 4 days afterward.

C. **Infections:**

1. Illness usually begins 9 to 11 days after exposure, with fever, cough, coryza, and conjunctivitis.
2. Koplik's spots, which are small gray-white spots surrounded by erythema on the buccal mucosa, occur early in the illness and are pathognomonic of measles.
3. Within several days after onset of illness, the typical rash begins, first over the head and progressing to the trunk and extremities.
4. Measles can be very severe, especially in malnourished or immunocompromised hosts.
5. Complications include bacterial superinfection, encephalitis, pneumonitis, and thrombocytopenic purpura. Subacute sclerosing panencephalitis can develop years later, particularly if measles has occurred at a young age.

D. **Diagnosis:**

1. Diagnosis of measles is usually based on clinical findings.
2. In atypical cases, laboratory confirmation by serologic testing (using complement fixation, hemagglutination in-

hibition, or indirect fluorescent antibody methods) may be necessary.

E. **Therapy:** No specific therapy is available.

F. **Prevention:** Measles vaccine is discussed in Chapter 1.

VII. MUMPS:

A. **Microbiology:**

1. Mumps is an enveloped, single-stranded RNA virus of the paramyxovirus family.
2. Only one antigenic type is known.

B. **Epidemiology:**

1. Mumps occurs most frequently during the late winter and spring months.
2. Patient is contagious from about 7 days before until 9 days after onset of illness.

C. **Infections:**

1. Typically mumps manifests with fever associated with swelling and tenderness of the salivary glands. Parotid glands are most commonly involved, and swelling may be unilateral or bilateral.
2. Complications of mumps can occur with or without parotitis. They include meningitis, encephalitis, transverse myelitis, pancreatitis, orchitis, myocarditis, and nephritis. These complications usually resolve without sequelae within several weeks.

D. **Diagnosis:**

1. Diagnosis is usually made on a clinical basis, which can be confirmed serologically (by complement fixation).
2. Mumps virus can also be isolated from the saliva, pharynx, urine, and other affected sites for growth in cell culture.

E. **Therapy:** No specific therapy is available.

F. **Prevention:** Effective, safe, and long-lasting mumps vaccine has been available since 1968 and is recommended for infants after the first year of life (see Chapter 1).

VIII. PARAINFLUENZA VIRUSES:

A. **Microbiology:**

1. Single-stranded RNA viruses belonging to the paramyxovirus group.

2. Four serotypes: Parainfluenza 1, 2, 3, and 4.

B. Epidemiology:

1. Spread is direct via droplet particles.
2. Outbreaks are most frequent during the fall months.

C. Infections:

1. Parainfluenza viruses (especially 1 and 3) are the major etiologic agents of acute croup.
2. Also associated with upper respiratory tract illness, pharyngitis, bronchitis, and pneumonia.
3. The illness may begin abruptly, as in acute croup, or as a mild upper respiratory tract (URI) illness with progression over several days. The duration of illness is usually 7 to 10 days.

D. Diagnosis: Diagnosis is made by virus isolation, direct immunofluorescence, or serology.

E. Therapy: There is no specific therapy at this time.

IX. PARVOVIRUS B19:

A. Microbiology: Small, single-stranded DNA viruses.

B. Epidemiology:

1. Transmission rate is high.
2. Virus is usually spread via the respiratory route.
3. Highest rate of infection occurs in children and young adults.

C. Infections:

1. Parvovirus B19 infection in patients with underlying hemolytic anemia often results in aplastic crisis because the virus infects erythroid precursors.
2. Erythema infectiosum, or fifth disease, also is caused by parvovirus B19. It is characterized by fever, malaise, headache, a lacy rash peripherally and an indurated rash on the face, with a "slapped cheek" appearance.
3. Parvovirus B19 infection during pregnancy can cause fetal hydrops and death; the risk of fetal death is less than 10% after proved maternal infection.

D. Diagnosis:

1. The diagnosis is supported by the presence of IgM-specific antibody or a fourfold or greater rise in IgG-specific antibody.

E. Therapy: No specific therapy is available.

X. POXVIRUSES:

A. Microbiology: Poxviruses are large DNA viruses responsible for variola (smallpox), vaccinia, molluscum contagiosum, and cowpox.

B. Smallpox (variola):

1. Smallpox has been eradicated; the last natural case occurred in 1977.
2. Smallpox manifested with fever, chills, myalgias, and a rash that progressed from papulovesicles to pustules, which were most prominent over the head and extremities.
3. The disease was highly contagious by respiratory exposure, direct contact, or by fomites.

C. Molluscum contagiosum:

1. **Poxvirus mollusci** is the causative agent of molluscum.
2. Infection occurs most frequently in young children.
3. It is usually acquired by direct contact.
4. Lesions of molluscum are painless, flesh-colored papules.
5. There are no associated systemic symptoms.
6. No specific therapy is usually required. Lesions that do not resolve spontaneously can be removed by cryotherapy, curettage, or electrodissection.

XI. RABIES:

A. Microbiology: Bullet-shaped, large, enveloped, single-stranded RNA virus of the rhabdovirus group.

B. Epidemiology:

1. Transmitted to humans from rabid animals. In the United States, one to five cases of human rabies are reported each year.
2. Rabies is most often associated with unimmunized dogs or cats, bats, skunks, raccoons, foxes, and wolves.

C. Infection:

1. Manifests as a fulminant and fatal encephalitis.
2. Disease begins as a nonspecific illness that progresses to hallucinations, combativeness, muscle spasms, seizures, and focal paralysis.
3. Median survival after onset of symptoms is 4 days.
4. Recovery is rare.

D. Diagnosis:

1. Viral antigen can be demonstrated in brain tissue by immunofluorescence.
2. Specific antibodies to rabies virus can be detected late in the disease.

E. Therapy:

1. Postexposure prophylaxis (consisting of rabies hyperimmune globulin and antirabies vaccine) should be given if rabies exposure is known or highly suspected. Vaccine consists of five doses on days 1, 3, 7, 14, and 28 (see Table 1–2).
2. Preexposure prophylaxis should be given to individuals at high risk of contact with rabies virus (i.e., animal handlers, some laboratory workers).

XII. RESPIRATORY SYNCYTIAL VIRUS (RSV):

A. Microbiology:

1. RSV is a single-stranded RNA virus of the paramyxovirus family.
2. There are at least two antigenic subgroups of RSV (A and B).

B. Epidemiology:

1. Outbreaks usually occur during the winter months.
2. Nosocomial infection with RSV is a major problem.
3. Careful hand washing between contacts with patients is crucial in controlling nosocomial spread.

C. Infections:

1. RSV is the most important cause of bronchiolitis and pneumonia in infants.
2. Incubation period is 1 to 4 days.
3. In infants, the illness begins with rhinitis, which progresses to coughing, wheezing, and respiratory distress.
4. Findings may include hypoxemia, hypercapnea, and pulmonary infiltrates.
5. The mortality rate in hospitalized infants is 0.5% to 1%; it is much higher in children with immunodeficiency, congenital heart disease, and chronic lung disease.
6. The clinical picture seen in older children and adults is that of a milder illness, including upper respiratory tract illness and croup.

D. Diagnosis: Diagnosis is usually made by direct immunofluorescent antibody detection of RSV antigen in nasopharyngeal epithelial cells.

E. Therapy:

1. Treatment is mainly supportive, and no vaccine is currently available.
2. Ribavirin should be considered in infants with RSV infection who have an underlying cardiac, pulmonary, or immunosuppressive illness or who are severely ill.

XIII. RETROVIRUSES:

A. Microbiology:

1. Enveloped, single-stranded RNA viruses that encode reverse transcriptase.
2. Most important representatives are the oncoviruses and the lentiviruses (human immunodeficiency virus type 1 [HIV-1] and type 2 [HIV-2]).

B. Infections:

1. Oncoviruses:
   a. Associated with cancers in animals.
   b. Human T-cell leukemia virus type I (HTLV-I) causes adult T-cell leukemia and may be associated with some chronic neurologic illnesses.
   c. HTLV-II has been associated with human leukemias, including hairy cell leukemia.
2. HIV-1 and HIV-2: Cause of AIDS (see Chapter 5).

C. Pathogenesis:

1. Oncoviruses are not usually cytolytic; instead they produce new virus indefinitely by transducing growth-promoting genes called **oncogenes** in the host cell.
2. HIV is characterized by a prolonged latent state.
3. HIV infects primarily cells with the CD4 surface antigen, especially CD4 lymphocytes.
4. The primary defect in acquired immunodeficiency syndrome (AIDS) is a result of reduction in numbers and functional impairment of CD4 helper-inducer lymphocytes.

D. Therapy: HIV treatment is discussed in Chapter 5.

XIV. RUBELLA:

A. Microbiology:

1. Single-stranded RNA virus of the togavirus family.
2. Only one serotype is known.

B. Epidemiology:

1. Rubella is highly contagious; however, only 30% to 60% of those infected develop clinical disease.
2. Patient is contagious from 7 days before to 7 days after the onset of rash.
3. Congenitally infected infants may be contagious for ≥ 6 months after birth.

C. Infections:

1. Illness is usually mild and consists of low-grade fever, lymphadenopathy, upper respiratory tract symptoms, and a macular rash most frequently over the head, neck, and trunk.
2. Complications include arthralgia and arthritis (most frequently in women), encephalitis, and thrombocytopenic purpura.
3. Rubella infection of pregnant women may result in severe fetal damage, especially if the infection occurs in the first trimester.
4. The major findings in congenital rubella syndrome include cardiac defects, eye defects such as cataracts, chorioretinitis and glaucoma, deafness, mental retardation, hepatosplenomegaly, intrauterine growth retardation, and thrombocytopenia (see Chapter 3).
5. The severity of defects varies greatly.

D. Diagnosis:

1. Diagnosis is usually made on clinical grounds and confirmed serologically with paired acute and convalescent samples.
2. IgM-specific antibody may be useful; however, it may be persistently positive (> 6 months) in some individuals with acquired infections, and some infants with congenital rubella may not produce IgM-specific antibodies.

E. Therapy: No specific therapy is available.

F. Prevention: Rubella vaccine is discussed in Chapter 1.

FUNGAL DISEASES

9

I. DEEP MYCOSES (see Table A–18):

A. Blastomycosis:

1. **Organism and pathogenesis:**
   a. *Blastomyces dermatitidis* is a dimorphic fungus (yeast and hyphal forms) found primarily in the eastern half of the United States. The yeast cells are larger than *Histoplasma capsulatum,* have thick walls, and form broad-based buds. Hyphae are septate and produce round to oval conidia.
   b. Primary pulmonary infection results from inhalation of conidia, which probably develop in soil, stimulating a mixed inflammatory response (neutrophils and/or granulomas with giant cells). Dissemination to skin and occasionally to bone may occur.
2. **Clinical manifestations:**
   a. Pulmonary involvement is often mild; asymptomatic cases probably occur frequently; pulmonary infection may produce cough, fever, chest pain, sputum production; hilar adenopathy and nodular pulmonary infiltrates may be present.
   b. Chronic skin lesions may develop; subcutaneous nodules ulcerate over weeks to months, most commonly in exposed areas.
   c. Bony involvement resembles chronic osteomyelitis.
   d. The classic triad: Lung, bone, and skin involvement.
3. **Diagnosis:**
   a. Skin tests are of no value.
   b. Serologic tests are of little value and cross-react with other fungi.
   c. Diagnosis requires biopsy demonstration of large yeasts with broad-based buds on hematoxylin and eosin or fungal stains and/or growth of *B. dermatitidis.*

4. **Treatment:**
   a. Treatment is limited to those with disseminated or severe progressive disease.
   b. Ketoconazole, 5 to 10 mg/kg po as a single daily dose, is the usual therapy. For patients with progressive infection despite therapy, those with very severe disease, and those with central nervous system (CNS) infection, intravenous amphotericin B is recommended. (See Table A–18.)

B. **Histoplasmosis:**
   1. **Organism and pathogenesis:**
      a. *H. capsulatum* is a dimorphic fungus (yeast and hyphal forms) found chiefly in the central U.S. areas drained by the Ohio and Mississippi rivers. Yeasts are smaller than blastomyces and form buds. Hyphae are septate and produce microconidia and macroconidia.
      b. Inhalation of conidia that are in soil contaminated with bird or bat droppings leads to primary pulmonary infection, asymptomatic in the majority of patients. Intracellular growth within macrophages is a hallmark of infection. An asymptomatic primary lung lesion with lymphatic spread (like tuberculosis) develops most often, leading to small calcifications. Very young children or immunocompromised hosts may develop progressive disseminated infection with hepatosplenomegaly, massive mediastinal adenopathy, and anemia.
   2. **Clinical manifestations:**
      a. Most cases are asymptomatic or only mildly symptomatic with brief cough and fever.
      b. More acute or severe pulmonary infection leads to chills, fever, cough, chest pain, dyspnea, and extensive infiltrates.
      c. Disseminated infection produces hepatosplenomegaly, generalized adenopathy, fever, anemia or pancytopenia, mucosal ulcers, and even CNS and adrenal involvement.
   3. **Diagnosis:**
      a. Histoplasmin skin test is of limited clinical value and boosts serum antibodies, leading to confusion.

b. Serologic demonstration of a fourfold or more rise in complement-fixation (CF) titer (or single titer >1:32) may be useful.
c. Histologic demonstration and/or growth of organisms from lung, bone marrow or other tissue is necessary for definite diagnosis.

4. **Treatment** (See Table A–18):
   a. Most patients require no therapy.
   b. Disseminated disease or chronic cavitary pulmonary infection without meningitis in an immunocompetent host: Ketoconazole, 5 to 10 mg/kg po as a single daily dose.
   c. Disseminated disease in an immunocompromised host, or meningitis in any host, or a patient failing to respond to ketoconazole: IV Amphotericin B, 0.5 to 0.7 mg/kg qd.

C. **Coccidiomycosis:**

1. **Organism and pathogenesis:**
   a. *Coccidioides immitis* is a dimorphic fungus with thick-walled **spherules** (instead of a yeast form), within which multiple endospores develop, and septate hyphae with barrel-shaped arthroconidia, the infectious form that is inhaled. *C. immitis* grows only in the Lower Sonoran life zone of the southwestern United States, particularly the San Joaquin Valley.
   b. Inhaled arthroconidia lodge in alveoli, convert to spherules, and incite an initial polymorphonuclear neutrophil (PMN) and macrophage response and a later granulomatous response. Spherule rupture releases hundreds of endospores, leading to acute inflammation. Most often, delayed hypersensitivity results, and infection is controlled. Occasionally progressive disease develops.
2. **Clinical manifestations:**
   a. The majority of those infected are asymptomatic.
   b. Others develop **valley fever** (malaise, cough, fever, chest pain, arthralgias) 1 to 3 weeks after infection; chest x-ray usually is normal or shows hilar adenopathy. *Erythema nodosum* may develop.
   c. Five percent or fewer develop a cavity, very few

progress to severe pneumonia or chronic lung disease, and < 1% disseminate (more in men, compromised hosts, and persons of non-European ancestry). Dissemination can involve bones, joints, skin, and meninges, with the latter being potentially fatal.

3. **Diagnosis:**
   a. Demonstration of spherules on potassium hydroxide preparation of skin or in visceral tissues (rarely in cerebrospinal fluid [CSF]).
   b. Culture from sputum, visceral lesions, and skin lesions; CSF rarely is culture positive; laboratories must take care to prevent spread of infection to personnel.
   c. Skin tests are useful in coccidiomycosis, with the coccidiodin skin test result becoming positive 1 to 4 weeks after primary infection and remaining positive for life.
   d. More than 50% of patients develop precipitating IgM antibody detected by gel diffusion within first 3 weeks of illness, lasting 2 to 4 months. IgG CF antibody develops later and disappears with resolution but persists with ongoing infection.
4. **Treatment:**
   a. Most patients require no therapy.
   b. For patients with severe primary disease or disseminated (non-meningeal) infection: Ketoconazole, 5 to 10 mg/kg as a single daily oral dose.
   c. For patients with meningitis: Amphotericin B given intravenously and intrathecally by a reservoir; fluconazole may be useful in this setting.

D. Cryptococcosis:

1. **Organism and pathogenesis:**
   a. *Cryptococcus neoformans* is a yeast that is characterized by a large capsule and grows in 2 to 5 days on a variety of media, including blood agar. It is found worldwide in soil contaminated with pigeon or other bird droppings.
   b. Inhalation of conidia generally leads to very mild pulmonary infection. In occasional patients (50% of whom are healthy, and 50% immunocompromised), lung infection progresses or spreads to the CNS. Tissue reaction to *C. neoformans* is highly variable.

2. **Clinical manifestations:**
   a. Pulmonary infection is almost always very mild or asymptomatic.
   b. Meningitis is the most common form of cryptococcosis. Intermittent headache, irritability, dizziness, and decreased mentation develop insidiously over weeks to months. Fever is usually present. Late manifestations include seizures, cranial nerve signs, and dementia.
3. **Diagnosis:**
   a. CSF examination may show organisms on india ink examination (the large capsule can be seen) or on culture. Lymphocytic pleocytosis and decreased glucose levels may be present in CSF. CSF may be normal.
   b. Detection of cryptococcal antigen by latex agglutination is more sensitive than india ink or culture.
4. **Treatment:**
   a. Amphotericin B, 0.3 to 0.6 mg/kg/day IV, usually with flucytosine, 100 to 150 mg/kg/day po divided q6h for 2 to 6 weeks. The value of adjunctive fluconazole is uncertain.
   b. Fluconazole, 6 mg/kg once daily, is useful for maintenance therapy to prevent relapses in compromised hosts.

II. OPPORTUNISTIC FUNGI:

A. Candidiasis:

1. **Organisms and pathogenesis:**
   a. *Candida albicans* and several other species (e.g., *Candida parapsilosis, Candida guilliermondii, Candida krusei, Candida tropicalis,* and *Candida glabrata*) are yeasts that grow as 4 to 6-μm budding round-oval cells and form pseudohyphae and hyphae under certain conditions. *C. albicans* forms germ tubes on 37°C incubation in serum. Most *Candida* species grow on blood agar and on fungal media.
   b. *C. albicans* is part of the normal flora of skin, lower gastrointestinal (GI) tract and female genital tract. Infection is associated with isolation from blood, CSF, urine, or viscera.

c. Factors that predispose to infection with *Candida* species include antibiotic or corticosteroid therapy, impaired T-cell function, diabetes, neutropenia, and breaches in physical barriers (e.g., indwelling lines and tubes and GI surgery). Tissue invasion is associated with a shift to formation of hyphae and pseudohyphae.

2. **Clinical manifestations:**
   a. *Thrush* (oropharyngeal candidiasis) is common in normal infants and in individuals with impaired T-cell function. This is manifested by white mucosal patches that bleed when scraped. Glossitis may occur.
   b. *Diaper dermatitis* is commonly candidal and is characterized by satellite lesions. *C. albicans* also occurs in wet macerated areas of skin in other situations.
   c. *Vaginitis* is common in adolescents and adults, is characterized by pruritus and vaginal discharge, and does not necessarily imply underlying disease.
   d. *Esophagitis* in compromised hosts is manifested by painful swallowing, substernal pain, and a sensation that food is "sticking."
   e. *Urinary candidiasis* manifests with usual urinary tract infection symptoms or may be asymptomatic.
   f. **Systemic candidiasis** refers to disseminated infection involving more than one organ, usually a consequence of candidemia in compromised hosts with lines or instrumentation. Common sites include brain, liver, spleen, lungs, kidneys, and endophthalmitis. Symptoms may include only fever.
   g. **CNS candidiasis** usually is a result of candidemic spread. Symptoms range from none to meningeal and/or encephalitic symptoms.
   h. **Candidal endocarditis** is frequently associated with previous cardiac surgery. Blood cultures often are negative, unlike bacterial endocarditis.
3. **Diagnosis:**
   a. Superficial infections can be diagnosed clinically, by culture and/or examination of Gram's stain or KOH preparation of scraped material.
   b. Deep infections may be difficult to diagnose. Esoph-

agitis is most often diagnosed on the basis of esophagoscopic appearance with or without biopsy and culture. Endocarditis is diagnosed by echocardiography and/or operative findings. Tracheal secretions, urine or other nonsterile fluids may be culture positive, demanding distinction between colonization and infection. Imaging procedures (computed tomography, magnetic resonance imaging) may demonstrate multiple small visceral lesions of systemic candidiasis.

4. **Therapy** (See Table A–18):
   a. Superficial infections: Topical nystatin, clotrimazole, econazole, or miconazole.
   b. Esophagitis: Fluconazole, 3 to 6 mg/kg once daily **or** ketoconazole, 5 to 10 mg/kg/day divided q12h to q24h, **or** clotrimazole, 10 mg troche po q4h for 7 days; if no response, amphotericin B IV.
   c. Deep infections: IV amphotericin B, 0.5 to 1.0 mg/kg/day followed by qod therapy for a total of 6 weeks, with or without oral 5-flucytosine (5-FC), 100 to 150 mg/kg/day divided q6h. The role of fluconazole in these infections needs to be defined.

B. Aspergillosis:

1. **Organisms and pathogenesis:**
   a. *Aspergillus* species are rapidly growing (1–2 days) molds with septate hyphae and asexual conidia. The most important species are *Aspergillus flavus* and *Aspergillus fumigatus,* which are worldwide and ubiquitous. Building construction, remodeling, and hospital air and ducts are associated with increased numbers of *Aspergillus*.
   b. *Aspergillus* is inhaled and can lead to **allergic bronchopulmonary aspergillosis** (ABPA), to the development of an **aspergilloma** in those with previous pulmonary disease (e.g., forming a fungus ball within a pre-existing cavity), or to **acute invasive pulmonary aspergillosis** in neutropenic or other compromised hosts. Indolent pulmonary or osseous aspergillosis can develop in children with chronic granulomatous disease.

2. **Clinical manifestations:**
   a. **ABPA** is manifested by recurrent acute wheezing, bronchial plugging, and is associated with fleeting infiltrates and eosinophilia.
   b. An **aspergilloma** is usually asymptomatic or associated with symptoms of the underlying disease.
   c. **Invasive pulmonary aspergillosis** is associated with fever, dyspnea, and hemoptysis, with rapidly progressing lesions on chest x-ray film and erosion of blood vessels.
3. **Diagnosis:**
   a. **ABPA** is diagnosed by typical history, eosinophilia, and elevated specific IgG and IgE antibodies.
   b. **Aspergilloma** is diagnosed radiologically.
   c. Diagnosis of **invasive aspergillosis** requires obtaining tissue by biopsy to demonstrate organisms with branching septate hyphae; culture is diagnostic.
4. **Treatment** (See Table A–18):
   a. **ABPA** is treated with corticosteroids.
   b. **Aspergilloma** is treated surgically if associated with hemoptysis; itraconazole may be useful in those without hemoptysis.
   c. **Invasive or extrapulmonary aspergillosis** requires aggressive therapy with 6 weeks of IV amphotericin B at 0.7 to 1.0 mg/kg/day. Surgical drainage or excision of an extrapulmonary focus may be necessary. The role of itraconazole is under investigation.

C. **Mucormycosis (Zygomycosis):**
   1. **Organisms and pathogenesis:**
      a. The **Mucorales** order (or zygomycetes) includes several ubiquitous saprophytic diphasic fungi that cause human disease (*Mucor, Rhizopus,* and *Absidia*) in the immunocompromised and in diabetic acidosis. These agents are found in soil and on foodstuffs.
      b. Inhalation of conidia leads to colonization of the nasal passages and the lower respiratory tract. **Pulmonary mucormycosis** is seen occasionally in severely immunocompromised hosts as a rapidly progressive pneumonitis that invades blood vessels. In acidotic diabetic adults, spores germinate in the sinuses and

nasal cavity and cause a devastating infection that invades posteriorly into cerebral tissue **(rhinocerebral mucormycosis).**

2. **Clinical manifestations:**
   a. Pulmonary infections are rapidly progressive, and patients are acutely ill with fever, dyspnea, and hypoxia.
   b. Rhinocerebral mucormycosis is associated with black eschar in the nasal cavity, proptosis, and orbital involvement.
3. **Diagnosis:**
   a. In lungs, diagnosis requires biopsy demonstration of large nonseptate hyphal elements usually invading blood vessels.
   b. Rhinocerebral infection can be diagnosed on clinical grounds and often by nasal biopsy.
4. **Therapy** (See Table A–18): Aggressive surgical debridement and IV amphotericin B is essential for these extremely serious infections.

D. ***Pneumocystis carinii*** **Pneumonia (PCP):**

1. **Organism and pathogenesis:**
   a. Although it was thought previously to be a protozoan, recent data reveal that the ribosomal RNA sequence of *P. carinii* corresponds more closely with those of fungi than with protozoa.
   b. The organism exhibits cystic, as well as noncystic, pleomorphic forms (termed **trophozoites),** which can be demonstrated in tissue with phase or fluorescence microscopy.
   c. *P. carinii* is a relatively nonvirulent, ubiquitous organism that seldom produces disease in those with normal T-cell function. PCP in immunocompromised patients is thought to represent reactivation of latent infection.
2. **Epidemiology:**
   a. Serum antibodies to *P. carinii* are present in most normal children, indicating that subclinical infection occurs commonly.
   b. Epidemics of PCP were first reported in Europe after World War II among debilitated and premature infants.

c. Sporadic cases occur in immunocompromised patients:
   1) The disease is associated with congenital immunodeficiencies in infants.
   2) PCP generally occurs as a complication of immunosuppressive therapy in older children and adults.
   3) Acquired immunodeficiency syndrome (AIDS) is now the most common predisposing condition for development of PCP. At least 80% of AIDS patients eventually develop PCP, with a mortality rate of 30% to 50%.

3. **Clinical manifestations:**
   a. The onset of illness is often insidious. The most common symptoms initially are fever, nonproductive cough, chills, and weight loss.
   b. Over the next several weeks, the patient develops tachypnea and dyspnea.
   c. Clinical signs of pneumonia (other than tachypnea) are usually absent.
   d. Patients with PCP have decreased arterial oxygen saturation, diffusion capacity of the lung, and vital capacity.
   e. Chest roentgenograms generally show diffuse, bilateral interstitial or alveolar infiltrates.
4. **Diagnosis:** Diagnosis depends on demonstration of the organism in clinical specimens. The organism may be found in respiratory secretions obtained by the following methods:
   a. Induced sputum: Reported to have > 50% sensitivity in adults with AIDS.
   b. Bronchial lavage and endobronchial brush biopsies: > 90% sensitivity.
   c. Open lung biopsy: Should be considered when previously listed methods do not yield a diagnosis.
5. **Therapy** (See Table A–20):
   a. Trimethoprim-sulfamethoxazole (TMP-SMX) is the drug of choice for PCP:
      1) The dose is 20 mg/kg/day (of the TMP component) in four divided doses. IV therapy should

be used for moderately to severely ill patients; they may be switched to oral therapy after clear clinical improvement.

2) The optimal duration of therapy is considered to be 21 days.

3) Adverse reactions occur frequently; they include rash, fever, leukopenia, and thrombocytopenia.

b. Pentamidine is the drug of choice for patients with PCP unable to tolerate TMP-SMX.

1) Pentamidine is given intravenously at 4 mg/kg/day for 21 days.

2) Adverse reactions are also frequent with pentamidine and include nephrotoxicity, glucose instability, fever, and leukopenia.

c. A number of therapeutic agents are currently undergoing trial, including TMP and dapsone, primaquine and clindamycin, trimetrexate and folinic acid, and aerosolized pentamidine.

d. Prednisone added to antimicrobial treatment decreases the incidence of respiratory deterioration and death in patients with moderate or severe PCP.

6. **Prophylaxis:**

a. The following human immunodeficiency virus (HIV)–infected patients should be given PCP prophylaxis:

1) Any child who has had an episode of PCP.

2) Those with CD4+ count < 20% of total lymphocytes.

3) Those ≥ 6 years old with CD4+ count < 200/mm^3.

4) Those aged 24 months to 5 years with CD4+ count < 750/mm^3.

5) Those aged 12 to 23 months with CD4+ count < 1,000/mm^3

6) Those aged 1 to 11 months with CD4+ count < 1,500/mm^3.

b. Those with depressed T-cell function secondary to malignancy and chemotherapy should also receive PCP prophylaxis.

c. TMP-SMX has been shown to be effective oral prophylaxis (TMP 5 mg/kg/day once daily or 3 times/week).

d. Aerosolized pentamidine (300 mg inhaled every 4 weeks) or dapsone is used in older children and in adults who are unable to tolerate TMP-SMX.

III. OTHER FUNGAL INFECTIONS:

A. Sporotrichosis:

1. **Organism and pathogenesis:**
   a. *Sporothrix schenkii* is a dimorphous fungus that grows as a cigar-shaped yeast in tissues and at 37°C and as a mold with thin septate hyphae and clusters of conidia at 25°C. This fungus is found in soil and on plants and decaying vegetation.
   b. Infection of subcutaneous tissue usually follows puncture by a thorn. This is relatively rare in children.
2. **Clinical manifestations:**
   a. A painless ulcerating red papule develops over weeks to months at the inoculation site, and granulomatous nodular lesions occur along the draining lymphatics.
   b. Extracutaneous involvement is rare and involves bones and joints.
3. **Diagnosis:**
   a. Demonstration of organisms in tissue is difficult.
   b. Diagnosis depends on culture of infected tissue on standard fungal media, with growth in 2 to 5 days.
4. **Treatment:**
   a. Cutaneous infections are treated with local heat and oral potassium iodide (1–2 drops/year of age tid, up to 30 drops tid, until resolved). Itraconazole has been used.
   b. Extracutaneous infection: IV amphotericin B for 6 weeks. The role of itraconazole is being defined.

B. Dermatophytoses:

1. **Organisms and pathogenesis:**
   a. A number of these fungi cause superficial skin, nail and hair infections, including *Microsporum, Trichophyton,* and *Epidermophyton* spp. These agents grow slowly, best on Sabouraud's media at 25°C. Hyphae are septate.
   b. These infections begin when fungi come in contact with minor traumatic skin lesions. After penetration

of the stratum corneum, the organism can proliferate to involve the skin and its appendages (nails, hair). Lesions are often the result of inflammatory reactions to infection and are frequently termed "ringworm."

2. **Clinical manifestations:**
   a. Infections cover the full range, from inapparent colonization to chronic progressive eruptions.
   b. Common syndromes include **tinea capitis** (scalp involvement), **tinea pedis** (athlete's foot), **tinea manuum** (hands), **tinea cruris** ("jock itch," groin,) **tinea barbae** (hair), and **tinea unguium** (nail beds), **tinea corporis** (body). Tinea capitis is particularly common in prepubertal children, whereas tinea pedis and tinea cruris are noted more often in adolescence.
   c. Tinea capitis manifests with patchy hair loss with inflammation. Its most severe manifestation is a **kerion,** an elevated, sharply circumscribed boggy scalp mass with loose, broken hairs and associated suppurative folliculitis.
   d. Dermatophytic involvement elsewhere manifests as annular lesions with erythematous, pruritic, scaly lesions with a tendency to central clearing.
3. **Diagnosis:**
   a. KOH preparations of scales scraped from the advancing margin of a lesion demonstrate septate hyphae, with broken hair shafts.
   b. Some dermatophyte species fluoresce on exposure to an ultraviolet lamp (Wood's lamp).
4. **Treatment** (See Table A–18):
   a. Topical tolnaftate, miconazole, econazole, or clotrimazole resolve most dermatophyte infections.
   b. Recalcitrant or more serious infections (e.g., kerion) require oral griseofulvin 15 mg/kg daily for 1 to 2 months or oral ketoconazole 5 to 10 mg/kg/day divided q12h or q24h.

PARASITIC DISEASES

10

I. PROTOZOA (see Table A–20):

A. Amebiasis:

1. **Pathogenesis:**
   a. Amebiasis is caused by the protozoan *Entamoeba histolytica,* which exists in trophozoite and cyst forms.
   b. The disease occurs worldwide but is more prevalent in the tropics.
   c. Transmission in humans is by the fecal-oral route. A small, noninvasive trophozoite form found mainly in the cecum and proximal colon gives rise to cysts excreted in feces. The environmentally resistant cysts are then ingested, perpetuating the life cycle.
   d. In symptomatic cases, a larger trophozoite form leads to tissue invasion. Events leading to development of the invasive trophozoite form are poorly understood.
   e. Certain bacteria, especially *Escherichia coli,* may be important in host colonization with *E. histolytica* and in production of invasive trophozoites. Cholesterol and iron also play a role in this process.
2. **Clinical findings:**
   a. Asymptomatic intraluminal colonization is the most common type of amebic infestation and places individuals at risk for invasive amebiasis.
   b. Amebic dysentery, the most common form of invasive disease, usually manifests with gradual onset of abdominal pain and stools with blood and mucus, with or without fever. Intussusception, necrotizing colitis, or intestinal perforation with peritonitis may develop.
   c. Direct extension of invasive intestinal amebiasis may lead to cutaneous involvement in the perianal, perineal, and genital areas.
   d. Amebic liver abscess is the most common complication of invasive intestinal amebiasis, particularly in

males and involving the right lobe of the liver. Patients typically have fever, hepatomegaly, and right upper quadrant tenderness. Pain may be referred to the right shoulder.

e. Extension of amebic liver abscesses into the thorax may lead to empyema, bronchohepatic fistulas, or pericardial amebiasis.

3. **Diagnosis:**
   a. Amebiasis should be considered in any child with bloody stools, particularly with history of recent travel to the tropics.
   b. The initial diagnostic test is microscopic examination of three stool samples. However, failure to visualize the organism does not exclude amebiasis.
   c. Typical proctoscopic findings include multiple small ulcerations and friable mucosa, and amebae are usually present in samples of mucus obtained.
   d. Serologic studies may be done when stool and proctoscopic examinations are negative and the diagnosis is still suspected:
      1) Enzyme-linked immunosorbent assay (ELISA) tests of serum and stool are very sensitive but are of somewhat limited availability.
      2) Indirect fluorescent antibody (IFA) assays are also sensitive for detection of active disease.
   e. Screening for hepatic involvement is essential in all cases. An elevated white blood cell (WBC) count is consistent with amebic liver abscess. Serum liver enzyme levels are elevated only in a minority with hepatic amebiasis. Ultrasound of the liver is very sensitive for detection of amebic liver abscesses.
4. **Therapy:**
   a. Asymptomatic carriage: Iodoquinol (diiodohydroxyquin), 30–40 mg/kg/day (maximum = 2 g) po divided q8h for 20 days, **or** diloxanide furoate (Centers for Disease Control, CDC), 20 mg/kg/day po divided q8h for 10 days, **or** paromomycin (CDC), 25–30 mg/kg/day po divided q8h for 7 days.
   b. Intestinal amebiasis:
      1) Metronidazole, 35 to 50 mg/kg/day po divided q8h for 10 days, is the preferred therapy. This should

be given intravenously in severe cases. Alternates are paromomycin for 7 days or dehydroemetine (CDC), 1.0 to 1.5 mg/kg/day (maximum 90 mg) IM divided q12h for 5 days.

2) After initial treatment, patients may have asymptomatic intestinal colonization with passage of cysts and thus should be treated with diloxanide furoate (CDC), 20 mg/kg/po q8h for 10 days. Iodoquinol, 30–40 mg/kg/day in three divided doses po for 20 days, is another alternative.

c. Extraintestinal amebiasis:

1) Intravenous (IV) metronidazole, 35 to 50 mg/kg/day divided q8h for 10 days is the treatment of choice, followed by iodoquinol, 30–40 mg/kg/day (maximum 2 g) po divided q8h for 20 days. An alternate regimen is dehydroemetine (CDC), followed by chloroquine plus iodoquinol. Patients who remain asymptomatic cyst passers after treatment should be treated as outlined earlier.

2) Large hepatic abscesses should be aspirated.

B. Babesiosis:

1. **The organism:**

a. Babesiosis is caused by two species of the protozoan genus *Babesia: Babesia divergens,* a parasite of cattle, which is a rare cause of human disease and infects only immunocompromised individuals; and *Babesia microti,* a North American parasite of rodents and deer.

b. *B. divergens* is transmitted chiefly by the cattle tick *Ixodes ricinus. B. microti* is transmitted by the tick *Ixodes dammini,* which feeds on rodents and deer.

c. The organisms multiply asexually in red blood cells (RBCs), with RBC rupture and infection of new RBCs occurring in a cyclical but nonsynchronized manner.

2. **Clinical findings:**

a. The incubation period is 1 to 4 weeks.

b. *B. divergens* infection occurs only in splenectomized individuals (particularly in Massachusetts) but is frequently fatal. Infection manifests abruptly with high fever, nausea, and severe hemolysis, typically progressing to hepatorenal failure and death.

c. *B. microti* infection occurs in normal individuals but is much milder, often clinically inapparent. It manifests with gradual onset of fever, chills, and myalgias, with mild to moderate hemolysis and hepatosplenomegaly. Spontaneous recovery is usual but may require months. Later relapse does not occur.

3. **Diagnosis:**
   a. Rare organisms may be seen intracellularly on stained thick smears of peripheral blood.
   b. Various serologic tests are available but are not entirely reliable.
4. **Therapy:**
   a. No specific treatment exists for *B. divergens* infections.
   b. *B. microti* infections are also difficult to treat. Quinine (25 mg/kg/day po for 7 days) and clindamycin (30 mg/kg/day po for 7 days) have been used with some success, and exchange transfusion may be helpful.

C. Cryptosporidiosis:

1. **The organism:**
   a. Disease is caused by various species of the protozoan *Cryptosporidium*.
   b. Infection may be transmitted by animal-human or human-human spread, occurring when oocysts are ingested. Sporozoites are liberated and attach themselves to intestinal epithelial cells, predominantly in the small bowel. The parasite lies in the brush border of intestinal villi, where it impairs absorption. Mature organisms liberate oocysts into the intestinal lumen, some of which may release sporozoites while still in the host intestine, causing autoinfection.
   c. *Cryptosporidium* was formerly thought to be only an animal parasite, but it is now recognized as an important cause of diarrhea in children (particularly in daycare settings) and in immunocompromised individuals, particularly those with acquired immunodeficiency syndrome (AIDS).
2. **Clinical findings:**
   a. Symptoms begin 1 to 2 weeks after infection, consisting of frequent watery, frothy diarrheal stools.

   b. Diarrhea is usually self-limited in normal individuals but occasionally may be relatively severe, producing marked dehydration in some children.
   c. In immunocompromised individuals, *Cryptosporidium* produces severe, unremitting chronic diarrhea with malabsorption and weight loss. It is a common cause of death in adults and in children with AIDS.
3. **Diagnosis:**
   a. Oocysts can be identified in stool using acid-fast stains.
   b. There are no useful serologic tests for diagnosis.
4. **Therapy:**
   a. There is no effective drug therapy for cryptosporidiosis. Octreotide and paromomycin are experimental agents.
   b. Treatment, if required, is supportive with provision of parenteral fluids to maintain hydration and electrolyte homeostasis.

D. Giardiasis:

1. **The organism and pathogenesis:**
   a. Giardiasis is caused by the flagellated protozoan *Giardia lamblia,* which exists in two forms: the trophozoite, found in the proximal small bowel of infected individuals, and the cyst, found in stool.
   b. Transmission is by the fecal-oral route. Spread is usually person-to-person but may also occur from contaminated food or water. Contaminated toys are important for transmission in day-care centers.
   c. The ingested cyst undergoes excystation in the stomach. The trophozoite then colonizes the proximal small bowel, causing malabsorption either by physically impairing nutrient absorption or by disrupting the intestinal environment.
2. **Clinical findings:**
   a. Most infections are asymptomatic.
   b. The most common symptom is diarrhea, but abdominal pain, bloating, nausea, and behavioral changes also occur.
   c. Failure to thrive may occur in chronically infected chil dren.

   d. Laboratory features include microcytic hypochromic anemia, steatorrhea, decreased serum carotene, and impaired D-xylose absorption.

3. **Diagnosis:**
   a. Examination of stool for cysts is the usual means of diagnosis. Several specimens may be required to detect cysts.
   b. Swallowing a weighted capsule on a string followed by retrieval (the "string test" or "entero test") enables sampling of duodenal mucus, often revealing trophozoites on microscopic examination. This test is probably more sensitive than stool examination.
   c. Jejunal biopsy is the gold standard for establishing the diagnosis but is relatively expensive and difficult to perform.
   d. ELISA and fluorescent antibody tests may assist in certain cases.
   e. A positive response to a therapeutic trial may confirm the diagnosis.
4. **Therapy** (See Table A–20):
   a. Metronidazole, 15 mg/kg/day divided q8h for 5 to 7 days, is the preferred treatment. Alternatives are furazolidone, 6–8 mg/kg/day po divided q6h for 7 to 10 days, **or** quinacrine, 6 mg/kg/day po divided q8h for 5 to 7 days.
   b. Symptoms recur in 10% to 20% of treated patients but usually respond to retreatment.

E. Leishmaniasis:

1. **The organism and pathogenesis:**
   a. Disease is caused by species of the protozoan genus *Leishmania:*
      1) Visceral leishmaniasis **(kala-azar)** is caused by *Leishmania donovani,* occurring in Central and South America, the Mediterranean region, and parts of Africa and Asia.
      2) Old World cutaneous leishmaniasis is caused by *Leishmania tropica major, Leishmania tropica minor,* and *Leishmania tropica aethiopica*. It occurs in the Mediterranean, the Middle East, parts of Africa, India, and Southwest Asia.

   3) New World (American) cutaneous leishmaniasis is caused by members of the *Leishmania mexicana* and *Leishmania braziliensis* species complexes and is found in Central and South America.
  b. Leishmaniasis is transmitted to humans by the bite of the sandfly:
   1) The amastigote form is ingested by the sandfly when biting an infected host.
   2) After replication in the sandfly's alimentary tract, the promastigote form of the organism may infect the sandfly bite wound.
   3) After phagocytosis, the organism reproduces in macrophages and reticuloendothelial cells.

2. **Clinical findings:**
  a. Visceral leishmaniasis:
   1) The latency period between infection and onset of symptoms varies widely, from 2 weeks to > 6 months. A primary skin nodule is seen in a minority of cases before the onset of symptoms.
   2) Disease onset may be sudden, with high fevers and vomiting, or insidious, with development of pneumonia or diarrhea.
   3) Massive splenomegaly is characteristic and is usually accompanied by some degree of hepatomegaly and lymphadenopathy.
   4) Pancytopenia is often seen, and anemia, frequently severe, is a universal finding. Nonspecific polyclonal IgG production occurs, with IgG levels as high as 5 g/dL.
   5) If untreated, this disease usually progresses to death within several months. A generalized bleeding diathesis often occurs terminally.
  b. Old World cutaneous leishmaniasis:
   1) Disease begins with a localized vesicular papule weeks to months after the infecting sandfly bite. The papule gradually enlarges and ulcerates, with a raised, indurated margin. If untreated, healing occurs over ≥ 1 year, leaving a characteristic depressed scar.
   2) Leishmaniasis recidiva and diffuse cutaneous leish-

maniasis are chronic forms that may persist for decades and lead to extensive scarring.

c. New World (American) cutaneous leishmaniasis:
   1) Disease caused by the *L. mexicana* complex is generally mild, with development of a single cutaneous ulcer that heals over several months. Infection and ulceration of the external ear with cartilage involvement may produce a chronic lesion (Chiclero's ulcer).
   2) Manifestations of disease caused by the *L. braziliensis* complex vary with the causative subspecies:
      a) *L. braziliensis braziliensis* produces destructive ulceration of the nasopharynx, "espundia."
      b) *L. braziliensis guyanesis* may spread along lymphatics, resulting in multiple cutaneous ulcers without nasopharyngeal involvement, *"pian bois,"* or "forest yaws."
      c) Other subspecies produce one or more cutaneous ulcers that spontaneously resolve.

3. **Diagnosis:**
   a. Visceral leishmaniasis:
      1) The organism can be found on bone marrow aspirate, liver biopsy, splenic aspirate, and sometimes in peripheral blood monocytes. The organism may be grown on special media.
      2) ELISA and fluorescent antibody techniques are available for serologic diagnosis.
      3) The leishmanin, or Montenegro, skin test, analogous to the tuberculin skin test, measures delayed hypersensitivity. However, results are negative in active visceral leishmaniasis, becoming positive only when disease begins to resolve.
   b. Old World and American cutaneous leishmaniasis:
      1) Diagnosis is best made by direct visualization of parasites on smears from ulcers, by culture of ulcer material on special media, or by biopsy.
      2) Results of the leishmanin skin test become positive within 3 months of appearance of lesions.
      3) Serology is of little diagnostic use in Old World

cutaneous leishmaniasis but is very helpful in American cutaneous leishmaniasis caused by the *L. braziliensis* complex.

4. **Therapy** (See Table A–20):
   a. Visceral leishmaniasis:
      1) The pentavalent antimonial sodium stibogluconate (CDC) is the drug of choice, given parenterally (preferably intravenously) at 20 mg/kg/day (maximum 800 mg) for 20 to 28 days.
      2) Pentamidine isethionate, 4 mg/kg/day for 14 days, is an acceptable alternate.
      3) Splenectomy may be necessary in patients with multiple treatment failures or with severe hypersplenism.
   b. Old World cutaneous leishmaniasis:
      1) Most lesions heal spontaneously and do not require treatment.
      2) Sodium stibogluconate, 10 to 20 mg/kg/day (maximum 600 mg) for 6 to 10 days, may be needed.
   c. American cutaneous leishmaniasis: This is usually treated with stibogluconate, 20 mg/kg/day (maximum 800 mg) IV or IM for 20 days or with amphotericin B, 0.25 to 1.0 mg/kg/day, up to 8 weeks.

F. Malaria

1. **The organism and pathogenesis:**
   a. Four species of *Plasmodium* cause malaria in humans:
      1) *Plasmodium vivax* (vivax or tertian malaria).
      2) *Plasmodium ovale* (ovale or tertian malaria).
      3) *Plasmodium malariae* (quartan malaria).
      4) *Plasmodium falciparum* (falciparum or malignant tertian malaria).
   b. Pathogenesis of human infection is closely related to the parasitic life cycle:
      1) Sexual phase (sporogony) occurs in female *Anopheles* mosquitoes, with production of **sporozoites** that enter the human circulation when the mosquito bites.
      2) Sporozoites enter hepatocytes, where they form **tissue schizonts,** which, in turn, divide to form **merozoites.** Merozoites rupture infected hepato-

cytes after 6 to 14 days, enter the bloodstream, and infect RBCs. *P. vivax* and *P. ovale* may form dormant tissue schizonts in liver **(hypnozoites),** which can later reactivate.

3) In RBCs, merozoites develop into **ring forms,** then **trophozoites.** Trophozoites divide to produce many merozoites, which are released by cell rupture and infect more RBCs. The periodicity of RBC infection and rupture produces the characteristic fever patterns. Some merozoites give rise to **gametocytes,** which are ingested by female *Anopheles* mosquitoes with a blood meal, completing the life cycle.

2. **Clinical findings:**
   a. Falciparum (malignant tertian) malaria:
      1) This is the most severe form of malaria.
      2) Fever, headache, arthralgias, emesis, and mild diarrhea appear after a 9- to 14-day incubation period. Fever is initially irregular but then develops a tertian pattern (spikes q48h). If untreated, tertian fevers may persist for several weeks. Relapses initially are frequent and severe but gradually lessen and usually cease by 1 year.
      3) Severe hemolytic anemia is a hallmark of primary falciparum malaria, with gross hemoglobinuria **(blackwater fever).** Endothelial cell damage and small-vessel vasculitis is also characteristic and may result in cerebral involvement.
      4) Figure 10–1 shows the geographic areas where chloroquine-resistant and chloroquin-sensitive falciparum malaria are found.
   b. Vivax and ovale (tertian) malaria:
      1) Less severe than falciparum malaria.
      2) Initial symptoms appear after a 12- to 14-day incu-

FIG 10–1.
Malarious areas with *Plasmodium falciparum* resistant and sensitive to chloroquine, 1990. (From *MMWR* 39(8):140–142, 1990.)

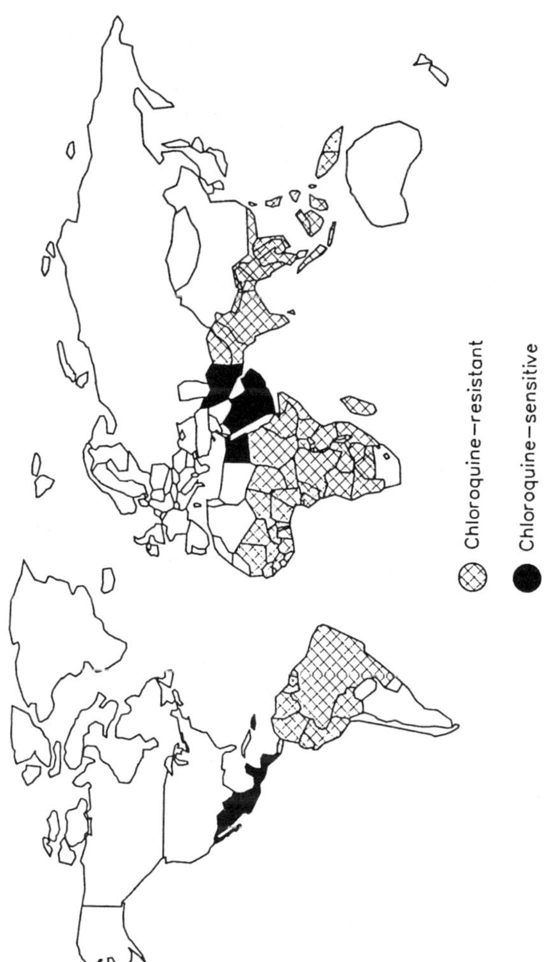
Chloroquine–resistant
Chloroquine–sensitive

bation period. Fever is irregular for 2 to 4 days but then develops a tertian pattern that persists for ≥ 1 week. Particularly with vivax, relapses may occur years after initial infection because of activation of tissue hypnozoites.

c. Quartan malaria *(P. malariae):*
   1) Relatively mild form of malaria.
   2) Initial symptoms appear after an 18- to 40-day incubation period. Fever pattern is quartan (spikes q72h). Relapses are common in the first year, then become infrequent, but may occur for many years because of persistent low-grade parasitemia.
   3) Splenomegaly is common. Anemia is less severe than in other forms of malaria.

3. **Diagnosis:**
   a. Detection of the ring form of the parasite in a thick smear of peripheral blood is the best diagnostic test.
   b. Retrospective diagnosis may be made by serologic test (CDC).
4. **Prophylaxis** (see Table A–19 for dosages):
   a. **Chloroquine phosphate** once weekly, beginning 1 to 2 weeks before arrival in endemic area and continued for 4 weeks after leaving endemic area.
   b. For areas with chloroquine-resistant *P. falciparum:*
      1) **Mefloquine hydrochloride** once weekly, beginning 1 to 2 weeks before arrival in endemic area and continued for 4 weeks after leaving endemic area.
      2) **Or chloroquine phosphate** plus **pyrimethamine-sulfadoxine (Fansidar);** the latter is taken only in the event of a febrile illness when medical care is not immediately available.
      3) **Or doxycycline.**
5. **Therapy** (See Table A–19):
   a. For all except chloroquine-resistant *P. falciparum:*
      1) **Oral: Chloroquine phosphate** plus **primaquine phosphate** (to prevent relapses of *P. ovale, P. vivax*).
      2) **Parenteral: Quinidine gluconate** IV or **quinine dihydrochloride** IV plus **primaquine phosphate.**

b. For chloroquine-resistant *P. falciparum:*
   1) **Oral:**
      a) **Quinine sulfate** plus **pyrimethamine-sulfadoxine.**
      b) **Or mefloquine hydrochloride.**
      c) **Or halofantrine** 8 mg/kg (max 500 mg) q6h for three doses.
   2) **Parenteral: Quinidine gluconate** IV or **quinine dihydrochloride** IV.

G. **Toxoplasmosis (Acquired Form):**

NOTE: Congenital toxoplasmosis is discussed in Chapter 3, section I.C.4.

1. **The organism:**
   a. *Toxoplasma gondii* is a protozoan parasite with three forms: the proliferative (tachyzoite) form, the encysted (bradyzoite) form, and the oocytic form.
   b. The cat family are the definitive hosts. Acquired human infection occurs when infective oocysts, present in the feces of infected cats, are ingested, or when undercooked meat containing *Toxoplasma* cysts is ingested.
2. **Clinical findings:**
   a. Acquired infection is asymptomatic in roughly 90% of infected individuals.
   b. When symptoms occur, the most common are lymphadenopathy (local or generalized) and fatigue. Fever is uncommon. Hepatitis may occur in severe cases.
   c. Immunosuppressed patients are more severely affected and may develop pneumonitis, myocarditis, or encephalitis. Adult or older childhood AIDS patients may develop reactivation of previously quiescent foci from a primary infection, most commonly mass(es) in the brain.
   d. Chorioretinitis may develop, but this complication is more frequently seen in congenital toxoplasmosis.
3. **Diagnosis:**
   a. Measurement of IgG anti-*Toxoplasma* antibody is the mainstay of diagnosis. When measured using reliable reagents and procedures, antibody appears in the first week of infection and reaches peak titers in 4 to 8 weeks.

b. A negative IgG titer essentially excludes acute acquired *Toxoplasma* infection in the immunocompetent individual. Diagnosis of acute acquired infection in the presence of a high IgG titer requires demonstration of a concomitantly elevated IgM anti-*Toxoplasma* titer.
c. Serologic diagnosis may be more difficult in immunocompromised individuals. In these patients, biopsy of involved tissue may be necessary for diagnosis.

4. **Therapy** (See Table A–20):
   a. Most immunocompetent patients with acquired toxoplasmosis do not require treatment unless their symptoms are severe or persistent, or significant vital organ involvement is present. All immunocompromised patients with acquired toxoplasmosis should be treated.
   b. In patients requiring treatment, a combination of pyrimethamine and sulfadiazine is used. The dosage of pyrimethamine is 1/mg/kg bid (up to 100 mg/day) po for three days, followed by 0.5 mg/kg bid until symptoms resolve (at least 4 weeks in immunocompetent individuals, at least 8–12 weeks in immunocompromised patients). Sulfadiazine is given concomitantly at a dose of 25 to 50 mg/kg qid. Supplemental folinic acid, 5 to 10 mg/day, should be given to prevent hematologic toxicity secondary to pyrimethamine.
   c. Corticosteroid therapy may also be indicated in severe cases of ocular toxoplasmosis.

H. African Trypanosomiasis (Sleeping Sickness):

1. **The organism:**
   a. Disease is caused by the protozoa *Trypanosoma brucei gambiense* and *Trypanosoma brucei rhodesiense*.
   b. The organism is transmitted to humans by the bite of tsetse flies *(Glossina)*. Humans are the main reservoir for *T. b. gambiense,* whereas antelopes are the main reservoir for *T. b. rhodesiense*.
2. **Clinical findings:**
   a. A local lesion (trypanosomal chancre) at the site of a tsetse fly bite is the first sign of infection. One to 3 weeks later, intermittent fever begins, correlating with parasitemia. Fever may recur irregularly for months, accompanied by malaise, severe headache, and arthralgias.

b. Lymphadenopathy and hepatosplenomegaly are common. Posterior cervical adenopathy is characteristic of *T. b. gambiense* infection. Other findings include signs of myocarditis and facial edema.
c. Markedly elevated serum IgM levels are characteristic.
d. Chronic meningoencephalitis produces the terminal "sleeping sickness" stage of African trypanosomiasis. Initial signs are increasing lethargy and speech difficulties, followed by tremors, seizures, and sometimes choreoathetoid movements. If untreated, the disease progresses gradually to coma over some years in *T. b. gambiense* infection but over a few months in *T. b. rhodesiense* infection.

3. **Diagnosis:**
   a. Trypanosomes can usually be visualized in peripheral blood in the early febrile stages.
   b. Serologic testing may be useful.
   c. In *T. b. gambiense* infections, trypanosomes are reliably seen in aspirates of enlarged lymph nodes.
   d. Cerebrospinal fluid (CSF) findings in the meningoencephalitic stage include pleocytosis and elevated protein levels; very high CSF protein levels correlate with more advanced disease. An elevated CSF IgM level is a reliable indicator of central nervous system (CNS) infection. Organisms are rarely visualized in CSF.
4. **Therapy** (See Table A–20):
   a. Tsetse fly repellents are useful for prophylaxis. Routine chemoprophylaxis is not recommended for travelers to endemic areas, given the low risk of infection.
   b. Suramin (CDC) is the usual treatment for early infection and is given intravenously slowly. After a test dose of 2 mg/kg, 20 mg/kg is given on days 1, 3, 7, 14, and 21. Pentamidine (4 mg/kg/day IV or IM for 10 days) is an alternative, especially in *T. b. gambiense* infections.
   c. CNS infection requires IV treatment with melarsoprol (CDC), a trivalent arsenical, with doses gradually increasing from 0.36 to 3.6 mg/kg IV for a total of ten doses (18–25 mg/kg) over 1 month.

I. American Trypanosomiasis (Chaga's Disease):

1. The organism and pathogenesis:

a. Disease is caused by the protozoan *Trypanosoma cruzi* and is limited to the Western hemisphere. It is prevalent in South America, Central America, and Mexico.

b. The organism is transmitted to humans by the reduviid (triatomine) bug, which ingests the organism in a blood meal. The organism reproduces in the insect's alimentary tract, and the infective metacyclic trypomastigote form is excreted in feces. Human infection occurs when infectious feces contaminates abraded or broken skin. Transfusion with contaminated blood and congenital (vertical) transmission are also important routes of infection.

2. Clinical findings:

a. The majority of individuals infected with *T. cruzi* are asymptomatic. Those who develop disease are usually infants and children < 10 years of age.

b. The first sign of infection is formation of a swelling (chagoma) at the site of infection, resulting from local proliferation of the tissue (amastigote) form of the organism. Chagomas often appear around the eye, producing a characteristic unilateral periorbital edema and conjunctivitis (Romana's sign).

c. In the acute phase, fever, malaise, and headache appear about 14 days after infection, with generalized lymphadenopathy and hepatosplenomegaly. Seizures may occur, especially in younger infants. Myocarditis occurs in almost all patients but is usually mild; however, early cardiac arrhythmia is a poor prognostic sign. Although the majority of patients recover from the acute phase, young infants often die of severe meningoencephalitis.

d. After the acute phase, a long latent phase begins, lasting 10 to 40 years. Most infected individuals never develop clinical evidence of chronic disease, even though *T. cruzi* may be isolated from the blood for decades by special techniques.

e. Chronic Chagas' disease is manifested by cardiac and gastrointestinal (GI) involvement, including congestive heart failure and conduction disturbances, and megaesophagus and megacolon resulting from destruction of ganglion cells in the myenteric plexus.

3. **Diagnosis:**
   a. *T. cruzi* may be visualized directly in peripheral blood smears during the acute phase.
   b. Several serologic tests aid in diagnosis. An assay that detects IgM antitrypanosome antibodies may document acute congenital infection.
4. **Therapy** (See Table A–20):
   a. No uniformly effective therapy exists.
   b. Nifurtimox (CDC) has been used with limited success. For children 1 to 10 years of age, the recommended dose is 15 to 20 mg/kg/day in four divided doses for 90 days. For children 11 to 16 years of age, the dosage is 12.5 to 15 mg/kg/day for 90 days. For adults the dosage is 8 to 10 mg/kg/day in four doses for 120 days.
   c. Benznidazole, 6 mg/kg/day for 30 to 120 days, has also been used.

II. HELMINTHS:

A. Ascariasis:

1. **The organisms:**
   a. The helminth *Ascaris lumbricoides* is highly prevalent worldwide, particularly in parts of Africa, Central and South America, and rural areas of the southern United States.
   b. Human infection occurs with the ingestion of eggs that hatch into larvae in the small intestine. The larvae penetrate the intestinal wall, enter venules or lymphatics, and are carried to the lungs. In the lungs, larvae leave the capillaries, migrate up the bronchial tree to the glottis, and pass over the epiglottis into the esophagus. They are then carried into the small intestine, where they mature into adult worms. The entire life cycle lasts 60 to 70 days.
2. **Clinical findings:**
   a. Light to moderate infections are usually asymptomatic.
   b. The most notable laboratory finding is peripheral eosinophilia, especially during the migratory phase.

c. Heavy intestinal infestation may result in mechanical obstruction by a bezoar or intertwined mass of worms. Intussusception or volvulus may also occur.
d. Aberrant migration of the adult worm may lead to intestinal perforation with peritonitis, biliary obstruction, appendicitis, or other symptoms, depending on the site of migration.

3. **Diagnosis:**
   a. Diagnosis is readily made by visualization of eggs in stool.
   b. Serologic tests are available but not reliable.
4. **Therapy** (See Table A–20): A single dose of pyrantel pamoate, 11 mg/kg, is highly effective, even in cases of intestinal obstruction because it paralyzes the adult worms, leading to relaxation of the tangled worm mass. Alternate therapy is mebendazole, 100 mg bid for 3 days.

B. Cutaneous Larva Migrans:

1. **The organism and pathogenesis:**
   a. Disease is caused by infective larvae of *Ancylostoma braziliense, Ancylostoma caninum,* and *Strongyloides* species.
   b. Infection occurs when bare human skin, usually hands or feet, is exposed to damp soil containing the larvae. The larvae burrow into the skin but are unable to penetrate beyond the stratum germinativum. They persist and migrate within the skin without further development.
   c. Cutaneous larva migrans (CLM) occurs in most humid tropical and subtropical areas. It is especially common in the southern United States.
2. **Clinical findings:**
   a. Symptoms appear within a few hours after infection and are remarkable for intense pruritus along the migratory tracks of the larvae.
   b. An erythematous papule is usually noted at the site of entry. The larvae migrate several millimeters to a few centimeters daily and leave erythematous, indurated tracks. Scratching may produce secondary infection.
3. **Diagnosis:**
   a. Diagnosis is clinical.

b. Peripheral eosinophilia is not seen, and it is usually not possible to isolate the larva from its track.

4. **Therapy:**

a. If untreated, infection spontaneously resolves in a few weeks to months.

b. If treatment is desired, topical or oral thiabendazole can be given. The oral dose is 25 mg/kg bid for 2 to 5 days.

C. **Hookworms (Ancylostomiasis):**

1. **The organisms and pathogenesis:**

a. In the Mediterranean region, Asia, India, and parts of South America, disease is chiefly caused by the nematode *Ancylostoma duodenale*. In Africa, the southern United States, the Caribbean, and Central and South America, *Necator americanus* is the chief cause of hookworm infestation.

b. Infection occurs when infective larvae, found in damp soil contaminated by human feces, burrow through exposed skin and gain access to the venous circulation. They are carried to the lungs where they penetrate the alveoli and crawl up the bronchial tree. The larvae then pass over the epiglottis, down the esophagus, and reach the small intestine 1 week after initial infection, where they mature into adult worms and attach themselves to the mucosa. Eggs appear in stool about 6 weeks after initial infection, completing the life cycle.

c. Pathology is largely the result of bleeding induced by adult worms, which secrete an anticoagulant to facilitate blood ingestion. Heavy infestations can result in profound iron deficiency anemia secondary to chronic blood loss. In addition, chronic loss of serum protein may lead to hypoproteinemia and edema, mimicking a protein-losing enteropathy.

2. **Clinical findings:**

a. Initial skin penetration by larvae is accompanied by transient pruritus at the site.

b. The migratory phase may be accompanied by pneumonitis and peripheral eosinophilia.

c. The acute intestinal phase may be accompanied by abdominal pain and diarrhea.

d. Symptoms of chronic infection are those of iron-deficiency anemia, which may be accompanied by hypoalbuminemia and edema.

3. **Diagnosis:**
   a. Diagnosis is made by finding eggs in the stool.
   b. There are no effective serologic tests.
4. **Therapy** (See Table A–20):
   a. Pyrantel pamoate at 11 mg/kg (maximum 1 g) once daily for 3 days is the drug of choice in areas where *N. americanus* is the prevalent hookworm species. Mebendazole, 100 mg bid for 3 days, is equally effective.
   b. For *A. duodenale,* mebendazole is more effective and should be the initial drug.

D. Pinworms (Enterobiasis):

1. **The organism:**
   a. Disease is caused by the nematode *Enterobius vermicularis*. Enterobiasis is the most common of all human helminthic infections, and children are most commonly infected.
   b. Infection occurs when eggs are ingested, most commonly by direct transmission from the perianal area via the finger. Eggs hatch in the duodenum and the larvae migrate through the small intestine. Adult worms live in the cecum. Females migrate down to the rectum and emerge to lay eggs on the perianal skin, completing the 4- to 6-week life cycle.
2. **Clinical findings:**
   a. Anal pruritus, sometimes severe, is the main symptom. Vulvar itching and vaginal discharge occasionally occur when an adult worm migrates into the vagina.
   b. Other symptoms, such as anorexia and weight loss, are reported in association with enterobiasis, but a true causal relationship has not been established.
   c. Adult worms have been reported to invade the peritoneal cavity very rarely, causing granulomata of various abdominal organs or peritonitis.
3. **Diagnosis:**
   a. Diagnosis is readily made by the "tape test," in which transparent adhesive tape is applied to the perianal skin and then examined microscopically for eggs.

b. Eggs are found in the feces of < 5% of infected individuals.

4. **Therapy** (See Table A–20):
   a. A single dose of pyrantel pamoate, 11 mg/kg (maximum 1 g), is highly effective, as is a single 100-mg dose of mebendazole. Retreatment in 2 to 3 weeks may be necessary.
   b. All household members should be treated.

E. Strongyloidiasis

1. **The organism:**
   a. Disease is caused by the nematode *Strongyloides stercoralis*. It is found worldwide, but is most prevalent in tropical and subtropical areas, particularly in parts of South America and Southeast Asia.
   b. Infection results when skin is exposed to infective larvae found in contaminated soil. The larvae burrow through the skin, enter the venous system, and are carried to the lungs. In the lungs the larvae enter the alveoli, migrate up the bronchial tree to the glottis, pass over the epiglottis, and are carried to the small intestine. In the intestine the maturational process is completed. Mature females lay eggs, which develop into noninfective larvae, in the intestine. These larvae are passed in the stool and undergo a molt to the infective form after passage, completing the 1-month life cycle.
   c. The noninfective larvae that hatch from eggs in the intestine instead may molt to the infective form while still in the intestine, thus completing the life cycle entirely within the host. This process is the autoinfective cycle and is responsible for persistence of infection in the untreated host. It is especially likely to occur in immunocompromised persons, and may lead to fatal overwhelming infection.
2. **Clinical findings:**
   a. Patients with light infection usually are asymptomatic.
   b. Patients with heavier infections usually have severe diarrhea and steatorrhea.
   c. For patients with massive infection resulting from the autoinfective cycle, infective larvae can penetrate all body tissues in a life-threatening process. Signs and

symptoms depend on the organ system involved. Overwhelming pulmonary infestation is not rare.

d. Marked peripheral blood eosinophilia is characteristic and helps to distinguish strongyloidiasis from other infectious and inflammatory causes of diarrhea.

3. **Diagnosis:**
   a. Diagnosis is made by visualization of larvae on microscopic stool examination or wet mount examination of bronchial secretions.
   b. There are no useful serologic tests.
4. **Therapy** (See Table A–20):
   a. The treatment of choice is thiabendazole 25 mg/kg twice a day for 2 to 3 days (5 days in massive infection).
   b. Albendazole 400 mg/day for 3 days or ivermectin also have been used, but are less effective.

F. Toxocariasis (Visceral Larva Migrans):

1. **Organism:**
   a. Visceral larva migrans (VLM) is caused by the nematode *Toxocara canis,* which is a common intestinal parasite of dogs. It occurs worldwide.
   b. Infection results when infective eggs are ingested. The eggs hatch in the stomach and small intestine, and larvae penetrate the bowel, entering the venous system. They may lodge in the liver or can be carried via the circulation to any organ in the body. Because humans are an aberrant host, the larvae do not mature further but continue to migrate through tissue until they are killed by the host's immune system.
2. **Clinical findings:**
   a. Retinal invasion produces a distinct syndrome of ocular toxocariasis, with granuloma formation. This is easily confused with retinoblastoma. Endophthalmitis and iridocyclitis may also occur.
   b. Systemic infection may produce myriad symptoms, depending on the organ predominantly affected. Common findings include fever and hepatosplenomegaly.
   c. Typical laboratory findings include marked eosinophilia and hyperglobulinemia.

3. **Diagnosis:**
   a. Definitive diagnosis is difficult and can be made only by direct visualization of larvae in tissues. Liver biopsy is probably the best means of diagnosis, but the yield is low.
   b. No reliable serologic tests exist. Isohemagglutinin titers (anti-A, anti-B) are generally very elevated in patients with visceral larvae migrans (VLM).
4. **Therapy** (See Table A–20):
   a. Most patients gradually recover with symptomatic treatment.
   b. Anti-infective therapy is generally unsatisfactory. Thiabendazole, 25 mg/kg bid for 5 days, is reported to have some efficacy. Diethylcarbamazine, 2 mg/kg tid for 7 to 10 days, has also been used. Corticosteroids are sometimes added for severe disease or ocular disease.

G. Trichinosis:

1. **Organism:**
   a. Disease is caused by the nematode *Trichinella spiralis*. Trichinosis occurs worldwide, although its incidence in the United States has markedly declined in the last 50 years.
   b. Human infection occurs when undercooked meat containing viable encysted larvae is ingested. In the United States, the usual sources of infection are pork and bear meat. Cysts are digested in the proximal small intestine, where the released larvae penetrate the mucosa and mature within 2 to 3 days. After copulation, the female produces many larvae that enter the mesenteric circulation and are carried by the systemic circulation throughout the body. Although larvae travel through various tissues, including heart and brain, they encyst only in striated skeletal muscle, mainly in the diaphragm, intercostal muscles, deltoids, and certain muscles of the head and neck. Cysts reach maturity about 3 months after infection and eventually calcify.
   c. Pathology results mainly from larval encystation in skeletal muscle, although passage of larvae through the

myocardium may result in an inflammatory myocarditis that may cause significant morbidity and mortality. Other organs uncommonly involved include the CNS, liver, lungs, and kidneys.

2. **Clinical findings:**
   a. Most infections are asymptomatic. In symptomatic cases, symptoms appear 1 day to 2 weeks after ingestion of infective larvae.
   b. The initial enteric phase may be asymptomatic. Symptoms, if present, appear during the first week after infection and consist of diarrhea, abdominal pain, nausea, and vomiting.
   c. The second phase of disease is the invasive (migratory) phase, which usually begins 1 to 2 weeks after infection. Facial and eyelid edema are characteristic of this phase and may provide a useful diagnostic clue. Other symptoms include fever, myalgias, weakness, and headache. Peripheral eosinophilia typically appears during this phase.
   d. In untreated patients, symptoms gradually resolve, and a convalescent stage begins during the second month after infection.
   e. Myocarditis is the main cause of mortality in trichinosis and usually manifests as congestive heart failure 4 to 8 weeks after infection.
3. **Diagnosis:**
   a. The diagnosis is suggested by a clinical picture encompassing fever, peripheral eosinophilia, facial and eyelid edema, and muscle pain with elevated muscle enzyme levels.
   b. Definitive diagnosis is made by muscle biopsy that demonstrates encysted larvae. Although seldom necessary, this procedure has a higher yield if performed on a tender muscle at least 14 days after infection.
   c. Diagnosis can be made serologically, although titers are usually not positive until 3 weeks after infection. Current recommendations are to use two different tests, because no single method is highly reliable.
4. **Therapy** (See Table A–20):
   a. The drug of choice is mebendazole, which is active

against both intestinal and extraintestinal organisms. However, treatment is not always successful, and dosing recommendations vary widely. A dose of 5 mg/kg tid daily for 14 days has been recommended, as has adult dosing of 200 to 400 mg tid for 3 days, then 400 to 500 mg tid for 10 days. Some recommend another agent, thiabendazole, 25 mg/kg bid for 7 days.

b. Simultaneous treatment with 1 to 2 mg/kg/day of prednisone is advisable, particularly in severe disease, to blunt the Jarisch-Herxheimer-like reaction that may occur with initiation of therapy. Corticosteroids may also be beneficial in treating CNS trichinosis and *Trichinella*-induced myocarditis.

III. FLATWORMS

A. Cysticercosis

1. **Organism:**
   a. Disease is caused by the larval stage (cysticercus) of the pork tapeworm *Taenia solium*.
   b. Human infection occurs when *T. solium* eggs are ingested, either in contaminated foodstuffs or by autoinoculation (transmission of eggs from anus to mouth in a patient harboring an adult worm).
   c. Embryos are released from ingested eggs in the intestine, enter the bloodstream, and migrate to various tissues, where they encyst and mature into the larval form over 3 to 4 months. The parasite dies after a variable period.
2. **Clinical findings:**
   a. Onset of infection usually is subclinical.
   b. Painless subcutaneous nodules of various sizes, mainly on the trunk, usually are the first sign of infection, appearing several weeks after infection.
   c. The central nervous system is the most common and serious site of involvement, with symptoms usually appearing several years after infection. The most common symptom is seizures. Basal meningeal cysts or cysts in the region of the fourth ventricle may cause obstructive hydrocephalus. Single or multiple parenchymal cysts may appear as a space-occupying lesion,

sometimes with signs of increased intracranial pressure. Psychosis with delirium and hallucinations may occur. Spinal cord cysts produce findings suggestive of transverse myelitis, arachnoiditis, or a mass lesion.

d. Ocular involvement may be manifested by uveitis, retinitis or conjunctivitis.

3. **Diagnosis:**
   a. Neurocysticercosis is best diagnosed radiographically, either by cranial computed tomography (CT) or magnetic resonance imaging (MRI) or by skull radiographs demonstrating calcified cysts. However, negative radiographs do not rule out early intracranial infection or infection elsewhere.
   b. Serologic testing of CSF and serum is often useful for diagnosis.
   c. Peripheral white blood cell and eosinophil counts usually are normal.
   d. Spinal fluid from patients with CNS cysticercosis shows variable pleocytosis, moderate increase in protein, and a sometimes profound hypoglycorrhachia, which may incorrectly suggest a diagnosis of tuberculous meningitis. Organisms are seen rarely.
   e. Examination of stools for evidence of infection with the adult organism is indicated.
4. **Therapy** (See Table A–20):
   a. Praziquantel is the drug of choice in cysticercosis and neurocysticercosis, although it is of no benefit when cysts are calcified. The usual dosage is 50 mg/kg/day given in three divided doses daily for 14 days. Close monitoring for signs of increased intracranial pressure is mandatory during therapy, and corticosteroids are given from 1 day before to 3 days after therapy to suppress cerebral edema and inflammation, triggered by dying cystercerci. Many limit praziquantel therapy to patients with lesions that appear active by CT and to patients with multiple lesions. Praziquantel is contraindicated in patients with ocular involvement.
   b. Alternate treatment is albendazole 15 mg/kg/day in three doses for 8 days, repeated as needed.
   c. Surgery is the treatment of choice for intraocular and most intraventricular cysts.

B. Echinococcosis (Hydatid Disease):

1. **Organism:**

   a. Disease is caused by species of the cestode *Echinococcus*. *E. granulosus* produces unilocular disease, the most common form, while *E. multilocularis* produces multilocular or alveolar disease. Other species produce polycystic disease, which is rare. Endemic areas correspond to sheep-raising areas, including Australia, New Zealand, Africa, and Southern South America.

   b. Life cycle of the organism:

      1) There are two strains of *E. granulosus*. Dogs are the usual definitive host for adult tapeworms of the pastoral strain; wolves are definitive hosts for adult organisms of the sylvatic strain. Ungulates (sheep, deer, moose) ingest eggs and become intermediate hosts in which the larval form develops. Human infection occurs when a person ingests eggs and becomes an accidental intermediate host.

      2) Foxes, and sometimes cats and dogs, are definitive hosts for adult *E. multilocularis;* rodents are the usual intermediate hosts. Humans may ingest eggs and become accidental intermediate hosts.

   c. Pathology:

      1) Unilocular disease results when ingested eggs hatch within the intestine, gain access to the portal circulation, and are deposited in the liver or lungs. The organism then forms a *hydatid cyst,* with a fibrous outer layer and a cellular inner layer, from which *brood capsules* develop. Larval scolices develop from the brood capsules, which grow inward and break free into the cyst cavity. Cysts typically are a few millimeters in diameter 1 month after infection, usually grow 1 to 5 cm in diameter per year, and may reach 30 to 40 cm in the liver. Symptoms are related to compression of surrounding normal tissues. Cysts occur most often in liver or lung, but may be found in any organ.

      2) *E. multilocularis* embryos are deposited in the liver after gaining access to the portal circulation via the intestine. They also form hydatid cysts, but

the brood capsule develops outward into surrounding normal tissue, an invasive pattern of growth that eventually may destroy the entire liver. Metastasis to lung or other organs may occur.

2. **Clinical findings:**
   a. Unilocular disease *(E. granulosus):*
      1) Pulmonary and hepatic involvement may present with fever, cough, hemoptysis, right upper quadrant pain, or jaundice. Pulmonary cysts that rupture into a bronchus result in the classic clinical finding of "coughing up grapeskins." Intrahepatic cyst rupture into the biliary tract may mimic ascending cholangitis.
      2) CNS cysts are much more common in children than in adults and may manifest as space-occupying intracranial mass lesions.

   b. Multilocular disease *(E. multilocularis)* usually is asymptomatic in children, but may manifest as tender hepatomegaly or a hepatic mass, sometimes accompanied by jaundice.
3. **Diagnosis:**
   a. Pulmonary hydatid disease may be suspected based on characteristic chest x-ray findings: hepatic cysts may be imaged using ultrasound or CT scans.
   b. Serologic tests exist, but are not entirely reliable.
   c. Definitive diagnosis usually is not made until surgery. Percutaneous needling of cysts to obtain fluid for diagnostic purposes is contraindicated because fluid spillage may lead to anaphylactic shock.
4. **Therapy** (See Table A–20):
   a. Surgery is the treatment of choice for all forms of hydatid disease. Surgical removal of unilocular cysts requires great care, because spillage of cyst contents may lead to anaphylactic shock and later disseminated echinococcosis. Multilocular disease is often not resectable because of its invasive nature.
   b. Inoperable cysts may be treated with albendazole 15 mg/kg/day for 28 days (repeat as needed), usually with limited success.

C. Schistosomiasis

1. **Organism:**
   a. Schistosomiasis is caused by the trematode species *Schistosoma mansoni, S. japonicum,* and *S. hematobium*. Other species capable of human infection are clinically unimportant.
   b. *S. japonicum* is found only in the Orient; *S. mansoni* in Africa, Southwest Asia, South America, and the Caribbean; and *S. hematobium* in Africa and Southwest Asia. Disease is not transmitted in North America because of the absence of the intermediate snail host, but large numbers of immigrants from endemic areas are infected.
   c. Adult *S. japonicum* and *S. mansoni* flukes usually inhabit the human intestinal venous system, whereas *S. hematobium* are found in veins that drain the urinary bladder. Adult flukes undergo sexual multiplication at these sites, and release large numbers of eggs. Eggs stimulate inflammation, and may be passed in feces or urine. Excreted eggs that reach fresh water release **miracidia,** which then infect certain aquatic snails, the intermediate hosts. Asexual replication occurs in the snail with release of **cercariae,** free-swimming forms capable of infecting humans by directly penetrating skin immersed in fresh water. After skin penetration, cercariae develop into schistosomula, which migrate to lungs, to liver, and then to the intestinal or vesical venous system, completing the life cycle.
2. **Clinical findings:**
   a. Schistosomal dermatitis ("swimmer's itch") results from cercarial penetration of skin. The first cercarial infection may be asymptomatic or associated with mild pruritus and a transient maculopapular rash. More intense local reactions may occur in previously exposed persons.
   b. The onset of egg production 2 to 8 weeks after initial skin penetration may be accompanied by **Katayama fever,** an acute serum sickness–like illness most common and most severe with *S. japonicum*. Symptoms include high spiking fever, abdominal pain, diarrhea,

generalized lymphadenopathy, and hepatosplenomegaly. Marked peripheral eosinophilia is characteristic. Katayama fever usually remits after a few weeks, but may persist for months.

c. Ongoing infection produces characteristic involvement of several organs:
    1) Granulomatous inflammation around eggs in the bowel wall leads to fibrosis, often asymptomatic but occasionally resulting in abdominal discomfort, anorexia, diarrhea, and growth retardation.
    2) Embolization of eggs to the liver via the portal circulation results in hepatic granulomatous inflammation and scarring, which may lead to portal hypertension. Liver function and serum transaminase levels usually are normal.
    3) Eggs also may embolize to the lungs via collaterals, resulting in pulmonary granulomas. Rarely this may cause pulmonary arteriolar obstruction, leading to pulmonary hypertension. This occurs nearly exclusively in patients with advanced hepatosplenic disease.
    4) Deposition of eggs in the walls of the bladder and ureter by *S. hematobium* causes inflammation and fibrosis, which may lead to hydroureter and hydronephrosis. Cancer of the bladder is more common in patients with *S. hematobium* infection.
    5) Cerebral involvement, manifested by diffuse encephalitis or focal granuloma formation, occurs rarely and only with *S. japonicum*. Transverse myelitis secondary to egg-induced granulomas in the spinal cord may occur with *S. mansoni* and *S. hematobium*.

3. **Diagnosis:**
    a. Definitive diagnosis is by demonstration of eggs in urine, stool, or biopsy specimens from rectum, bladder, or liver.
    b. Various serologic tests exist, but results generally are unsatisfactory.
4. **Therapy** (See Table A–20):
    a. Praziquantel is the drug of choice for all schistosomal

infections. The dosage is 60 mg/kg/day po in three doses for 1 day. *S. mansoni* and *S. hematobium* may be treated with a 20 mg/kg/dose bid for 1 day.

b. An alternative for *S. mansoni* is oxamniquine 20 mg/kg/day given in two doses for 1 day.

OTHER PATHOGENS AND DISEASES

11

I. SPIROCHETES:

Spirochetes are gram-negative helical organisms with flexible cell walls and endoflagella. They are usually visualized by dark-field microscopy, electron microscopy, or special staining techniques. *Treponema, Leptospira,* and *Borrelia* are the causative agents of important human and zoonotic diseases—syphilis, leptospirosis, and Lyme disease, respectively.

A. *Treponema Pallidum* and syphilis:

1. **Epidemiology:** Almost all causes of non-congenital syphilis are acquired by sexual contact and are most common in individuals 18 to 24 years of age. The incidence in the U.S. is highest in urban areas and among homosexual or bisexual men. Approximately one third of the sexual contacts of individuals with primary or secondary syphilitic lesions develop the disease. Because of the frequency of association of syphilis and HIV infection, all sexually active patients with syphilis should be encouraged to be tested for HIV.
2. **Clinical manifestations:** Congenital syphilis is discussed in Chapter 3, section I,C,5.
   a. Primary syphilis: The primary lesion or chancre develops 2 to 10 weeks after infection. It is a painless ulcerated lesion of the penis, external genitalia, anal region, or lips. The lesion is densely infiltrated with spirochetes, lymphocytes and plasma cells and is highly infectious. Bilateral, nonsuppurative, painless inguinal lymphadenopathy usually develops within 1 week of the chancre and may persist for months. Untreated, the primary lesion heals within 2 months.
   b. Secondary syphilis: Secondary syphilis develops 2 to 10 weeks after the primary lesion has healed. The de-

gree of severity is variable. Secondary lesions present as a skin rash, erosions of mucous membranes, and/or wartlike condyloma lata in moist areas (e.g., external female genitalia or perianal areas). These lesions are also highly infectious. Systemic manifestations such as fever, malaise, lymphadenopathy, and alopecia may be present. The infection resolves spontaneously in one third of untreated patients. In another 40% to 50%, serologic tests remain positive but no further clinical manifestations appear. The remaining untreated patients develop tertiary manifestations several months to 30 years later.

c. Tertiary syphilis:
   1) Tertiary syphilis manifests as cardiovascular syphilis, neurosyphilis, or gummatous lesions affecting the skin, bone, joints, oral and nasal cavities, parenchymal organs, the cardiovascular system, and the nervous system.
   2) The most characteristic lesion of cardiovascular syphilis is the development of aortitis and aortic dilatation resulting from gummatous changes in the media of the aorta leading to loss of elasticity.
   3) Neurosyphilis is manifested as meningovascular syphilis (most often presenting with personality changes), general paresis, or tabes dorsalis. Tabes dorsalis involves demyelination of the posterior columns and dorsal roots and damage to dorsal root ganglia, thereby producing ataxia, wide-based gait, foot slap, and loss of sensation.
   4) Late manifestations probably involve delayed-type hypersensitivity responses to the spirochete or an autoimmune reaction to host tissues in areas in which spirochetes persist. Late disease is not infectious.

3. **Diagnosis:**
   a. *T. pallidum* can be detected in primary and secondary lesions by dark-field microscopy or by direct fluorescent antibody (DFA) staining. Organisms can not be cultured on artificial media.

b. Most cases of syphilis are diagnosed serologically.
   1) Nontreponemal (anti-cardiolipin) tests such as the VDRL and RPR become positive in the early stages of the primary lesion, remain positive during the secondary stage, and slowly decline in the late stage.
   2) Treponemal tests involve direct detection of antibody to *T. pallidum*. The two most frequently used treponemal tests are the fluorescent treponemal antibody absorption test (FTA-ABS) and microhemagglutination test for *T. pallidum* antibody (MHA-TP).
   3) Treponemal tests are highly specific but remain positive after successful treatment. Nontreponemal tests are less specific; however, the titers reflect the activity of disease, thereby enabling them to be used as a test of cure. VDRL and other nontreponemal titers decrease fourfold or more after successful treatment of primary, secondary, or early latent syphilis.

4. **Therapy:**
   a. Penicillin is the drug of choice for syphilis; there is no evidence of resistance to penicillin. Erythromycin, tetracyclines, chloramphenicol, and cephalosporins are alternatives in penicillin-hypersensitive patients.
   b. Early syphilis (i.e., primary, secondary, or latent syphilis of less than 1 year duration) should be treated with IM benzathine penicillin G (50,000 U/kg, up to 2.4 million U).
   c. Syphilis of more than 1 year duration, excluding neurosyphilis, should be treated with benzathine penicillin G (50,000 U/kg up to 2.4 million U), given IM once weekly for 3 weeks.
   d. Any child thought to have neurologic involvement should be treated with 200,000 to 300,000 U/kg/day of parenteral aqueous crystalline penicillin G every 6 hours for 10 to 14 days.
   e. Jarisch-Herxheimer reactions occur in fewer than 10% of patients treated for primary or secondary syphilis and consist of fever, arthralgia, myalgia, increased

lymphadenopathy, and worsening of secondary lesions. The value of corticosteroids in controlling these reactions is unknown.

5. **Follow-up:**
   a. All patients with early syphilis should have repeat nontreponemal tests at 3, 6, and 12 months after treatment. The VDRL (or RPR) titer should decline fourfold by 3 months and eightfold by 6 months. Ninety-seven percent of effectively treated patients with primary syphilis are seronegative 2 years after therapy.
   b. Patients with latent syphilis have less predictable serologic responses.
   c. All patients with neurosyphilis should have repeat CSF examinations within 3 months of treatment, at 6-month intervals until the CSF is normal, and then annually for 3 years.
   d. Retreatment should be considered if clinical signs and symptoms persist or recur; if there is a fourfold or greater increase in nontreponemal titer; or if the initial nontreponemal test fails to decline at least fourfold within a year.

B. Lyme Disease:

1. **Etiology:**
   a. Lyme disease (LD) is a zoonosis (a disease transmitted from animals) that is named for the town in Connecticut where cases were first recognized.
   b. The causative agent is a spirochete, *Borrelia burgdorferi*. It is a large, gram-negative spirochete easily visualized with Giemsa, Wright's, or acridine orange stain.
2. **Epidemiology:**
   a. In the United States, LD is transmitted by *Ixodes dammini* deer ticks in the eastern and central states and by *Ixodes pacificus* in the West. *Ixodes* ticks attach to, feed, and mate on deer; therefore, LD occurs in areas where deer are present. LD is most prominent in the northeastern states, Wisconsin, Minnesota, and parts of California and Oregon.
   b. The disease usually occurs between May and September, and is most common in children.

3. **Pathogenesis:**
   a. The exact pathogenesis is not yet established.
   b. In the early stage of LD, spirochetes are sometimes isolated from involved tissues, especially from the primary skin lesion.
   c. In the later stages, spirochetes are rarely present in affected tissues, suggesting that autoimmune responses may be responsible for the clinical manifestations.
4. **Clinical manifestations:** As with syphilis, clinical LD can be divided into stages. Stage 1 consists of a localized skin lesion, followed within days or weeks by stage 2, disseminated infection. Stage 3 occurs at least 1 year after initial infection.
   a. **Stage 1:**
      1) The primary skin lesion, known as **erythema chronicum migrans** (ECM), occurs at the site of a tick bite 3 to 14 days after the bite. About 60% to 80% of those infected have a history of ECM:
         a) The lesion begins as a macule or papule that becomes an expanding red-bordered circular lesion with central clearing. The center may become necrotic.
         b) Approximately one half of untreated patients develop other skin lesions resembling the primary one.
      2) The patient frequently may develop fever, malaise, headache, muscle and joint pains, and mild neck stiffness.
      3) In the untreated patient, ECM usually disappears over several weeks; however, constitutional symptoms may persist for months.
   b. **Stage 2:** Stage 2 usually begins weeks to months after resolution of ECM and involves the nervous system, heart, or both.
      1) About 15% of patients develop neurologic abnormalities, which may include aseptic meningitis, cranial or peripheral neuropathy, or encephalitis.
      2) About 10% of patients have cardiac involvement. The most common abnormalities are atrioventricu-

lar block, myopericarditis, and left ventricular dysfunction.

3) Neurologic and cardiac abnormalities usually resolve completely within a period of weeks to several months.

c. **Stage 3:** Stage 3 is manifested by arthritis, which develops weeks to years after the onset of infection:
   1) Large joints are usually affected.
   2) Recurrent attacks of arthritis are common.
   3) In a small percentage of patients, the arthritis becomes chronic, with erosion of cartilage and bone.

5. **Pregnancy:** *B. burgdorferi* infection during pregnancy can cause infection of the fetus, but it is unclear whether it produces fetal abnormalities.
6. **Diagnosis:**
   a. Diagnosis is made clinically when ECM is present.
   b. In patients lacking a rash, the diagnosis is usually made serologically.
      1) Enzyme-linked immunosorbent assay (ELISA) and indirect fluorescent antibody (IFA) tests are available. ELISA is used more often because of greater sensitivity and specificity. Antibody tests for LD are poorly standardized, and considerable variability from laboratory to laboratory exists.
      2) Antibodies may be absent in the first 3 weeks of infection or if antibiotic therapy is given early in the course of illness.
      3) Most untreated patients with stage 2 or 3 have a positive antibody titer.
7. **Therapy:**
   a. Stage 1 disease is treated with oral tetracycline (250 mg qid) or doxycycline (100 mg bid) in children $\geq$ 7 to 8 years and with oral penicillin V or oral amoxicillin (each 25–50 mg/kg/day tid) in children $<$ 7 or 8 years. Therapy is given for 10 to 21 days, depending on clinical response.
   b. Isolated Bell's palsy, acute arthritis, and mild carditis may be treated with the same oral regimen as stage 1 disease.

c. Persistent arthritis or severe carditis should be treated with parenteral ceftriaxone, 75 to 100 mg/kg once daily, or intravenous (IV) penicillin G, 300,000 to 400,000 U/kg/day for 14 to 21 days.
d. Meningitis or encephalitis is treated with parenteral ceftriaxone, 75 to 100 mg/kg once daily for 14 to 21 days.
e. Appropriate therapy for Lyme disease during pregnancy has not been determined.

8. **Prevention:**
   a. Patients in tick-infested areas should be advised to cover as much of their arms and legs with clothing as possible. Tick repellents are effective but must be applied frequently.
   b. Ticks should be removed promptly from the body.
   c. Empiric treatment of asymptomatic patients who have been bitten by ticks is not recommended.

II. CHLAMYDIA:

A. Microbiology:

1. Species include *Chlamydia trachomatis* (chiefly responsible for human oculogenital and infantile pneumonitis), *Chlamydia psittaci* (etiologic agent of psittacosis, chiefly a zoonosis), and *Chlamydia pneumoniae* (TWAR), a cause of atypical pneumonia.
2. The chlamydiae cannot generate adenosine triphosphate (ATP) and are therefore obligate intracellular bacteria.
3. The 48-hour developmental cycle of chlamydiae involves an infectious but metabolically inactive extracellular form (elementary body), which is taken into cells by endocytosis and differentiates into a noninfectious, metabolically active intracellular form (reticulate body). The reticulate bodies undergo binary fission, redifferentiate into elementary bodies, and are released by cytolysis or exocytosis.

B. Epidemiology:

1. Perinatal infection:
   a. Rates of cervical colonization with *C. trachomatis* during pregnancy vary among different populations. The overall rate in pregnant U.S. women is about 8%, with rates usually higher in younger women.

   b. Thirty percent to 70% of infants born through a colonized birth canal acquire chlamydial infection; of these, 50% to 75% develop conjunctivitis, and 10% to 30% develop pneumonia.
   c. Women with chlamydial infection may have a higher incidence of premature or low birth weight infants.
2. Childhood infection:
   a. *C. trachomatis* rarely causes significant respiratory tract infection in childhood after infancy, but *C. pneumoniae* is being increasingly recognized as an important pathogen.
   b. Rectogenital infection or colonization may occur after exposure at birth or from sexual abuse and may persist for several years. In cases of sexual abuse, *Chlamydia* and *Neisseria gonorrhoeae* are often coinfecting organisms.
3. Adolescent infection:
   a. The rate of genital chlamydial infection in adolescents ranges from 8% to 37%. It is the most common sexually transmitted pathogen in adolescents.
   b. Infected females may be asymptomatic or may have mucopurulent cervicitis, which can evolve into acute salpingitis.
   c. Infected males usually have urethritis, which may be asymptomatic. Infection may result in acute epididymitis.

C. Clinical Features:

1. **Neonatal infections:**
   a. Inclusion conjunctivitis: Signs of conjunctivitis occur within several days to 2 weeks after birth without systemic signs.
   b. Chlamydial pneumonitis: Afebrile pneumonitis manifesting when the patient is 3 weeks to 3 months of age, with a staccato cough, rales, and wheezing; it is associated with mild eosinophilia and elevated serum immunoglobulin levels.
2. **Childhood infections:**
   a. *C. pneumoniae* (TWAR) may be important as a cause of "atypical" pneumonitis with mild respiratory and systemic symptoms.

b. Genital infections (urethritis, cervicitis, vaginitis) in prepubertal children may reflect sexual abuse.

3. **Adolescent infections:**
   a. Salpingitis and pelvic inflammatory disease manifest as in adults, with fever, lower abdominal pain, and discharge, and may lead to particularly severe scarring of the fallopian tubes in teenagers.
   b. Nongonococcal urethritis in males manifests with penile discharge and dysuria.
   c. Lymphogranuloma venereum (LGV) manifests as inguinal adenopathy that frequently becomes suppurative with drainage.

D. Diagnosis:

1. Growth of the organism in culture is fairly difficult and requires cultivation in cell cultures.
2. Existing antigen detection tests include a direct fluorescent antibody assay and an enzyme immunoassay. Both demonstrate good sensitivity and specificity in evaluating cervical and urethral specimens from adolescents and conjunctival and nasopharyngeal specimens from young children. However, sensitivity is highly dependent on the quality of specimen collection. These tests are not approved for use on specimens obtained from sites other than those already mentioned.

E. Therapy:

1. Men and nonpregnant women with rectogenital chlamydial infection should receive tetracycline or doxycycline for 7 days. Pregnant women should receive erythromycin (base or ethylsuccinate). Sexual partners of infected adults should also be treated. LGV requires at least 3 weeks of tetracycline (> 7 or 8 years) or erythromycin therapy.
2. Chlamydial conjunctivitis in infants should be treated with a 10- to 14-day course of oral erythromycin. Topical therapy alone has an unacceptably high failure rate.
3. Infants with chlamydial pneumonia should be treated with 14 days of erythromycin therapy.
4. Parents of infants with chlamydial infection should also be offered treatment.

III. RICKETTSIAL DISEASES:

A. The Organisms and Pathogenesis:

1. Rickettsiae:
    a. Small coccobacilli that resemble both viruses and bacteria, the latter more closely.
    b. Grow only intracellularly (like viruses), but resemble bacteria by mode of replication, by possessing both RNA and DNA, Krebs cycle, electron transport, and protein synthetic enzymes, and by susceptibility to certain antibiotics.
    c. Naturally occur in insects (lice, fleas) and arachnids (ticks and mites), which are major modes of transmission to humans (except for *Coxiella burnettii*).
2. Rickettsial diseases:
    a. Spotted fevers: include Rocky Mountain spotted fever (RMSF) due to *Rickettsia rickettsii*, the tick typhuses, and rickettsialpox *(Rickettsia akari)*.
    b. Typhus group: includes epidemic typhus and Brill-Zinsser disease (both *Rickettsia prowazekii*) and murine typhus *(Rickettsia typhi)*.
    c. Scrub typhus: *Rickettsia tsutsugamushi*.
    d. Q fever: *C. burnettii*.
    e. Ehrlichiosis: *Ehrlichia sennetsu, E. canis, E. chafearsis*.
    f. Trench fever: *Rochalimaea quintana*.
3. Pathogenesis:
    a. After the bite of an infected vector, rickettsiae invade small vessel endothelial cells, multiply within those cells, and disseminate hematogenously.
    b. Focal areas of endothelial damage and proliferation with perivascular mononuclear cell infiltration lead to focal hemorrhage and thrombosis.
    c. Vascular lesions are most prominent in skin, myocardium, and brain, correlating with most symptoms.
    d. Only *C. burnettii* is most often transmitted by inhalation of rickettsiae, leading to prominent respiratory symptoms.

B. Clinical Disorders:

1. **Spotted fevers** (Rocky Mountain spotted fever):
    a. General features:
        1) Rocky Mountain spotted fever is by far the most

important and most severe; all spotted fevers except rickettsialpox *(R. akari)* are tick transmitted.

2) Untreated, the disease has a 20% to 25% fatality rate; early treatment lowers mortality; overall U.S. mortality is 5% to 7%.

b. Epidemiology:

1) The majority of cases now occur from Virginia to Georgia, the Ohio River Valley, Oklahoma, Arkansas, and Missouri.

2) Infections occur April to September coinciding with tick prevalence. Rickettsiae are passed transovarially in ticks (*Dermacentor* and *Amblyomma*), and ticks require a blood meal, usually from a dog, horse, or sheep. Humans are incidental hosts, with rickettsial transmission from saliva of an infected adult tick after several hours of attachment.

c. Clinical features:

1) Mean incubation period after tick bite is 7 days (range 2–14 days).

2) Fever, rash, toxicity, headache, myalgia, and confusion, all of variable severity.

3) Rash usually develops by day 3 or 4, first on wrists and ankles and spreading to trunk; rash on palms and soles is highly characteristic; rash begins as small blanching red macules and progresses to petechial-purpuric lesions.

4) Persistent headache and toxic appearance are common, and signs of meningoencephalitis may develop.

5) Differential diagnosis includes meningococcal infection, atypical measles, leptospirosis, enteroviral infection, toxic shock syndrome, secondary syphilis, systemic lupus erythematosus, thrombotic thrombocytopenic purpura, and other rickettsioses.

d. **Diagnosis:**

1) Laboratory tests are of limited value early in RMSF; therefore, one must make a clinical diagnosis.

2) Nonspecific features: Leukopenia, hyponatremia, and thrombocytopenia.

3) Weil-Felix serologic reactions (Table 11–1) are rarely useful until the second week of illness, with rising *Proteus* OX-19 and OX-2 titers.
4) Specific complement fixation titers in acute and convalescent sera are useful for retrospective diagnosis.

e. **Treatment:**
1) Must be instituted in the first week of illness to be effective.
2) Agents of choice are chloramphenicol, 50 to 100 mg/kg/day po or IV divided into four doses, or tetracycline (for those > 7 or 8 years of age), 25 to 50 mg/kg/day po or 15 to 25 mg/kg/day IV, continued until the patient is afebrile at least 48 hours; these agents are rickettsiostatic, not rickettsiocidal.

f. Rickettsial pox *(R. akari):*
1) The second most common spotted fever rickettsiosis in the United States.
2) Occurs primarily in New York City and elsewhere in the Northeast United States.
3) Human infection occurs when the natural cycle be-

TABLE 11–1.
Rickettsial Serologic Responses

	Weil-Felix Reactions			Complement Fixation Tests		
	OX-19	OX-2	OX-K	Typhus	Spotted Fever	Q Fever
Typhus fevers						
Epidemic louse-borne	+++	+	0	+++	0	0
Brill-Zinsser disease	+++/0	0	0	+++	0	0
Murine typhus	+++	+	0	+++	0	0
Spotted fevers						
Rocky Mountain spotted fever	+++	+++	0	0	+++	0
Tick typhuses	+++	+++	0	0	+++	0
Rickettsial pox	0	0	0	0	+++	0
Scrub typhus	0	0	+++	0	0	0
Q fever	0	0	0	0	0	+++

tween the mite vector and the house mouse is disrupted by a paucity of mice, leading mites to seek alternative human hosts.

4) **Clinical features:** After a 9- to 14-day incubation period, a papule develops at the mite bite site, evolving to a black eschar; regional adenitis and temperature 37.8° C to 39.5° C occur with headache. Within a few days of fever onset, 5 to 100 scattered macules appear rapidly to become maculopapules and then vesiculopapules, resembling chickenpox. This illness is benign and self-limited; therapy is not required.
5) Weil-Felix reactions are negative.

2. **Typhus fevers:**
   a. Three illnesses caused by two rickettsial species.
   b. **Classic louse-borne epidemic typhus:**
      1) A severe acute infection by *R. prowazekii* transmitted from the human body louse *(Pediculus humanus corporis)*.
      2) Associated with war, famine, and other catastrophes; reported fatality rates are 60% to 70% in those >50 years of age, about 10% in young adults and children.
      3) In the United States, flying squirrels serve as a reservoir.
      4) Clinical features: One to 2 weeks after bite of infected louse, high fever, rash, myalgia, and headache abruptly develop. Small vessel vasculitis results in various manifestations, including renal failure, myocardial and central nervous system (CNS) dysfunction, pneumonia, gastrointestinal (GI) disease, and a characteristic rash beginning on the trunk and spreading to the extremities (opposite of RMSF), sparing the face, palms and soles; rash progresses from macules to papules to hemorrhagic or necrotic lesions.
      5) Diagnosis depends on clinical and epidemiologic features; serologic tests are useful after the first week of illness.
      6) Therapy is as for RMSF.

c. **Brill-Zinsser disease:**
   1) Relapses of louse-borne typhus years after the initial attack, reflecting reactivation of dormant rickettsiae in the reticuloendothelial system.
   2) Clinical features resemble louse-borne typhus but are milder and of shorter duration.
   3) Occurs if the initial attack was not treated or < 5 days of treatment was taken.

d. **Murine (endemic) typhus:**
   1) *R. typhi* infection transmitted from rats by the oriental rat flea when humans are incidentally bitten by an infected flea.
   2) Most U.S. cases have occurred in Texas and Gulf Coast areas.
   3) Clinical features resemble louse-borne typhus but are milder and of shorter duration; mortality is < 1%, and complications are rare.
   4) Therapy is as for other rickettsioses.

3. **Scrub typhus:**
   a. This mite-borne infection by *R. tsutsugamushi* is limited to Japan, Southeast Asia, and the southwestern Pacific; it was common in western troops in World War II.
   b. Clinical features are similar to other rickettsioses with the addition of generalized adenopathy.
   c. Treatment is as for other rickettsioses.
4. **Q (query) fever:**
   a. This rickettsial infection by *C. burnettii* is unique in that it is transmitted by inhalation of contaminated aerosols, and there is no rash.
   b. Epidemiology: Subclinically infected cattle, goats, sheep, and ticks serve as reservoirs; transmission occurs as result of excretion of *C. burnettii* in milk, urine, placental tissue, and feces; *C. burnetti* is very resistant to desiccation, heat, and physicochemical agents, surviving for many months in dried dust particles.
   c. Clinical features: After a 20-day (14- to 39-day range) incubation period, abrupt onset of fever, rigors, severe headache, myalgias, retrobulbar pain but no rash;

cough, chest pain, and patchy or round pulmonary infiltrates are common, as is hepatosplenomegaly with little hepatitis or jaundice. It is generally a mild and self-limited illness lasting 1 to 2 weeks, with <1% mortality.

d. Diagnosis: Clinical; no Weil-Felix reactions.
e. Therapy as for other rickettsioses.

5. **Ehrlichiosis:** Intraleukocytic rickettsiae: *E. canis:* This agent causes tropical canine pancytopenia, and human infection is increasingly recognized. The brown dog tick is the vector. Clinical features resemble those of RMSF, and patients seronegative for RMSF should be considered for erlichiosis.

IV. MYCOPLASMAS:

A. Mycoplasma Pneumoniae:

1. **Organism and pathogenesis:**
   a. Mycoplasmas are the smallest free-living organisms, lacking cell walls, and growing slowly in enriched liquid media and on special agar. *M. pneumoniae* colonies demonstrate hemadsorption (binding to red blood cells) mediated by a surface adhesin that also mediates attachment to respiratory epithelium.
   b. *M. pneumoniae* is acquired by droplet spread, attaches to respiratory epithelium, interferes with ciliary activity, and leads to mucosal desquamation and to lymphocytic inflammatory reaction. Organisms are shed in upper respiratory tract secretions from 2 to 8 days before symptoms to as long as 14 weeks after infection. Local and systemic antibody and cellular immune responses develop, and clinical manifestations may be the result of cellular immune responses.
2. **Clinical manifestations:**
   a. **Primary atypical pneumonia** is the classic illness caused by *M. pneumoniae* in school-aged children and young adults. This is less severe than usual bacterial pneumonia, infrequently requiring hospitalization. Insidious onset of fever, headache, and malaise precedes nonproductive cough by several days. Chest x-ray usually shows a lower lobe infiltrate, sometimes with a

small pleural effusion. Particularly severe pneumonitis occurs in patients with sickle cell disease.

b. **Upper respiratory tract infection** is more common in preschool-aged children, and presents with cold symptoms. Pharyngitis may occur at any age.

c. Meningoencephalitis, rash, hemolytic anemia, and allergic reactions such as Stevens-Johnson syndrome and erythema multiforme are other clinical manifestations of mycoplasmal infection.

3. **Diagnosis:**
   a. Cultures are impractical for routine use.
   b. Fourfold rise in serum CF titer to *M. pneumoniae* or a single high ($\geq$ 1:128) titer is highly suggestive of infection.
   c. Cold hemagglutinins (anti-I) are somewhat nonspecific but may be helpful in establishing a diagnosis of mycoplasmal infection.
4. **Treatment:**
   a. Antibiotics shorten the clinical illness, but organisms are shed for prolonged periods.
   b. Erythromycin, 30 to 40 mg/kg/day (maximum 2 g) divided q8h is preferred. Alternate in those $>$ 7 or 8 years old is tetracycline, 25 to 50 mg/kg/day (maximum 2 g) divided qid.

B. Ureaplasma urealyticum:

1. **Organism and pathogenesis:**
   a. *U. urealyticum* was formerly termed T (for tiny)– mycoplasma and is distinguished from mycoplasmas by production of urease.
   b. *U. urealyticum* colonizes the genital tract of sexually active men and women, probably as a direct result of sexual activity. Transmission to infants may occur during passage through the birth canal.
2. **Clinical manifestations:**
   a. *U. urealyticum* causes up to 50% of nongonococcal, nonchlamydial urethritis in men and chorioamnionitis and postpartum fever in women.
   b. Although data are incomplete, *U. urealyticum* (and *Mycoplasma hominis,* another inhabitant of the geni-

tourinary tract) may be responsible for an uncertain proportion of neonatal lower respiratory tract disease.

3. **Diagnosis:**
   a. Because of high colonization rates in normals, it is difficult to diagnose accurately those infections caused by these genital mycoplasmas.
   b. Neonatal nonbacterial lower respiratory tract infections may be related to these agents.
4. **Treatment:**
   a. Indications for neonatal therapy for these agents are unclear.
   b. Erythromycin would appear to be the best choice if one wishes to institute therapy for possible neonatal infection.

POSTINFECTIOUS SYNDROMES 12

I. ACUTE RHEUMATIC FEVER:

A. Etiology and Pathogenesis:

1. Acute rheumatic fever (ARF) results from untreated group A β-hemolytic streptococcal (GAS) pharyngitis. Infection with GAS elsewhere does not lead to ARF. It is quite likely that there are strains of GAS that are particularly highly "rheumatogenic."
2. The pathogenesis of ARF appears to be immune-mediated, resulting in an inflammatory reaction in various connective tissues, particularly the heart, joints, and arteries. The precise inciting streptococcal antigen(s) and immune mechanisms remain unknown. GAS antigens that are antigenically related to components of human tissues may induce formation of cross-reactive antibodies.
3. Fewer than 3% of individuals with untreated GAS pharyngitis develop ARF, but the precise host determinants of susceptibility are unknown.
4. GAS produce extracellular substances such as streptolysin S and O, DNAses, and proteinases that could be potentially involved in pathogenesis.

B. Epidemiology:

1. In the United States, ARF was extremely common in the 19th-century. Its incidence declined after 1900, increased briefly during World War II, and then continued to decline sharply. By the late 1970s, ARF had become a rare disease in the United States; however, rates increased in the mid-1980s in a number of U.S. areas. ARF remains a very common problem in many developing countries.
2. Crowding, which facilitates spread of streptococcal pharyngitis, and poor medical care contributed strongly to the former prevalence of ARF. Timely detection and treatment of streptococcal pharyngitis, use of penicillin prophylaxis to prevent recurrences of ARF, and improved

living conditions all have contributed to the decline in prevalence. Fluctuations in prevalence of rheumatogenic strains may also be important.

3. The ARF outbreaks in the United States since 1985 usually have been associated with middle-class suburban populations. Unique mucoid GAS strains, previously associated with ARF, have been seen with these outbreaks, raising interesting questions about pathogenesis.

C. **Clinical Findings:**

1. Diagnosis of ARF is based on a constellation of signs and symptoms summarized in the recently modified Jones criteria (Table 12–1). At least two major criteria, or one major and two minor criteria, **plus** evidence of antecedent streptococcal infection are required for diagnosis.
2. Acute RF usually occurs 2 to 4 weeks after an episode of untreated GAS pharyngitis in selected individuals. Symptoms include fever, malaise, and migratory polyarthritis involving at least one large joint. Carditis may be manifested by mitral and/or aortic insufficiency murmurs, pericarditis with chest pain, or myocarditis with tachycardia and congestive heart failure (CHF). Subcutaneous nodules (or erythema marginatum) are seen rarely. Chronic arthritis does not develop.
3. Sydenham's chorea may be the only manifestation of ARF, most often in prepubertal girls. It is manifested by emotional lability, slurred speech, clumsy fine motor skills, and purposeless movements accentuated by stress.

TABLE 12–1.
Modified Jones Criteria for Diagnosis of ARF

Major Criteria	Minor Criteria
Carditis	Fever
Migratory polyarthritis	Arthralgia
Chorea	Elevated ESR or positive CRP
Erythema marginatum	Prolonged P-R interval
Subcutaneous nodules	
Plus	
Evidence of antecedent streptococcal infection	

Chorea develops insidiously and may appear 2 to 6 months after the streptococcal infection. Therefore, evidence of steptococcal infection often cannot be documented. Permanent neurologic sequelae are not seen.

4. Long-term sequelae of ARF are limited to the heart; mitral and/or aortic valve damage (very rarely tricuspid or pulmonary) may occur, leading to valvar insufficiency. Mitral and/or aortic stenosis may develop years after ARF, more rapidly in Third World areas in which juvenile mitral stenosis is common.
5. ARF patients are at great risk for recurrent episodes of ARF unless given prophylactic antibiotics (see section I,E).
6. ARF outbreaks since 1985 in the United States have been notable for high incidence of carditis, often severe, and of Sydenham's chorea.

D. Laboratory Findings:

1. Throat cultures are seldom (20%) positive for GAS at presentation with ARF. Antecedent streptococcal infection is usually documented by elevated antibody titers. Antistreptolysin O (ASO) titers are used most commonly, with >250 Todd units indicative of prior infection. Other titers used include anti-DNase B, anti-DPNase, anti-NADase, antihyaluronidase, and anti-streptokinase. Streptozyme is less useful as it is poorly standardized.
2. A very elevated erythrocyte sedimentation rate or C-reactive protein level, mild anemia, and mild leukocytosis are usually seen.
3. The electrocardiogram may show a prolonged P-R interval, which is not indicative of carditis. Cardiomegaly may be seen on chest x-ray.

E. Therapy and Prevention:

1. ARF is treated with anti-inflammatory agents. High-dose (70–100 mg/kg/day) aspirin is used most often. Prednisone (2 mg/kg/day) is indicated in those with moderate or severe carditis (cardiomegaly, CHF), but neither corticosteroids nor salicylates affect the ultimate incidence of residual heart disease.
2. Patients with ARF should receive 1.2 million units of intramuscular (IM) benzathine penicillin even if the throat culture is negative.

3. ARF can be prevented in most susceptible individuals by adequate antibiotic treatment of GAS pharyngitis.
4. Recurrences of ARF are effectively prevented by IM benzathine penicillin G, 1.2 million units q4wk (600,000 units for those <60 lb). Patients at unusual risk may receive injections every 3 weeks. Oral penicillin V, 250 mg bid, or sulfadiazine, 500 mg bid (250 mg bid for those <60 lb), is also effective.

II. REACTIVE ARTHRITIS (RA):

A. Definition, Etiology, and Pathogenesis:

1. RA is joint inflammation following an infection at a distant site (usually GI or genitourinary). Affected joints are not infected. **Reiter's syndrome,** a form of reactive arthritis, is the triad of reactive arthritis, urethritis, and conjunctivitis.
2. RA generally results from a cross-reactive host immune response to cell wall or extracellular antigens of an infecting organism.
3. A majority of RA patients are positive for HLA-B27, indicating a genetic predisposition.
4. Certain organisms are associated with RA in susceptible individuals:
   a. Most pediatric cases of RA follow a diarrheal illness by *Salmonella, Yersinia, Campylobacter,* or *Shigella flexneri* (no other *Shigella*).
   b. Genital infections with *Chlamydia* are associated with RA, mostly in sexually active adolescents.
   c. RA may occur in 1% to 2% of children recovering from meningococcal or *Hemophilus influenzae* meningitis, which occurs later than does pyogenic arthritis.
   d. Rubella vaccination leads to short-lived RA in 1% to 2% of recipients, particularly in women. Arthritis may be recurrent in 0.1% of vaccinated children.
   e. Enteroviral infections induce RA in about 0.1% of those infected.
   f. The chronic arthritis of Lyme disease may represent, in part, RA.

B. Clinical and Laboratory Findings:

1. Primarily large joints are involved. Elbows and knees are most frequently affected in postmeningitis RA.

2. Some patients with postdiarrheal RA or postgenital Chlamydia infection RA have the complete triad of Reiter's syndrome (conjunctivitis, urethritis, RA).
3. RA is generally self-limited, lasting a few weeks to a few months. It is only rarely recurrent in children.
4. Synovial fluid aspiration is often required to distinguish RA from septic arthritis (see Table 6–15). Synovial fluid in RA contains neutrophils but is not grossly purulent and is sterile. In meningitis-associated RA, microbial antigens can be detected by latex agglutination or counterimmunoelectrophoresis (CIE) in synovial fluid, but culture is sterile.
5. An elevated ESR and mild leukocytosis are usual.

C. Therapy:

1. A nonsteroidal anti-inflammatory agent is used until symptoms subside.
2. Bacterial infections that trigger RA should be treated with appropriate antibiotics.

III. POSTSTREPTOCOCCAL GLOMERULONEPHRITIS (PSGN):

A. Etiology and Pathogenesis:

1. PSGN is an immune complex–mediated disorder that follows either pharyngeal or skin infection with certain nephritogenic strains of GAS.
2. The latent period between pharyngeal GAS infection and PSGN averages 10 days and averages about 4 weeks between GAS skin infection and PSGN.
3. Pathologic findings include subepithelial deposition of immune complexes, resulting in diffuse proliferative or exudative glomerular changes.

B. Epidemiology:

1. PSGN occurs at any age but is most common in young children and in males.
2. Recurrences of PSGN are unusual.

C. Clinical Findings:

1. PSGN typically manifests with acute onset of edema, hematuria, proteinuria, oliguria or anuria, hypertension, and azotemia.
2. Marked hypocomplementemia, with depressed total hemo-

lytic complement, C3, and properdin levels, is present. This typically resolves within 6 to 8 weeks.

3. Serologic and/or culture evidence of recent or active GAS infection usually confirms the diagnosis in the appropriate clinical setting. Serologic tests for detection of antecedent GAS infection are discussed in the section on RF.
4. PSGN is usually self-limited in children but may lead to chronic renal disease in 20% of adults with PSGN.

D. Therapy:

1. Penicillin or erythromycin is given to eradicate any residual streptococci. Diuretics and antihypertensive agents may be required.
2. PSGN, unlike ARF, probably cannot be prevented by prompt therapy of GAS infection. In addition, because recurrences are rare, prophylactic antibiotics to prevent recurrences are not recommended.

IV. NEUROLOGIC SYNDROMES:

A. Postinfectious encephalomyelitis (ECM) secondary to measles, varicella, or rubella:

1. Disease process involves myelin destruction without neuronal damage and is thought to represent an autoimmune hypersensitivity phenomenon triggered by the antecedent infection.
2. Incidence is about 1:1000 cases of measles, 1:10,000 cases of varicella, and 1:20,000 cases of rubella.
3. In all three infections, symptoms of ECM usually appear within 10 days of onset of the rash. Clinical findings associated with ECM include irritability and drowsiness. Focal neurologic signs, seizures, and coma occur in more severe cases. The CSF may be normal or may show a lymphocytosis and an elevated protein level. Although rare, postrubella ECM tends to be severe, with one half of all cases progressing to coma. Postmeasles ECM is somewhat less severe, but nearly one half of all patients experience seizures. Postvaricella ECM is the least severe of the three and typically manifests with hypotonia and ataxia.
4. Postinfectious ECM is a self-limited disease, but survivors may be left with major neurologic sequelae, particularly after postmeasles ECM.
5. Aside from symptomatic treatment, no therapy exists.

B. Transverse myelitis (TM):

1. TM occurs in association with or after a variety of infections, including Epstein-Barr virus, influenza, measles, mumps, rubella, hepatitis B, and herpes.
2. The disease probably results from a cell-mediated autoimmune response that produces a focal, transverse infiltration and necrosis of one or more spinal cord segments. TM usually manifests with back or extremity pain or sensory loss, followed by rapidly progressive paraparesis that may be ascending. Loss of sphincter tone is present. CSF pleocytosis and elevated protein level are seen in about one half of cases.
3. The disease is self-limited, and about 60% of patients have good return of function. No therapy exists except for supportive care.

C. Guillain-Barré Syndrome:

1. This syndrome typically begins within 2 weeks after an often nonspecific viral infection.
2. The disease may involve both cellular and humoral immune responses triggered by an infectious agent. This response results in Schwann cell damage and segmental demyelination at all levels of the peripheral nervous system.
3. The initial symptom is usually lower extremity weakness, which ascends and is usually symmetric. Respiratory muscle involvement occurs in more severe cases. Proprioception may be impaired. Cranial nerve palsies may appear at any point; the facial nerve is most commonly involved. The most characteristic laboratory finding is an elevated CSF protein level without pleocytosis (albumino-cytologic dissociation). Symptoms often evolve rapidly and plateau within 1 to 2 weeks. Complete recovery, usually within 2 months, is seen in most pediatric cases.
4. No proved therapy exists, although plasmapheresis is frequently used.

D. Acute cerebellar ataxia:

1. This disease occurs after a variety of viral infections, most commonly varicella.
2. Pathophysiology may involve direct viral invasion of the cerebellum or an autoimmune response triggered by the infecting agent.

3. Clinical findings include the acute onset of severe truncal ataxia with deterioration of gait. Nystagmus occurs in about one half of cases, and speech is often affected. The CSF is either normal or demonstrates a mild pleocytosis. The disease is self-limited in about two thirds of cases and lasts for 1 week to 2 months. Neurologic deficits persist in about one third of cases.
4. No effective therapy is available.

PREVENTION OF INFECTIONS ASSOCIATED WITH INTERNATIONAL TRAVEL 13

I. SOURCES OF INFORMATION:

The most comprehensive information on medical issues relating to foreign travel is found in the booklet *Health Information for International Travel,* which is published by the Centers for Disease Control (CDC). State and local health departments may be consulted for updated information before travel. In addition, information is available from the CDC at 404-639-1610.

II. EVALUATION:

A. **When evaluating a child** who will be traveling to another country, the physician should assess the patient's current status and then decide what precautions need to be taken considering the risks associated with travel to that area.

B. **If ongoing care will be necessary,** a detailed history and management plan should be prepared for the parent(s) to take.

C. **The physician should review the itinerary,** noting whether the points of destination are rural or urban areas and noting the length of stay at each location. The physician should then determine what (if anything) is required by the countries to be visited and what precautions (i.e., vaccinations, immune globulin, prophylactic antibiotics) should be taken.

III. GENERAL PRECAUTIONS:

A. Food and water are the most common vectors of infectious agents that can be spread by the fecal-oral route (hepatitis A, non-A, non-B hepatitis, typhoid fever, etc.):

1. In areas where sanitation is poor, one should not consume beverages (including ice) made from water that has not been boiled first.
2. Water (including that used to brush teeth) should be boiled first.
3. Carbonated bottled or canned drinks, beer, and wine are usually safe to drink.
4. **It is not safe** to eat raw vegetables, unpeeled fruit, or undercooked seafood.

B. Those planning to hike or camp in rural areas should be advised about local hazards:

1. Clothing should cover as much of the body as possible to minimize the risk of contact with mosquitoes, ticks, snakes, or hazardous plants.
2. Because rabies is endemic in many parts of the world (Asia, Europe, Central and South America, Africa), one should avoid touching wild animals.
3. Swimming may be risky in certain areas where leptospirosis or schistosomiasis (Puerto Rico, the Nile Valley, Central Africa, India, the Middle East, Southeast Asia) is endemic.

IV. IMMUNIZATION AND PROPHYLAXIS:

A. Routine immunizations should be up to date, including all required boosters:

1. The prevalence of vaccine-preventable illnesses may be higher in the countries to be visited than in the United States.
2. Measles vaccine should be given to infants 6 to 11 months of age before departure. They should be revaccinated with measles-mumps-rubella (MMR) at 15 months (or 12 months if they reside in a high-risk area).

B. Special immunizations:

1. Yellow fever vaccine:
   a. This vaccine is available only at official yellow fever vaccination centers; locations can be provided by local state departments of health.

   b. Yellow fever vaccine is recommended for those traveling to areas where this disease is present (certain African countries, Central and South America, China).
   c. The vaccine is highly effective and may provide protection for as along as 30 to 40 years.
   d. Yellow fever and cholera are the only diseases for which some countries require vaccination.
2. Cholera vaccine:
   a. Cholera vaccine is of limited value and is thought to be about 50% effective for a 3- to 6-month period.
   b. Cholera immunization is required by some countries in Asia, the Middle East, and Africa.
   c. Primary series consists of two doses at least 1 week apart. Dosing is as follows:

6 mo–4 yr:	0.2 mL SQ or IM
5–10 yr:	0.3 mL
>10 yr:	0.5 mL

   Immunization of children <6 months of age is not recommended.
   d. Yellow fever and cholera vaccines should not be given concurrently. Ideally they should be separated by at least 3 weeks.
3. Typhoid vaccine should be given to those traveling to areas where typhoid fever is endemic and to those who will be consuming food and water at nontourist facilities. Dosing is two doses of 0.5 mL SQ 3 weeks apart for those ≥10 years old and two doses of 0.25 mL SQ 3 weeks apart for those 6 months to 10 years of age. A new live attenuated oral typhoid vaccine (Ty21a) has recently become available.
4. Meningococcal vaccine should be considered for those traveling to endemic areas in central Africa and Brazil or to countries with active meningococcal A or C epidemics.
5. Hepatitis B virus (HBV) vaccination should be considered for persons who plan to reside > 6 months in areas in which HBV infection is highly endemic and who will have close contact with the local population. Ideally vaccination should begin ≥ 6 months before travel to enable completion of the full series; however, partial series offer some protection against HBV infection.

6. Hepatitis A virus:
   a. TravelerS to developing areas should receive 0.02 mL/kg of immune globulin for stays ≤ 3 months.
   b. For longer stays, 0.06 mL/kg should be given q5mo.
   c. Travelers should be counseled about avoiding potentially contaminated food or water.

V. MALARIA (see Table A–19):

A. Malaria is probably the greatest threat to foreign travelers.

B. The following precautions should be taken to minimize the risk of malaria:
1. Reduce outdoor activities in the evening and nighttime hours, because *Anopheles* mosquitoes feed during these hours.
2. Wear clothing that covers as much of the body as possible when outdoors.
3. Use insect repellents.
4. Sleeping quarters should be screened, and mosquito nets should enclose the bed.

C. The proper prophylactic regimen for malaria is dependent on the following factors: The risk of malaria in a given area, the presence of chloroquine-resistant *Plasmodium falciparum* (CRPF), the length of stay, and history of allergies to any of the medications to be used:
1. For travel to areas with little or no CRPF:
   Chloroquine phosphate (5 mg base/kg) once weekly starting 1 week before departure and continuing for 4 weeks after last exposure.
2. For travel to areas where CRPF is endemic, one of the following regimens should be given:
   a. Chloroquine given as listed earlier, plus a treatment dose of pyrimethamine-sulfadoxine (Fansidar), the latter to be taken **only** if a febrile illness develops. In this situation, chloroquine should be continued and medical care sought to evaluate the patient. Pediatric dosage for pyrimethamine-sulfadoxine is as follows:
      <2 mo: Contraindicated
      2 mo–1 yr.: ¼ tablet
      1–3 yr: ½ tablet
      4–8 yr: 1 tablet

9–14 yr: 2 tablets
>14 yr: 3 tablets

b. Mefloquine is an effective alternative, given once weekly, starting 1 week before travel and continuing for 4 weeks, then every other week until 4 weeks after last exposure. Mefloquine is not recommended in children weighing <15 kg. Dosage is as follows:
   15 to 19 kg: ¼ tablet/week
   20 to 30 kg: ½ tablet/week
   31 to 45 kg: ¾ tablet/week
   >45 kg: 1 tablet/week

BIBLIOGRAPHY

American Academy of Pediatrics: *Report of the Committee on Infectious Diseases,* ed 22, Elk Grove Village, Ill, 1991, The Academy.

American Medical Association: *Drug evaluations, 1991,* Chicago, 1991, The Association.

Bartlett JG: *Pocketbook of infectious disease therapy,* Baltimore, 1991, Williams & Wilkins.

Feigen RD, Cherry JD: *Textbook of pediatric infectious diseases,* ed 2, Philadelphia, 1987, WB Saunders.

Gantz NM, Gleckman RA, Brown RB, et al: *Manual of clinical problems in infectious disease,* Boston, 1986, Little, Brown.

Hoeprich PD, Jordan MC: *Infectious diseases,* ed 4, Philadelphia, 1989, JB Lippincott.

Krugman S, Katz SL, Gershon AA, et al: *Infectious diseases of children,* ed 9, St Louis, 1992, Mosby–Year Book.

Mandell GL, Douglas RG, Bennett JE: *Principles and practice of infectious diseases,* ed 3, New York, 1990, Churchill Livingstone.

Manson-Bahr PEC, Bell DR: *Manson's Tropical Diseases,* ed 19, London, 1987, Bailliere Tindall.

Moffet HL: *Pediatric infectious diseases,* ed 3, Philadelphia, 1989, JB Lippincott.

Nelson JD: *1991–1992 Pocketbook of pediatric antimicrobial therapy,* ed 9, Baltimore, 1991, Williams & Wilkins.

Nelson JD, editor: *Current therapy in pediatric infectious disease,* ed 2, Toronto, 1988, BC Decker.

Reese RE, Betts RF: *A practical approach to infectious diseases,* ed 3, Boston, 1992, Little, Brown.

Remington JS, Klein JO: *Infectious disease of the fetus and newborn infant,* ed 3, Philadelphia, 1990, WB Saunders.

Sanford JP: *Guide to antimicrobial therapy 1991,* Bethesda, Md, 1991, Antimicrobial Therapy.

Sherris JC: *Medical microbiology: an introduction to infectious diseases,* ed 2, New York, 1990, Elsevier.

Shulman ST, Phair JP, Sommers HM: *The biologic and clinical basis of infectious diseases,* ed 4, Philadelphia, 1992, WB Saunders.

Appendix

LOWE'S TABLES OF ANTIMICROBIAL AGENTS

I: NEONATAL USE OF ANTIMICROBIALS

TABLE A–1.
Antibacterial Drugs for Newborn Infants

Antibiotics (mg/kg)	Routes	Wt <1,200 g (Age 0–4 wk)	Wt 1,200–2,000 g		Wt >2,000 g	
			<1 wk. old	>1 wk. old	<1 wk old	>1 wk old
Amikacin	IV, IM	7.5 q12h	7.5 q12h	7.5 q8h	7.5 q12h	7.5 q8h
Ampicillin	IV, IM					
Meningitis		50–100 q12h	50–100 q12h	50–100 q8h	50–100 q8h	50–100 q6h
Nonmeningitis		25–50 q12h	25–50 q12h	25–50 q8h	25–50 q8h	25–50 q6h
Aztreonam	IV, IM	30 q12h	30 q12h	30 q8h	30 q8h	30 q6h
Cefotaxime	IV, IM	50 q12h	50 q12h	50 q8h	50 q12h	50 q8h
Ceftazidime	IV, IM	50 q12h	50 q12h	50 q8h	30 q8h	50 q8h

Ceftriaxone	IV, IM	50 q24h	50–75 q24h	50 q12h or 75q 24h	50–75 q12–24h	50q 12h or 75 q24h
Cephalothin	IV	20 q12h	20 q12h	20 q8h	20 q8h	20 q6h
Chloramphenicol	IV, PO	25 q24h	25 q24h	25 q24h	25 q24h	25 q12h
Clindamycin	IV, IM, PO	5 q12h	5 q12h	5 q8h	5 q8h	5 q6h
Erythromycin	PO	10 q12h	10 q12h	10 q8h	10 q12h	10 q8h
Gentamicin	IV, IM	2.5 q 18-24h	2.5 q12h	2.5 q8h	2.5 q12h	2.5 q8h
Metronidazole	IV, PO	7.5 q48h	7.5 q24h	7.5 q12h	7.5 q12h	15 q12h
Nafcillin	IV	25 q12h	25 q12h	25 q8h	25 q8h	25 q6h
Penicillin G	IV					
Meningitis		50,000 U/kg q12h	50,000 U/kg q12h	75,000 U/kg q8h	50,000 U/kg q8h	50,000–100,000 U/kg q6h
Nonmeningitis		25,000 U/kg q12h	25,000 U/kg q12h	25,000 U/kg q8h	25,000 U/kg q8h	25,000–50,000 U/kg q6h
Ticarcillin	IV, IM	75 q12h	75 q12h	75 q8h	75 q8h	75 q6h
Vancomycin	IV	15 q24h	10–15 q12h	10 q8h	15 q12h	10 q8h

TABLE A–2
SELECTED CLINICAL APPLICATIONS OF ANTIBIOTICS IN NEONATAL INFECTIONS

Drug	Application
Penicillin G	Group B streptococcal sepsis/meningitis Pneumococcal infections Congenital syphilis
Ampicillin	Empiric therapy of suspected bacterial infection (with aminoglycoside or third generation cephalosporin) Group B streptococcal sepsis/meningitis Listeriosis
Nafcillin/methicillin	Susceptible staphylococcal infections
Ticarcillin/piperacillin	*Pseudomonas aeruginosa* infections Susceptible proteus infections
Cephalothin/cefazolin	Limited usefulness; use only in non-CNS infections caused by susceptible organisms
Cefotaxime	Aminoglycoside-resistant gram-negative enteric bacilli Meningitis caused by susceptible organism Empiric therapy of suspected bacterial infection (with ampicillin)
Ceftriaxone	Aminoglycoside-resistant gram-negative enteric bacilli Meningitis caused by susceptible organism Gonococcal ophthalmia neonatorum Empiric therapy of suspected bacterial infection (with ampicillin)
Ceftazidime	Invasive infection with *P. aeruginosa* or other gram-negative organisms
Vancomycin	*Staphylococcus epidermidis* and other methicillin-resistant staphylococcal infections
Gentamicin/amikacin	Invasive infection with gram-negative bacilli (for meningitis, consider broad-spectrum cephalosporin)
Erythromycin	Chlamydial conjunctivitis and pneumonitis Pertussis
Clindamycin	Infection with anaerobic organisms

TABLE A–3.
Placental Transfer of Antibiotics

I. Agents readily passed to infant (infant/maternal serum levels >50%):
- Acyclovir
- Carbenicillin
- Cefoxitin
- Chloramphenicol*
- Griseofulvin
- Isoniazid*
- Methicillin
- Metronidazole
- Mezlocillin
- Nitrofurantoin*
- Sulfonamides*
- Tetracyclines*
- Trimethoprim-sulfamethoxazole*
- Zidovudine (AZT)

II. Agents passed moderately well (infant/maternal serum levels 30%–50%):
- Amphotericin B*
- Ampicillin
- Cefoperazone
- Cefuroxime
- Clindamycin
- Gentamicin*
- Kanamycin*
- Penicillin G
- Rifampin
- Streptomycin*

III. Agents passed poorly transplacentally (infant/maternal serum levels <30%):
- Amikacin*
- Aztreonam
- Cefazolin
- Cefotaxime
- Ceftriaxone
- Cephalothin
- Cephradine
- Dicloxacillin
- Erythromycin
- Nafcillin
- Oxacillin
- Tobramycin*

*Potential adverse effect on fetus.

TABLE A–4.
Antibiotics in Breast Milk

I. Agents readily excreted into milk (milk/serum level >50%):
- Acyclovir
- Amikacin
- Ampicillin
- Carbenicillin
- Chloramphenicol
- Erythromycin
- Gentamicin
- Isoniazid
- Metronidazole
- Sulfonamides
- Tetracyclines
- Trimethoprim

II. Agents poorly excreted into milk (milk/serum level <50%):
- Amantadine
- Azlocillin
- Aztreonam
- Cephalexin
- Cefazolin
- Cefoperazone
- Cefotaxime
- Cefoxitin
- Ceftriaxone
- Cephalothin
- Clindamycin
- Kanamycin
- Methicillin
- Mezlocillin
- Nafcillin
- Nalidixic acid
- Nitrofurantoin
- Oxacillin
- Penicillin G and V
- Pyrimethamine
- Streptomycin

II: ANTIBIOTIC DOSAGES

TABLE A–5.
Summary of Commonly Used Antibiotics

Generic Name	Spectrum of Activity	Route	Standard Pediatric Dosage*	Comments
Amikacin	Gram-negative aerobes(*Pseudomonas, Escherichia coli, Proteus, Klebsiella, Enterobacter, Serratia, Citrobacter, Providencia)*	IV, IM	5–7.5 mg/kg/dose q8–12h	Follow levels (see Table A–16)
Amoxicillin	Gram-positives (not β-lactamase-positive *Staphylococcus aureus*); Active vs. many enterococci; gram-negatives (some *E. coli, Proteus, Klebsiella, Salmonella,* β-*lactamase-negative Hemophilus influenzae)*	PO	30–50 mg/kg/day q8h	Better oral absorption than ampicillin; not as effective as ampicillin in shigellosis

(Continued.)

TABLE A–5 (cont.).

Generic Name	Spectrum of Activity	Route	Standard Pediatric Dosage*	Comments
Amoxicillin-clavulanate	Gram-positives (active vs. β-lactamase-positive *S. aureus*, not MRSA†); gram-negatives (active vs. β-lactamase-positive *H. influenzae, Moraxella catarrhalis, E. coli, Proteus, Klebsiella);* anaerobes (including *Bacteroides fragilis*)	PO	30–40 mg/kg/day (amoxicillin component) q8h	
Ampicillin	Same as amoxicillin; also active vs. most *Shigella* spp.	PO	50 mg/kg/day q6h	Rash particularly with infectious mononucleosis; frequently causes diarrhea
		IV, IM	Mild-moderate infections: 50–100 mg/kg/day q6h Severe infections: 200–400 mg/kg/day q6h	
Ampicillin-sulbactam	Same as amoxicillin-clavulanate	IV, IM	See Ampicillin	

Azlocillin	Gram-positives (not β-lactamase-positive or MRSA); gram-negatives (including *Pseudomonas, Enterobacter, Providencia; Serratia, Klebsiella,* and *Acinetobacter* variable); anaerobes including *B. fragilis*	IV	300–450 mg/kg/day q4–6h	Antipseudomonal activity
Aztreonam	Gram-negatives (Neisseria, *H. influenzae, Enterobacter, Pseudomonas aeruginosa;* not *Acinetobacter, Xanthomonas maltophilia,* or *Pseudomonas cepacia)*	IM, IV	90–120 mg/kg/day q6h	Safe in penicillin allergic individuals; spectrum very similar to that of aminoglycosides (without nephrotoxicity)
Bacampicillin	Same as ampicillin	PO	As per ampicillin	Hydrolyzed to ampicillin
Carbenicillin	Gram-positives (not β-lactamase-positive or MRSA); gram-negatives *(Pseudomonas, Proteus, E. coli, Enterobacter, H. influenzae, M. catarrhalis;* not *Klebsiella) Bacteroides* spp. at high doses	IV PO	400–600 mg/kg/day q4–6h 30–50 mg/kg/day q6h	$4.7\ mEqNa^{+}/g$ Few indications for this agent now

(Continued.)

TABLE A–5 (cont.).

Generic Name	Spectrum of Activity	Route	Standard Pediatric Dosage*	Comments
Cefaclor	Gram-positives (not enterococci; variable vs. β-lactamase-positive *S. aureus* and *Neisseria*, not MRSA; gram-negatives (especially *H. influenzae, M. catarrhalis;* most *E. coli, Proteus, Klebsiella;* variable vs. *Salmonella* and *Shigella;* not *Enterobacter, Pseudomonas* or *Acinetobacter)*	PO	30–40 mg/kg/day q8h	May cause serum sickness–like reaction
Cefadroxil	Similar to cefaclor; variable vs. *H. influenzae* or *M. catarrhalis*	PO	30 mg/kg/day q12h	Twice daily dosing is convenient
Cefamandole	Gram-positives (not enterococci, MRSA); gram-negatives *(E. coli, Proteus, Klebsiella, Citrobacter, H. influenzae;* variable vs. *Enterobacter;* not *Pseudomonas, Serratia* or *Acinetobacter);* anaerobes (not *B. fragilis*)	IV, IM	100–150 mg/kg/day q4–6h	Inadequate CSF concentrations for meningitis

Cefazolin	Gram-positives (not enterococci, MRSA); gram-negatives (*E. coli, Proteus mirabilis, Klebsiella, H. influenzae;* not indole-positive *Proteus, Enterobacter, Pseudomonas, Serratia,* or *Acinetobacter*)	IV, IM	50–150 mg/kg/day q8h	Parenteral first-generation cephalosporin
Cefixime	Gram-positives (Not *S. aureus,* enterococci, *Listeria*); gram-negatives (not *Pseudomonas, Acinetobacter,* or *Bacteroides*)	PO	8 mg/kg/day q12–24h	Therapeutic role remains to be defined
Cefoperazone	Gram-positives (not enterococci, MRSA, *Staphylococcus epidermidis, Listeria*); gram-negatives (*E. coli, Proteus, Klebsiella, Enterobacter, Citrobacter, Providencia, H. influenzae;* variable vs. *Serratia, Pseudomonas;* not *Acinetobacte);* anaerobes; variable vs. *B. fragilis*	IV, IM	100–150 mg/kg/day q8–12h	70% elminated in bile unchanged; inadequate CSF concentrations for meningitis
Ceforanide	Similar to cefamandole	IV, IM	20–40 mg/kg/day q12h	Not approved for infants <1 yr

(Continued.)

TABLE A–5 (cont.).

Generic Name	Spectrum of Activity	Route	Standard Pediatric Dosage*	Comments
Cefotaxime	Gram-positives (not enterococci, MRSA, *Listeria*); gram-negatives *(E. coli, Proteus, Klebsiella, Enterobacter, Citrobacter, H. influenzae, M. catarrhalis,* variable vs. *Pseudomonas;* not *Acinetobacter);* variable vs. *B. fragilis;* not *Clostridium difficile*	IV, IM	100–150 mg/kg/day (meningitis 200 mg/kg/day) q6–8h	Good CSF activity; parenteral third-generation drug
Cefoxitin	Gram-positives (not enterococci, MRSA, *Listeria*); gram-negatives *(E. coli, Klebsiella, H. influenzae, M. catarrhalis, Proteus;* not *Pseudomonas, Enterobacter, Serratia;* active vs. *B. fragilis*	IV, IM	80–160 mg/kg/day q4–8h	Parenteral second-generation agent with excellent anaerobic activity
Ceftazidime	Similar to cefotaxime; active vs. *Pseudomonas* and most *Acinetobacter* spp.; not *B. fragilis* or *C. difficile*	IV, IM	100–150 mg/kg/day q8h	Best antipseudomonal cephalosporin
Ceftizoxime	Similar to cefotaxime; active vs. most *Pseudomonas* and *Acinetobacter* spp.; active vs. *B. fragilis;* not *C. difficile*	IV, IM	150–200 mg/kg/day q6–8h	Good CSF activity

Ceftriaxone	Similar to cefotaxime	IV, IM	50–100 mg/kg/day c12–24h	A single daily dose of 80 mg/kg can be used for treatment of serious infections; excellent activity in CSF; long half-life
Cefuroxime	Similar to cefoxitin; more active vs. gram-positive and *H. influenzae;* not usually active vs. *B. fragilis* and *C. difficile*	IV, IM	100–150 mg/kg/day (meningitis 240 mg/kg/day) q8h	Excellent choice for respiratory tract, skin, soft tissue, bone, and joint infections
Cefuroxime Axetil	See cefuroxime	PO	30–40 mg/kg/day q12h	Oral second-generation
Cephalexin	Gram-positives (not enterococci, MRSA; variable vs. β-lactamase-positive staphylococci and neisseria); gram-negatives (most *E. coli, P. mirabilis,* some *Klebsiella, Salmonella,* and *Shigella,* spp.; not *Enterobacter, Pseudomonas, Acinetobacter*)	PO	25–50 mg/kg/day q6h	Oral first-generation
Cephalothin	Similar to cefazolin	IV, IM	75–125 mg/kg/day q6h	Parenteral first-generation
Cephapirin	Similar to cefazolin	IV, IM	40–80 mg/kg/day c6h	Parenteral first-generation
Cephradine	Similar to cephalexin	PO	25–50 mg/kg/day c6h	Oral first-generation
Chloramphenicol	Gram-positives; gram-negatives *Chlamydia;* rickettsiae; anaerobes (including *B. fragilis*)	IV, PO	50–100 mg/kg/day (IV); 50–75 mg/kg/day (PO)	Follow levels; use only for serious infections; bacteriostatic except for *H. influenzae*

(Continued.)

TABLE A–5 (cont.).

Generic Name	Spectrum of Activity	Route	Standard Pediatric Dosage*	Comments
Ciprofloxacin	Gram-positives (not enterococci, *Listeria;* variable vs. *Streptococcus pneumoniae* and group A streptococci); gram-negatives (including *Pseudomonas*); not *B. fragilis*	PO	20–30 mg/kg/day q12h	Not approved for patients <21 yr
Clindamycin	Gram-positives (Not enterococci); anaerobes; most *B. fragilis,* not *C. difficile;* parasites: *Plasmodium falciparum, Toxoplasma gondii*	IV, IM PO	25–40 mg/kg/day q6–8h. 20–30 mg/kg/day	Not to be used for CNS infections
Cloxacillin	Gram-positive, especially *S. aureus* (not MRSA)	PO	50–100 mg/kg/day q6h	
Colistimethate	Gram-negatives (especially *Pseudomonas,* not *Proteus*)	IV, IM	5 mg/kg/day q6–8h	Rarely used now
Colistin sulfate	See colistimethate	PO	10–15 mg/kg/day q8h	Nonabsorbable oral agent for GI infection
Dicloxacillin	Same as cloxacillin	PO	20–50 mg/kg/day q6h	Taste is a deterrent

Metronidazole	Anaerobes (including *B. fragilis*, clostridia, *Gardnerella vaginalis;* not *Propionobacterium, Actinomyces*); *C. jejuni, Entamoeba histolytica, Giardia, Trichomonas*	PO IV	15–35 mg/kg/day q8h 30 mg/kg/day q6h	Antabuse-like reactions; excellent anaerobic agent
Mezlocillin	Gram-positives (not β-lactamase-positive or MRSA) gram-negatives (including *Klebsiella, Enterobacter, H. influenzae, Providencia, Pseudomonas, Serratia*) anaerobes including *B. fragilis*	IV	200–300 mg/kg/day q4–6h	Almost 2 mEq Na*/g; similar to azlocillin
Minocycline	Gram-positives (more effective than other tetracyclines vs. *S. aureus*); gram-negatives (some *Acinetobacter, Chlamydia, Mycobacterium marinum*)	PO	4 mg/kg/day q12h	Patients >7 or 8 yr
Moxalactam	Gram-positives (not enterococci, *Listeria*, MRSA); gram-negatives (*E. coli, Citrobacter, Enterobacter, H. influenzae, M. catarrhalis, Klebsiella, Proteus;* few *Pseudomonas* spp; not *Acinetobacter, Campylobacter*); anaerobes: not *C. difficile*	IV	150–200 mg/kg/day q6–8h	Limited pediatric use at present

(Continued.)

TABLE A–5 (cont.).

Generic Name	Spectrum of Activity	Route	Standard Pediatric Dosage*	Comments
Mupirocin	Impetigo caused by *S. aureus*, group A streptococci; nasal *S. aureus* carriers	Topical	Apply to infected skin q8h	A pseudomonal product that is very active
Nafcillin	Gram-positives, especially *S. aureus*, not MRSA	IV, IM	50–200 mg/kg/day q6h	Phlebitis common
Nalidixic acid	Gram-negative UTI pathogens *(E. coli, Proteus, Klebsiella;* not *Pseudomonas)*	PO	50 mg/kg/day q6h	Used for UTI; resistance develops rapidly
Neomycin	Gram-negatives (not anaerobes)	PO	100 mg/kg/day q6–8h	Nonabsorbable; enteric infections
Netilmicin	Gram-positives (not *S. pneumoniae);* gram-negative *(E. coli, Enterobacter, Klebsiella, Proteus, Providencia, Pseudomonas, serratia,* some *Acinetobacter* spp.) not anaerobes	IV, IM	3–7.5 mg/kg/day q8h	Little used in United States Monitor levels (see Table A–16)
Nitrofurantoin	Gram-negative UTI pathogens except *Pseudomonas*	PO	5–7 mg/kg/day q6h	Used for UTI; ineffective in renal failure
Norfloxacin	All gram-positive and gram-negative urinary pathogens (including *Pseudomonas* and enterococci)	PO	400 mg q12h	Quinolone not approved for children

Oxacillin	Gram-positives, especially *S. aureus* (not MRSA)	IM, IV	150–200 mg/kg/day q6h	Like nafcillin, methicillin
Oxytetracycline	Gram-positives, gram-negatives; anaerobes: *Clostridia;* not *B. fragilis; Chlamydia, M. pneumoniae,* rickettsiae	PO	40–50 mg/kg/day q6h	Patients >7 or 8 yr
Penicillin G, benzathine	Group A streptococci; syphilis	IM	50,000 units/kg	Long-acting (~28 days) depot injection
Penicillin G, crystalline	Gram-positives (not β-lactamase-positive *S. aureus*); gram-negatives *(Neisseria)*	IM, IV	100,000–400,000 U/kg/day q4–6h	
Penicillin G	Same as Penicillin G	PO	25,000–50,000 U/kg/day q6–8h	1,600 U = 1 mg
Penicillin V	Same as Penicillin G	PO	25,000–50,000 U/kg/day q6–8h	Better absorbed than Penicillin G
Piperacillin	Gram-positives (not β-lactamase-positive or MRSA); gram-negatives (including *Enterobacter, Klebsiella, Pseudomonas, Providencia* variable, not *Serratia*); anaerobes including *B. fragilis*	IV	200–300 mg/kg/day q4–6h	Similar to ticarcillin
Polymyxin B	Gram-negatives (especially *Pseudomonas;* not *Proteus*)	IM, IV	3–4.5 mg/kg/day q6h	10,000 U = 1 mg; very limited use

(Continued.)

TABLE A–5 (cont.).

Generic Name	Spectrum of Activity	Route	Standard Pediatric Dosage*	Comments
Rifampin	Gram-positives (including MRSA; variable vs. enterococci); gram-negatives (*Neisseria, H. influenzae, L. pneumophila*); anaerobes: *C. difficile, B. fragilis;* also active vs. *Chlamydia, Mycobacterium tuberculosis*, some atypical mycobacteria (*M. kansasii, M. marinum, M. leprae*)	PO, IV	10–20 mg/kg/day q12–24h	Resistance develops rapidly, especially when used alone; penetrates tissues well
Spectinomycin	*Neisseria gonorrhoeae*, including penicillinase-producing strains	IM	40 mg/kg × 1 dose	
Streptomycin	Gram-negatives (*F. tularensis, Y. pestis, Brucella*) *M. tuberculosis*	IM	20–30 mg/kg/day q12h	Currently used as second-line drug for tuberculosis
Sulfadiazine	UTI pathogens (*E. coli, P. mirabilis;* some *Klebsiella, Proteus, Enterobacter*, and *Pseudomonas*-resistant spp.) *T. gondii, P. falciparum*	PO	120–150 mg/kg/day q4–6h	Stevens-Johnson, erythema multiforme reactions
Sulfamethizole	UTI pathogens	PO	30–45 mg/kg/day q6h	Stevens-Johnson, erythema multiforme reactions

Sulfamethoxazole	UTI pathogens	PO	50–60 mg/kg/day q12h	Stevens-Johnson, erythema multiforme reactions
Sulfasoxazole	UTI pathogens	PO	120–150 mg/kg/day q4–6h	Stevens-Johnson, erythema multiforme reactions
Tetracycline	Similar to oxytetracycline	PO IV	25–50 mg/kg/day q6h 20–30 mg/kg/day q8–12h	Patients >7 or 8 yr
Ticarcillin	Gram-positives (not MRSA); Gram-negatives (*Pseudomonas, Proteus, E. coli, Enterobacter, H. influenzae, M. catarrhalis;* not *Klebsiella*) *Bacteroides* at high doses	IV	200–300 mg/kg/day q4–6h	5.2–6.5 mEqNa*/g
Ticarcillin clavulanate	Gram-positives (not MRSA); gram-negatives (active vs. β-lactamase-positive *H. influenzae, M. catarrhalis, Klebsiella, Enterobacter, Pseudomonas, Proteus, E. coli;* effective vs. most *B. fragilis*	IV	200–300 mg/kg/day q4–6h (of Ticarcillin component)	Not yet approved for children
Tobramycin	Gram-positives (*S aureus;* not *S. pneumoniae);* gram-negatives *(P. aeruginosa, Acinetobacter, E. coli, Klebsiella, Enterobacter, Providencia, Proteus, Serratia);* not anaerobes	IV, IM	3–7.5 mg/kg/day q8h	Monitor levels (see Table A–16); Very similar to gentamicin

(Continued.)

TABLE A–5 (cont.).

Generic Name	Spectrum of Activity	Route	Standard Pediatric Dosage*	Comments
Trimethoprim	UTI pathogens (not *Pseudomonas*)	PO	4 mg/kg/day q12h	OK for those who are sulfa-allergic
Trimethoprim-sulfamethoxazole	Gram-positives (not enterococci or Group A streptococci); gram-negatives (*H. influenzae, S. typhi, Pseudomonas pseudomallei;* not *P. aeruginosa, Bacteroides*) variable vs. *Shigella dysenteriae, M. marinum, Nocardia asteroides;* effective vs. *Pneumocystis carinii*	PO, IV	6–12 mg TMP/kg/day q12h Pneumocystis: 20 mg TMP/kg/day q6h	Versatile and widely used drug
Vancomycin	Gram-positives, especially *S. aureus (including MRSA)* and *S. epidermidis,* enterococci, and clostridia	IV	40 mg/kg/day q6h (60 mg/kg/day for meningitis)	Monitor levels; nephrotoxic
		PO	10–50 mg/kg/day q6h	nonabsorbed

*MRSA = methicillin-resistant *S. aureus,* UTI = urinary tract infection.
*Up to maximal dosage as indicated in Table A–7.

TABLE A–6.
Systemic Infections

Site	Diagnosis	Circumstances	Etiologic Agents	Therapy	Comments
Central nervous system infections					
Meninges	Meningitis	Neonate (See Table A–1)	Group B streptococcus, *Escherichia coli*, *Listeria monocytogenes*, *Enterococcus*	Ampicillin and cefotaxime or ceftriaxone (IV), or ampicillin and aminoglycoside (IV) × 14–21 days	
		Infants and children	*Hemophilus influenzae* type b or unknown	Ceftriaxone or cefotaxime (IV) × 7–10 days or ampicillin and chloramphenicol (IV) × 7–10 days	Adjunctive dexamethasone may decrease deafness in *H. influenzae* meningitis
			Streptococcus pneumoniae	Penicillin G (IV) × 10–14 days or ceftriaxone × 10–14 days	
			Neisseria meningitidis	Penicillin G (IV) × 7 days or ceftriaxone (IV) × 7 days	

(Continued.)

TABLE A–6 (cont).

Site	Diagnosis	Circumstances	Etiologic Agents	Therapy	Comments
			Mycobacterium tuberculosis	Isoniazid (INH), 15 mg/kg/day (PO, IM), and rifampin, 15 mg/kg/day (PO, IV), and pyrazinamide 30 mg/kg/day (PO) × 2 mo initially; then INH and rifampin × 10 mo (total = 12 mo)	Some recommend addition of streptomycin; suspected highly resistant organism requires use of additional agents
Brain	Encephalitis		Herpes simplex (HSV)	Acyclovir 30 mg/kg/day (IV) × 21 days	Early diagnosis and treatment crucial
	Brain abscess	Otitis, sinusitis, mastoiditis and congenital heart disease are predisposing factors	Viridans streptococci, anaerobic streptococci, *Staphylococcus aureus,* Enterobacteriaceae, *Bacteroides*	Nafcillin or vancomycin and ceftriaxone and metronidazole (IV) × 6 wk (antibiotics alone) or × 10 day (if excision performed)	Surgical drainage or excision frequently required

Ventricles	Shunt infection	Presence of ventricular shunt	Coagulase-negative Staphylococci, *S. aureus*,	Nafcillin or vancomycin (IV) (therapy should be continued until cultures are negative) × 7–10 days	Removal of shunt apparatus mandatory
			Enterobacteriaceae	Ceftriaxone (IV) until cultures are negative × 10 days	
Eye Infections					
Eye	Conjunctivitis		*H. influenzae* (nontypable), group A streptococci, *S. pneumoniae*, adenovirus, enterovirus 70	Erythromycin or polymyxin bacitracin ointment	
	Hordeolum (sty) or Chalazion		*S. aureus*	No antibiotics	Warm compresses; incision and drainage when necessary
	Keratitis		HSV	Trifluridine 1% and prednisolone acetate 1% × 7–14 days	Ophthalmologic evaluation necessary

(Continued.)

TABLE A–6 (cont).

Site	Diagnosis	Circumstances	Etiologic Agents	Therapy	Comments
	Endophthalmitis	Postoperative, posttraumatic, or hematogenous	*Staphylococcus epidermidis, S. aureus, Streptococcus* spp., Enterobacteriaceae, *N. meningitidis*	Vancomycin or cephalothin plus aminoglycoside (IV and intravitreal) × 10–14 days	Most urgent of all primary ocular infections
	Retinitis	Immunocompromised patients	Cytomegalovirus	Ganciclovir or foscarnet (IV) × 14–21 days, then maintenance therapy	
	Ophthalmia neonatorum	Onset first day	Clemical (silver nitrate)	None	
		Onset age 2–5 days	*N. gonorrhoeae*	Ceftriaxone 125 mg (IV or IM) × 1 dose	
		Onset age 5–10 days	*Chlamydia trachomatis*	Erythromycin (PO) × 10–14 days	
		Onset age 1–16 days	HSV (usually type 2)	See above	
	Orbital cellulitis	Often history of sinusitis or posttraumatic	*S. aureus,* streptococci, anaerobes	Clindamycin or nafcillin (IV) × 2–3 wk	Ophthalmologic evaluation required; surgical intervention often necessary

	Periorbital cellulitis		*H. influenzae, S. pneumoniae, S. aureus*	Cefuroxime (IV) until clinical improvement, then cefaclor (PO) for total 7–10 days	
Upper respiratory infections					
Ear	External otitis		*S. aureus, Pseudomonas aeruginosa,* gram-negative enterics	Corticosporin (polymixin, neomycin, and hydrocortisone) 3 ×/day × 5–7 days	For recurrent "swimmer's ear," VoSol or alcohol-vinegar to ear canal after water exposure
	"Malignant" otitis externa	Usually in diabetics or immunocompromised host	*P. aeruginosa*	Tobramycin and ticarcillin (IV) or ceftazidime (IV) × 6 wk	
	Otitis media	Newborns	Pneumococci, *H. influenzae, Moraxella catarrhalis, S. aureus,* Enterobacteriaceae	Cefaclor or Augmentin (amoxicillin–clavulanate potassium) (PO) × 10 days	Aminoglycoside or ceftriaxone for enteric gram-negative infection

(Continued.)

TABLE A–6 (cont).

Site	Diagnosis	Circumstances	Etiologic Agents	Therapy	Comments
		Infants and children	*S. pneumoniae, H. influenzae, M. catarrhalis*	Amoxicillin, trimethoprim-sulfamethaxazole (TMP/SMX), erythromycin/sulfa, or Augmentin (PO) × 10 days	
Mastoid	Mastoiditis	Acute	*S. pneumoniae,* group A streptococci, *S. aureus, H. influenzae*	Cefuroxime IV × 10 days	Surgery if abscess formation or medical failure
		Chronic	*P. aeruginosa, Proteus* spp., *S. aureus,* anaerobes	Tobramycin and ticarcillin or ceftazidime (IV) × 10–14 days	Daily cleansing of ear; mastoidectomy if necessary
Sinus	Sinusitis	Acute	*S. pneumoniae, H. influenzae, M. catarrhalis, S. aureus*	Amoxicillin or Augmentin (PO) × 21 days	Sinus irrigations when necessary

		Chronic	Viridans streptococci, *S. aureus, H. influenzae, Bacteroides* spp., *Fusobacterium*	Augmentin or cefaclor (PO) × 3–4 wk	Ear-nose-throat (ENT) evaluation for anatomic abnormalities, sinus lavage or antrostomy
Mouth	Vincent's angina		Fusospirochetal organisms	Penicillin V (PO) × 1 wk	Chlorhexidine or hydrogen perioxide rinses
Pharynx	Exudative pharyngitis		Group A streptococci, Group C streptococci, *Arcanobacterium haemolyticum,* infectious mononucleosis	Penicillin V or erythromycin (PO) × 10 days	
	Diphtheria		*Corynebacterium diphtheriae*	Penicillin G (IV) or erythromycin (PO) × 10 days	Diphtheria antitoxin
	Retropharyngeal abscess		Group A streptococci, *S. aureus,* anaerobes (*B. fragilis, B. melanogenicus,* and *Fusobacterium*)	Clindamycin or ampicillin sulbactam (Unasyn) (IV) initially, then clindamycin or Augmentin (PO) × 10–14 days	Surgical (I&D)

(Continued.)

TABLE A–6 (cont).

Site	Diagnosis	Circumstances	Etiologic Agents	Therapy	Comments
Tonsil	Peritonsillar abscess (Quinsy)		Group A streptococci *S. aureus*, anaerobes, *H. influenzae*	Penicillin G or clindamycin (IV) initially, then penicillin V or clindamycin (PO) × 10–14 days	Surgical drainage
Epiglottis	Epiglottitis		*H. influenzae* type b	Cefuroxime (IV) × 7 days or Ampicillin and chloramphenicol	Provide airway
Lower Respiratory Tract Infections					
Bronchi	Bronchitis		Viral or *M. pneumoniae*	None or Erythromycin	
			H. influenzae, M. catarrhalis, S. pneumoniae	Augmentin or amoxicillin (PO) × 5–7 days	
Bronchioles	Bronchiolitis		Respiratory syncytial virus (RSV), parainfluenza	Ribavirin (aerosolized) × 3–5 days	Only in patients with underlying cardiopulmonary disease or immunodeficiency or with severe disease

Lungs	Pneumonia (nonbacterial)	Infants	*C. trachomatis*, RSV, parainfluenzae 3, influenza A and B	Erythromycin (PO) × 14d for chlamydial infection	
		Children	*Mycoplasma pneumoniae*, *C. pneumoniae*, parainfluenzae, influenzae, adenovirus	Erythromycin (PO) × 10 days for chlamydial or mycoplasma infection	
	Pertussis		*Bordetella* spp.	Erythromycin (PO) × 10 days	Hospitalize young infants
	Pneumocystis carinii pneumonia	immunocompromised patients	*P. carinii*	TMP-SMX or pentamidine (IV) × 21 days	Prednisone in moderate to severe cases
	Tuberculosis		*M. tuberculosis*	INH and rifampin (PO) × 9 mo, or INH and ethambutol (PO) × 9 mo, or INH, rifampin, and pyrazinamide (PO) × 2 mo, followed by INH and rifampin × 4 mo	

(Continued.)

TABLE A–6 (cont).

Site	Diagnosis	Circumstances	Etiologic Agents	Therapy	Comments
	Bacterial pneumonia	Neonates	Group B streptococci, *E. coli*, group A streptococci, *S. aureus*	Ampicillin or nafcillin and aminoglycoside or ceftriaxone (IV) × 14 days	
		Infants and Children	*S. pneumoniae, H. influenzae, S. aureus*	Cefuroxime IV × 10 days	
		Immunocompromised host	*L. pneumophila*	Erythromycin (IV) initially, then PO × 3 wk total	Rifampin may be added; rarely documented in children
		Cystic fibrosis	*Pseudomonas* spp.	Tobramycin and ticarcillin or ceftazidime or aztreonam (IV) × 7–10 days (or until clinical improvement seen)	Larger than usual doses often required

	Lung abscess	Common in patients with altered consciousness	*Bacteroides* spp., *Peptococcus, Peptostreptococcus, S. aureus, S. pneumoniae,* group A streptococci, gram-negative bacilli	Clindamycin or penicillin (IV) × 2–3 wk	Surgical drainage or resection may be necessary
Cardiac infections					
Pericardium	Purulent pericarditis		*S. aureus, H. influenzae* type b. *S. pneumoniae, N. meningitidis*	Nafcillin and ceftriaxone (IV) initially, then as indicated by identification and sensitivities of the isolated organism, × 2–4 weeks	Surgical drainage is necessary
Endocardium	Infective endocarditis	Preexisting structural heart disease usually present	Viridans streptococcus	Penicillin G and gentamicin (IV) × 2 wk; then penicillin for 2 wk (total = 4 wk) or vancomycin (IV) × 4 wk	Monitor serum bactericidal activity Longer course of therapy in presence of prosthetic material

(Continued.)

TABLE A–6 (cont).

Site	Diagnosis	Circumstances	Etiologic Agents	Therapy	Comments
			S. aureus, S. epidermidis	Nafcillin or vancomycin (IV) × 6 wk	Consider adding Rifampin or aminoglycoside for synergistic effect
			Enterococcus	Ampicillin or penicillin and gentamicin (IV)× 4–6 wk	Rare in children
	Fungal endocarditis	Immunocompromised patients, central hyperalimentation, prolonged antibiotic use	*Candida* spp., Aspergillus	Amphotericin B (IV) × at least 6 wk	Surgical excision of infected tissue required
	Culture-negative endocarditis			Nafcillin and gentamicin (IV) × 2 wk, then nafcillin (IV) × 4 wk (total = 6 wk)	
Gastrointestinal tract infections					
Gastrointestinal	Diarrhea, Dysentery		Rotavirus, Norwalk agent	None	
			Salmonella spp.	None, unless patient <3 mo or is compromised host	
			Shigella spp.	TMP-SMX (PO, IV) × 5 days	

Campylobacter spp.	Erythromycin (PO) × 5 days	
Vibrio cholerae	TMP-SMX or tetracycline (if > 7 yr) × 2 days	
Yersinia enterocolitica	None or TMP-SMX × 5 days	
Giardia lamblia	Furazolidone or quinacrine or metronidazole (PO) × 7–10 days	
Entamoeba histolytica	Metronidazole (PO) × 10 days, followed by iodoquinol × 20 days	
Cryptosporidium parvum	None	Spiramycin or po Immunoglobulin reported effective in case reports
E. coli		
Enterotoxigenic	None or TMP-SMX (PO) × 5 days	
Enteropathogenic	None or TMP-SMX (PO) × 5 days	
Enteroinvasive	TMP-SMX (PO) × 5 days	
Enterohemorrhagic	TMP-SMX (PO) × 5 days	

(Continued.)

TABLE A–6 (cont).

Site	Diagnosis	Circumstances	Etiologic Agents	Therapy	Comments
	"Turista"		Enterotoxigenic *E. coli*, *Shigella*, *Salmonella*, *G. lamblia*, rotavirus	TMP-SMX × 5 days	
	Pseudomembranous colitis	Associated with antibiotic use	*Clostridium difficile*	Vancomycin (PO) or metronidazole (po or IV) × 7 days	
Peritoneum	Peritonitis	Primary	*S. pneumoniae*	Pencillin G (IV) × 7–10 days	
		Following perforation	Enteric coliforms, *Bacteroides fragilis*, *Enterococcus* spp.	Clindamycin or metronidazole (IV) and aminoglycoside or ceftazidime × 10–14 days	Consider coverage for *Enterococcus;* surgical repair and drainage
		Continuous ambulatory peritoneal dialysis	*S. epidermidis*, *S. aureus*	Cefadyl or vancomycin in dialysate × 7–10 days	
Liver	Liver abscess		*S. aureus*, enteric coliforms, *Bacteroides* spp.	Nafcillin and aminoglycoside (IV) × 4–6 wk	Surgical drainage

Rectum	Perirectal abscess		*S. aureus*, enteric coliforms, anaerobes	Clindamycin and aminoglycoside × 10–14 days (or clinical improvement)	Surgical drainage
Genitourinary tract infections					
Bladder	Cystitis		*E. coli, Proteus* spp., *Klebsiella* spp.	Amoxicillin or TMP-SMX (PO) × 10 days	
Kidney	Pyelonephritis		Same as above	Ampicillin and aminoglycoside (IV) or TMP-SMX (IV) initially, then oral antibiotic (based on sensitivities) for total 10 days	
		Prophylaxis for severe reflux or frequent infections		Nitrofurantoin, 1–2 mg/kg PO q1–2d, or TMP-SMX (TMP 2 mg/kg/day), PO	
Genital tract	Vaginitis/cervicitis	Women taking oral contraceptive pills, antibiotics, corticosteroids	*Candida albicans*	Miconazole or clotrimazole (intravaginally) qhs × 3 days	
			Trichomonas vaginalis	Metronidazole, 40 mg/kg po × 1 or 15 mg/kg/day q8h × 7 days	Treat sex partners

(Continued.)

TABLE A–6 (cont).

Site	Diagnosis	Circumstances	Etiologic Agents	Therapy	Comments
		Referred to as bacterial vaginosis	*Gardnerella vaginalis* anaerobes	Metronidazole × 10–14 days	May or may not be acquired sexually
	Urethritis		*C. trachomatis*	Doxycycline or tetracycline (patients > 7 yr) or erythromycin × 10–14 days	Treat sex partners
	Chancroid		*Hemophilus ducreyi*	Cefriaxone, IM × 1 or TMP-SMX × 5–7 days	Treat sex partners
	Lymphogranuloma venereum		*C. trachomatis*	Tetracycline (doxycycline) or sulfisoxazole × 2 wk	Treat sex partners
	Gonorrhea	Uncomplicated urethral, endocervical or rectal infections	*N. gonorrhoeae*	(1) Ceftriaxone, IM × 1; or (2) amoxicillin, and probenecid, × 1; or (3) procaine penicillin G, IM, and probenecid × 1; or (4) cefuroxime IM × 1; or (5) spectinomycin, IM × 1	Treat also for *C. trachomatis;* treat sex partners

Pelvic inflammatory disease	Outpatient	*N. gonorrhoeae, C. trachomatis,* Enterobacteriaceae, anaerobes	Ceftriaxone, IM × 1 dose, plus tetracycline (or doxycycline) PO × 10 days	
	Inpatient	Same as above	Doxycycline and metronidazole and ceftriaxone (IV) × 10–14 days or doxycycline and cefoxitin (IV) × 10–14 days	
Syphilis	Congenital	*Treponema pallidum*	Aqueous crystalline penicillin G, q8–12h, or procaine penicillin G, IM daily × 10–14 days	Entire course restarted if 1 day of therapy missed
	Older infants and children:			
	Without neurologic involvement		Benzathine penicillin G, 50,000 U/kg IM (≤ 2.4 million U) × 1 dose (3 weekly doses if duration > 1 yr)	

(Continued.)

TABLE A–6 (cont.).

Site	Diagnosis	Circumstances	Etiologic Agents	Therapy	Comments
		With neurologic involvement		Aqueous crystalline penicillin G, 200,000–300,000 U/kg/day × 10–14 days	
Skin and soft tissue infections					
Skin	Impetigo		Group A streptococci, *S. aureus*	Mupirocin topically or erythromycin or clindamycin (PO) × 7–10 days	
	Acne vulgaris		*Propionibacterium acnes*	Topical benzoyl peroxide, erythromycin or clindamycin	
	Cellulitis		*S. aureus*, group A streptococci (erysipelas)	Nafcillin or cephalothin (IV) initially, then dicloxacillin or cephalexin (PO) × 10 days	Mild cases may be treated orally.
	Buccal cellulitis		*H. influenzae* type b	Cefuroxime (IV) initially, then cefaclor (PO) × 10 days	Meningitis associated in 5%–10%

	Scalded skin syndrome	*S. aureus*	Nafcillin or cephalothin (IV) initially, then dicloxacillin or cephalexin × 5–7 days	
	Human bites	Group A streptococci, viridans streptococci, *S. aureus*, anaerobes	Augmentin (PO) 5–7 days	
	Animal bites (cat or dog)	*Pasteurella multocida*, viridans streptococci, *S. aureus*, anaerobes,	Augmentin 5–7 days	Consider rabies prophylaxis
Muscle	Suppurative myositis	*S. aureus*, group A steptococci	Nafcillin × 10–14 days	Surgical drainage
	Gas gangrene	*Clostridia* spp.	Clindamycin, metronidazole, or penicillin (IV) × 10 days	Surgical drainage
Fascia	Necrotizing fasciitis	*S. aureus*, group A streptococci	Nafcillin (IV) × 10 days	Surgical debridement
Lymph Nodes	Lymphadenitis	*S. aureus*, group A streptococci	Dicloxacillin or cephalexin (PO) × 10–14 days	
	Mycobacterial adenitis	*M. tuberculosis*, Atypical mycobacteria	INH and rifampin (PO) × 9 mo; none or rifampin	Surgical excision

(Continued.)

TABLE A–6 (cont.).

Site	Diagnosis	Circumstances	Etiologic Agents	Therapy	Comments
Bone	Acute osteomyelitis	Newborn	*S. aureus*, group B streptococci, Enterobacteriaceae	Nafcillin and ceftriaxone (until culture results are known)	
		Infants	*S. aureus*, group A streptococci, *H. influenzae* type b	Cefuroxime (IV) × 3 wk	Surgical debridement if fever persists > 48–72 hr
		Children	*S. aureus*, group A streptococci	Nafcillin or cephalothin (IV) × 3 wk	
		Associated hemoglobinopathy	*S. aureus*, *Salmonella* spp.	Nafcillin and/or ceftriaxone (IV) × 3 wk	
		Nail puncture, foot	*Pseudomonas* spp.	Ceftazidime (IV) or gentamicin and ticarcillin (IV) × 7–10 days	Complete surgical debridement
	Chronic osteomyelitis		*S. aureus*	Nafcillin or cephalothin (IV) × 6 wk, then dicloxacillin or cephalexin (PO) × 6 mo	Surgical debridement

Joint	Suppurative arthritis	Newborn	*S. aureus*, group B streptococci, Enterobacteriaceae	Nafcillin and ceftriaxone (IV) × 3 wk	
		Infants	*H. influenzae* type b, group A streptococci, *S. aureus*	Cefuroxime (IV) × 14–21 days	Surgical drainage, especially of hips, is necessary
		Children	*S. aureus*, group A streptococci	Nafcillin or cephalothin (IV) × 14–21 days	
			N. gonorrhoeae	Ceftriaxone or penicillin (IV) × 7–10 days	
Systemic infections					
	Brucellosis	Associated with consumption of unpasteurized milk	*Brucella* spp.	TMP-SMX or tetracycline (if patient > 7 or 8 yr), and gentamicin (IM or IV) × first 5 days	Consider adding rifampin for relapses
	Kawasaki disease		Unknown	No antibiotics necessary; IV γ-globulin 2 g/kg × 1 dose and aspirin 80–100 mg/kg/day	Coronary aneurysms may occur

(*Continued.*)

TABLE A–6 (cont.).

Site	Diagnosis	Circumstances	Etiologic Agents	Therapy	Comments
	Leprosy	Asian and Hispanic immigrants	*Mycobacterium leprae*	Dapsone and clofazimine (PO, daily) and rifampin (po, monthly) × at least 2 yrs	Patients should be tested for G6PD deficiency before starting dapsone therapy
	Leptospirosis	Mammals serve as reservoirs	*Leptospira* spp.	Penicillin G (IV, IM) or tetracycline (PO) × 7–10 days	
	Lyme disease	Tick exposure	*Borrelia burgdorferi*	Early disease: penicillin V or ampicillin or tetracycline (PO) or doxycycline × 10–21 days; late disease (with severe carditis, arthritis or CNS disease): ceftriaxone (IV, IM) or penicillin (IV) × 14–21 days	Ceftriaxone is recommended for late CNS diseases

Relapsing fever	Western United States, North Africa	*Borrelia recurrentis*	Erythromycin or tetracycline (PO, IV) × 7–10 days	
Rocky Mountain spotted fever	Tick exposure	*Rickettsia ricketsii*	Chloramphenicol or tetracycline (PO, IV) × 10–14 days	
Tetanus	Associated with "dirty" wounds	*Clostridium tetani*	Penicillin G, IV 10 days and antitoxin	Sedation
Toxic shock syndrome	Associated with colonization or infection with *S. aureus*	*S. aureus*	Nafcillin (IV) × 7 days	Removal of the source of toxin production (e.g., tampon, abscess)
Tularemia	Tick exposure	*Francisella tularensis*	Gentamicin or streptomycin (IV, IM) × 7–10 days	
Typhoid fever	Common in developing countries	*Salmonella typhi*	Amoxicillin, ampicillin TMP-SMX, chloramphenicol, or ceftriaxone × 14–21 days	

TABLE A–7.
Maximum Daily Parenteral Antibiotic Doses

Penicillins	
Penicillin G	24 million U
Benzathine Penicillin G	2.4 million U
Procaine Penicillin G	4.8 million U
Ampicillin	12 g
Azlocillin	24 g
Carbenicillin	40 g
Methicillin	12 g
Mezlocillin	24 g
Nafcillin	12 g
Oxacillin	12 g
Piperacillin	24 g
Ticarcillin	24 g
Cephalosporins	
Cefotaxime	12 g
Ceftizoxime	12 g
Cefoxitin	12 g
Cephalothin	12 g
Cefoperazone	8 g
Cefazolin	6 g
Ceftazidime	6 g
Cefuroxime	6 g
Ceftriaxone	4 g
Cefonicid	2 g
Ceforanide	2 g
Aminoglycosides	
Amikacin	1 g
Gentamicin	300 mg
Kanamycin	1 g
Streptomycin	2 g
Tobramycin	300 mg
Aztreonam	8 g
Chloramphenicol	4 g
Clindamycin	2.7 g
Erythromycin	4 g
Imipenem	4 g
Metronidazole	2 g
Tetracyclines	2 g
Vancomycin	2 g

TABLE A–8. Bacteriostatic and Bactericidal Antibiotics

Bacteriostatic	Bactericidal
Chloramphenicol*	Aminoglycosides
Clindamycin	Aztreonam
Erythromycin	Cephalosporins
Sulfonamides	Imipenem
Tetracyclines	Metronidazole
Trimethoprim-sulfamethoxazole	Penicillins
	Quinolones
	Vancomycin

*Bactericidal against *Hemophilus influenzae.*

TABLE A–9. Classification of β-Lactam Antibiotics

CEPHALOSPORINS:

First generation

- Oral agents
  - Cephalexin (Keflex)
  - Cephradine (Velosef, Anspor)
  - Cefadroxil (Duricef)
- Parenteral agents
  - Cefazolin (Ancef, Kefzol)
  - Cephalothin (Keflin)
  - Cephapirin (Cefadyl)
  - Cephradine (Velosef)

Second generation:

- Oral agents
  - Cefaclor (Ceclor)
  - Cefuroxime axetil (Ceftin)
- Parenteral agents
  - Cefamandole (Mandol)
  - Cefoxitin (Mefoxin)
  - Cefuroxime (Zinacef)
  - Ceforanide (Precef)
  - Cefonicid (Monocid)
  - Cefotetan (Cefotan)
  - Cefmetazole (Zefazone)

(Continued.)

TABLE A–9 (cont.).

Third generation
- Oral agents
  - Cefixime (Suprax)
- Parenteral agents
  - Cefotaxime (Claforan)
  - Moxalactam (Moxam)
  - Cefoperazone (Cefobid)
  - Ceftizoxime (Cefizox)
  - Ceftriaxone (Rocephin)
  - Ceftazidime (Fortaz)
  - Cefmenoxime (Cefmax)
  - Cefsulodin (Monaspor)

PENICILLINS:

β-Lactamase susceptible, non-antipseudomonal:
- Penicillin G
- Phenoxymethyl penicillin (Penicillin V)
- Ampicillin
- Amoxicillin

β-Lactamase susceptible, antipseudomonal:
- Carbenicillin (Geopen)
- Azlocillin (Azlin)
- Mezlocillin (Mezlin)
- Piperacillin (Pipracil)
- Ticarcillin (Ticar)

β-Lactamase resistant
- Cloxacillin (Tegopen)
- Dicloxacillin (Dynapen)
- Flucloxacillin (Floxapen)
- Methicillin (Staphcillin)
- Nafcillin (Unipen)
- Oxacillin (Prostaphlin)

Combinations with β-lactamase inhibitors
- Ampicillin/sulbactam (Unasyn)
- Amoxicillin/clavulanate (Augmentin)
- Ticarcillin/clavulanate (Timentin)

MONOBACTAMS:
- Aztreonam (Azactam)

CARBAPENEMS
- Imipenem and cilistatin (Primaxin)

TABLE A–10.
Drug Interactions With Anti-infectives

Antibiotic	Interacting Agent	Effect
Acyclovir	Probenecid	Possible increased acyclovir toxicity
	Zidovudine	Marked lethargy
Amantadine	Anticholinergics	Toxic psychosis, hallucinations, confusion, nightmares
	Thiazides	Increased amantidine toxicity
Aminoglycosides (amikacin, gentamicin, kanamycin, tobramycin	Amphotericin	Increased nephrotoxicity
	Cephalosporins	Possible nephrotoxicity
	Cisplatin	Increased nephrotoxicity and ototoxicity
	Cyclosporine	Increased nephrotoxicity
	Loop diuretics (ethacrynic acid, furosemide)	**Increased ototoxicity, nephrotoxicity**
	Neuromuscular blockers, magnesium sulfate	Increased neuromuscular blockade, apnea
	Vancomycin	Increased nephrotoxicity
	Penicillins, with renal failure	Decreased efficacy of aminoglycosides
Amphotericin B	Aminoglycosides	Increased nephrotoxicity
	Corticosteroids	Increased hypokalemia
	Cisplatin	Increased nephrotoxicity
	Cyclosporine	Increased nephrotoxicity
	Digitalis	Increased cardiotoxicity related to hypokalemia

(Continued.)

TABLE A–10 (cont.).

Antibiotic	Interacting Agent	Effect
	Diuretics	Increased hypokalemia
	Neuromuscular blockers	Increased effect as a result of hypokalemia
	Vancomycin	Increased nephrotoxicity
Ampicillin, amoxicillin	Allopurinol	Increased frequency of rash
	Oral anticoagulants	Increased prothrombin time
	Oral contraceptives	Decreased contraceptive effectiveness
	β-Blockers	Decreased absorption of blockers
Cephalosporins (those with methyltetrathiazole side chain: moxalactam, cefamandole, cefotetan, cefoperazone, cefmetazole)	Alcohol	Antabuse (disulfiram) effect
	Oral anticoagulants	Increased anticoagulation
	Aminoglycosides	Possible increased nephrotoxicity
	Diuretics (ethacrynic acid, fusosemide)	Increased nephrotoxicity
Chloramphenicol	Barbiturates	Increased barbiturate effect, decreased chloramphenicol effect
	Phenytoin (Dilantin)	**Increased phenytoin effect**
	Oral anticoagulants	Increased anticoagulant effect
	Sulfonylureas (tolbutamide)	Increased sulfonylurea effect, hypoglycemia
	Acetaminophen	Increased chloramphenicol effect
	Rifampin	Decreased chloramphenicol effect
	Cyclophosphamide	Decreased effect of cyclophosphamide
Chloroquine	Cimetidine	Decreased metabolism of chloroquine
Clindamycin, lincomycin	Neuromuscular blockers	Increased neuromuscular blockade
	Theophylline	Increased level of antibiotic
Cloxacillin, dicloxacillin	Sulfonamides	Decreased effect of cloxacillin, dicloxacillin
	Warfarin	Decreased prothrombin time

Cycloserine	Ethionamide or isoniazid	CNS toxicity
	Phenytoin (Dilantin)	Increased phenytoin effect
Dapsone	Trimethoprim	Increased levels of both
Erythromycin	Oral anticoagulants	Increased anticoagulant effect
	Carbamazepine	**Neurotoxicity**
	Corticosteroids	Increased corticosteroid effect
	Cyclosporine	Increased cyclosporine levels, nephrotoxicity
	Digoxin	Increased digoxin effect
	Ergot alkaloids	Increased ergot effect, peripheral ischemia
	Theophylline	**Increased theophylline effect (toxicity)**
Fluconazole	Oral anticoagulants	Increased hypoprothrombinemia
Furazolidone (>4 cays)	**Amine-containing foods, amphetamines, ephedrine, α-adrenergics**	**Hypertension, headache, fever**
	Tricyclic antidepressants	Dizziness, excitability
	Insulin, sulfonylureas	Hypoglycemia
Ganciclovir	Probenicid	Increased levels of ganciclovir
	Pentamidine, amphotericin, trimethoprim-sulfamethoxazole	Increased toxicity of ganciclovir
	Imipenem	Seizures
Griseofulvin	Alcohol	Disulfiram reaction
	Barbiturates	Decreased griseofulvin levels
	Oral contraceptives	Decreased contraceptive effect
	Oral anticoagulants	Decreased anticoagulant effect
Imipenem	Cyclosporine	Increased cyclosporine levels, CNS effects
	Ganciclovir	Seizures

(Continued.)

TABLE A–10 (cont.).

Antibiotic	Interacting Agent	Effect
Isoniazid	Aluminum-containing antacids	Decreased isoniazid effect
	Oral anticoagulants	Increased anticoagulant effect
	Benzodiazepines	Increased effect of benzodiazepines
	Carbamazepine	**Increased toxicity of both drugs**
	Cycloserine, ethionamide	Dizziness, drowsiness
	Ketoconazole	Decreased absorption of isoniazid and increased metabolism of ketoconazole
	Phenytoin	**Increased phenytoin toxicity**
	Rifampin	Increased hepatotoxicity
Ketoconazole	Antacids, cimetidine	Decreased ketoconazole absorption
	Cyclosporine	Increased cyclosporine nephrotoxicity
	Oral anticoagulants	Increased hypoprothrombinemia
	Isoniazid, rifampin	Decreased ketoconazole activity
	Theophylline	Decreased theophylline levels
Mefloquine	Beta-blockers	Increased arrhythmias
	Anticonvulsants	**Decreased levels of anticonvulsants**
Metronidazole	Alcohol	Disulfiram reaction
	Oral anticoagulants	**Increased anticoagulant effect**
	Barbiturates, phenytoin	Increased metabolism of metronidazole with decreased levels
	Cimetidine	Increased metronidazole toxicity
	Disulfiram	Organic brain syndrome
	Lithium	Lithium toxicity

Nalidixic acid	Oral anticoagulants	Increased anticoagulant effect
Nitrofurantoin	Antacids, magnesium salts	Decreased absorption of nitrofurantoin
	Probenecid	Decreased nitrofurantoin effect
Penicillins	Allopurinol	Increased rash with ampicillin
	Oral anticoagulants	Decreased anticoagulant effect with nafcillin, dicloxacillin
	Oral contraceptives	Possible decreased effect with ampicillin or oxacillin
	Methotrexate	Possible increased methotrexate toxicity
	Probenecid	Increased concentrations of penicillins
	Cholestyramine	Decreased antibiotic absorption
	β-Blockers	Increased anaphylaxis
Pentamidine	Aminoglycosides	Increased nephrotoxicity
	Amphotericin B	Increased nephrotoxicity
	Foscarnet	Increased nephrotoxicity
Quinolones (ciprofloxacin, etc.)	Antacids with aluminum or magnesium	Decreased quinolone absorption
	Oral anticoagulants	Increased hypoprothrombinemia
	Caffeine	Increased caffeine effect
	Probenecid	Increased quinolone levels
	Theophylline	Increased theophylline levels
	Cyclosporine	Increased nephrotoxicity
Rifampin	Isoniazid	Increased hepatotoxicity
	Chloramphenicol	Decreased chloramphenicol effect
	Anticoagulants, barbiturates, benzodiazepines, **Cyclosporine,** β-blockers, **contraceptives,** estrogens, ketoconazole, corticosteroids, diazepam,	Decreased effect of all these agents

(Continued.)

TABLE A–10 (cont.).

Antibiotic	Interacting Agent	Effect
	dapsone, digoxin, hypoglycemic agents, quinidine, phenytoin, theophylline, verapamil	
Spectinomycin	Lithium	Increased lithium toxicity
Sulfonamides	Anticoagulants	Increased hypoprothrombinemia
	Barbiturates	Increased thiopental effect
	Cyclosporine	Decreased cyclosporine levels
	Digoxin	Decreased digoxin effect with sulfasalazine
	Hypoglycemics	Increased hypoglycemia
	Methotrexate	Possible increased methotrexate toxicity
	MAO inhibitors (phenelzine)	Increased sulfonamide toxicity
	Phenytoin (Dilantin)	Increased phenytoin effect
Tetracycline	Antacids, Pepto-Bismol, iron, zinc sulfate	Decreased tetracycline effect
	Phenytoin, carbamazepine, barbiturates, rifampin	Decreased doxycycline effect

	Oral contraceptives		Decreased contraceptive effect
	Digoxin		**Increased digoxin effect**
	Theophylline		Possible increased theophylline toxicity
Thiabendazole	Theophylline		Increased theophylline toxicity
Trimethoprim, trimethoprim-sulfamethoxazole	Azathioprine		Increased hepatotocxicity
	Cyclosporine		Increased nephrotoxicity
	Digoxin		**Possible increased digoxin effect**
	Phenytoin (Dilantin)		Increased phenytoin levels
	Oral anticoagulants		Increased hypoprothrombinemia
Vancomycin	Aminoglycosides		Increased nephrotoxicity and possibly increased ototoxicity
	Amphotericin B		Increased nephrotoxicity
	Cisplatin		Increased nephrotoxicity
	Digoxin		Possible decreased digoxin effect
Vidarabrine	Allopurinol		Nephrotoxicity
	Theophylline		Increased theophylline effect
Zidovudine (AZT)	Ganciclovir		Increased neutropenia & anemia
	Ribavirin	—	Decreased effect of AZT
	Probenecid		Increased levels of AZT
	Pyrimethamine		Decreased efficacy of pyrimethamine against toxoplasmosis

TABLE A–11.
Major Adverse Reactions to Antibiotics

Antibiotic	Major adverse reactions
Acyclovir	Phlebitis; rare CNS problems, including seizures, hallucinations; rare renal or hepatic toxicity
Aminoglycosides (amikacin, gentamicin, kanamycin, tobramycin)	Renal insufficiency (probably related to excessive serum trough concentrations); vestibular and auditory damage (usually related to prolonged or repeated courses); neuromuscular blockade
Amphotericin B	Renal insufficiency (reversible), phlebitis, hypokalemia, hypotension, fever, nausea and vomiting, hypomagnesemia, anemia
Aztreonam	Phlebitis, eosinophilia, elevated liver enzymes (safe in penicillin-allergic patients)
Cephalosporins	Phlebitis, allergic reactions, hypoprothrombinemia (cefamandole, cefoperazone, moxalactam, cefmetazole, cefotetan), eosinophilia, rare hepatic dysfunction, rare neutropenia or thrombocytopenia, hemolytic anemia
Chloramphenicol	GI intolerance (oral); dose-related marrow suppression (very common) and aplastic anemia (very rare); gray baby syndrome; rare optic neuritis
Clindamycin	Diarrhea, rare pseudomembranous colitis, rash, neutropenia, eosinophilia, neuromuscular blockade, phlebitis
Dideoxyinosine (ddl)	Pancreatitis in about 1%; peripheral neuropathy; nausea, vomiting, diarrhea; CNS changes
Erythromycin	GI intolerance after oral dosing; phlebitis; reversible cholestasis (with estolate); rare rash; transient ototoxicity in presence of renal failure
Ethambutol	Optic neuritis (usually reversible; monitor acuity and red-green perception); peripheral neuropathy; rash
Fluconazole	GI intolerance, rash, hepatitis, Stevens-Johnson syndrome
Flucytosine	GI intolerance, rash, hematologic problems (leukopenia, thrombocytopenia, especially in patients with renal insufficiency), hepatic dysfunction

Foscarnet	Renal impairment, headache, fatigue, anemia, electrolyte changes
Furazolidone	GI intolerance, rash, headache, pulmonary infiltrates
Ganciclovir	Hematologic changes (neutropenia, thrombocytopenia, anemia), fever, rash, neurologic changes, renal failure
Griseofulvin	Headache, photosensitivity, GI intolerance, rash, exacerbation of systemic lupus erythematosus
Imipenem/cilastatin	Phlebitis, rash, transient hepatic enzyme elevation, eosinophilia, rare marrow suppression or renal toxicity, nausea, vomiting, diarrhea, seizures
Isoniazid	Hepatitis (very rare in children); pyridoxine deficiency and peripheral neuropathy (not in prepubertal children); optic neuritis and other CNS reactions very rarely; allergic rashes
Ketoconazole	GI intolerance, hepatotoxicity (usually reversible), impaired corticosteroid and testosterone synthesis, headache, dizziness
Mefloquine	Vertigo, light-headedness, nausea, headache, diarrhea, pruritus, sinus bradycardia
Metronidazole	GI intolerance, metallic taste, headache, peripheral neuropathy, phlebitis
Nitrofurantoin	GI intolerance, allergic reactions, pulmonary infiltrates with eosinophilia, peripheral neuropathy, hepatitis
Penicillins	Hypersensitivity reactions common (rash, fever, wheezing, etc.); GI intolerance (orals); positive Coombs' response; phlebitis; Jarisch-Herxheimer reactions; hematologic reactions (leukopenia, thrombocytopenia); platelet dysfunction with carbenicillin and ticarcillin
Pentamidine	Local discomfort, hypotension, hypoglycemia, rash, nephrotoxicity, neutropenia, thrombocytopenia, hepatic dysfunction; bronchospasm after inhalation
Primaquine	Hemolysis with glucose-6-phosphate dehydrogenase (G-6-PD) deficiency, GI intolerance, leukocytosis
Pyrazinamide	Mild hepatitis, hyperuricemia, arthralgias, GI intolerance, rare photosensitivity
Pyrimethamine	Folate deficiency (dose-related, reversed by leucovorin); rare CNS reactions
Quinine	GI intolerance, tinnitus, headache, visual disturbances, hemolysis with G-6-PD deficiency, arrhythmias, hypoglycemia, hepatitis, thrombocytopenia
Quinolones	Contraindicated in children because of animal studies showing arthropathy in young animals

(Continued.)

TABLE A–11 (cont.).

Rifampin	Orange color of urine, tears, sweat; hepatitis, GI intolerance, pruritus with or without rash, thrombocytopenia, leukopenia
Sulfonamides	Allergic reactions common with fever, rash, pruritus, photosensitivity, Stevens-Johnson, periarteritis nodosa, serum sickness; crystalluria; GI intolerance; rare neurotoxocity (psychosis, neuropathy); hemolysis with G-6-PD deficiency; marrow suppression, usually neutropenia
Tetracyclines	GI intolerance; stains teeth in children <7 to 8 yr old, vertigo (minocycline), hepatotoxicity, phlebitis, photosensitivity, negative nitrogen balance
Trimethoprim	GI intolerance, rash, pruritus, glossitis, thrombocytopenia, neutropenia, megaloblastosis
Trimethoprim-Sulfamethoxazole	See trimethoprim. Patients with AIDS frequently cannot tolerate because of rash, leukopenia, fever
Vancomycin	Phlebitis; "red man syndrome" (flushing over neck and chest); hypotension (too rapid infusion); rash; fever; neutropenia; eosinophilia; ototoxicity and nephrotoxicity (dose-related)
Vidarabine	Phlebitis, GI intolerance, fluid overload, blood dyscrasias, CNS effects especially with renal failure
Zidovudine (AZT)	Anemia, leukopenia, headache, malaise, myalgias, myopathy, nausea, seizures, rash, very rare anaphylaxis

TABLE A–12.
Classification of Allergic Reactions to Penicillins

Type I: IgE-mediated
Immediate allergic reaction (within 2–30 min of exposure)
- Cutaneous erythema, pruritus
- Urticaria
- Angioedema
- Wheezing, rhinitis
- Hypotension

Accelerated allergic reaction (1–72 hr.): IgE-mediated (modified by IgG)
- Cutaneous erythema, pruritus
- Urticaria
- Angioedema
- Laryngeal edema
- Wheezing, rhinitis

Type II: IgG cytotoxic antibodies (complement-mediated)
- Hemolytic anemia

Type III: Immune complex-mediated with complement fixation (10–14 days)
- Serum sickness

Type IV: Cell-mediated (T-cell) reactions (>72 hr)
- Contact dermatitis

Type V: Late allergic reactions (>72 hr): Mechanism unknown (idiopathic)
- Maculopapular rashes
- Drug fever
- Interstitial nephritis
- Pulmonary infiltrates with eosinophilia
- Exfoliative dermatitis
- Stevens-Johnson syndrome
- Hematologic reactions: neutropenia, thrombocytopenia

TABLE A–13.
Modifications of Antibiotic Dosage With Renal Insufficiency

No adjustment needed (agents excreted extrarenally, primarily by liver)
- Cephalosporins
  - Cefoperazone, ceftriaxone, cefotaxime
- Penicillins
  - Nafcillin, cloxacillin, dicloxacillin, mezlocillin
- Chloramphenicol
- Erythromycin
- Tetracyclines
  - Doxycycline, minocycline
- Isoniazid
- Rifampin
- Ketoconazole
- Amphotericin B
- Metronidazole

Agents requiring moderate reduction in dosage
- Acyclovir
- Azlocillin
- Aztreonam
- Penicillins:
  - Carbenicillin, penicillin, ampicillin-sulbactam, ticarcillin, amoxicillin, methicillin, piperacillin, ampicillin
- Cephalosporins
  - Cefamandole, cefazolin, cefmenoxime, cefmetazole, cefotetan, cefoxitin, cefsulodin, ceftazidime, ceftizoxime, cefuroxime, cephalexin, cephalothin, cephapirin, cephradine, cefixime, moxalactam
- Imipenem
- Trimethoprim-sulfamethoxazole
- Ciprofloxacin
- Clindamycin
- Ethambutol, ethionamide
- Zidovudine (AZT)

Agents requiring major reduction in dosage
- Aminoglycosides (amikacin, gentamicin, kanamycin, streptomycin, tobramycin)
- Flucytosine
- Vancomycin
- Ganciclovir
- Fuconazole

Agents to be avoided
- Nalidixic acid
- Nitrofurantoin
- Norfloxacin
- Tetracycline

TABLE 1–14.
Antibiotics to be Avoided or Used With Caution in Patients With Severe Hepatic Dysfunction

Aztreonam	Mezlocillin
Carbenicillin*	Nafcillin*
Cefoperazone	Nitrofurantoin
Ceftriaxone*	Penicillin*
Chloramphenicol	Rifampin
Clindamycin	Ticarcillin-clavulanate*
Erythromycin	Ticarcillin*
Isoniazid	Vancomycin
Metronidazole	

*Avoid particularly if combined renal and hepatic insufficiency present.

TABLE A–15.
Clinically Significant CNS Penetration by Antibiotics*

Minimal, even with inflammation

- Amphotericin
- Cefoperazone
- First-generation cephalosporins
- Clindamycin
- Erythromycin
- Gentamicin
- Itraconazole
- Ketoconazole
- Lincomycin
- Streptomycin
- Tobramycin

Adequate only with inflammation

- Amikacin (erratic)
- Ampicillin
- Azlocillin, mezlocillin
- Aztreonam
- Carbenicillin, piperacillin
- Cefotaxime
- Cefoxitin

(Continued.)

TABLE A–15 (cont.).

Ceftazidime
Ceftriaxone
Cefuroxime
Ciprofloxacin
Ethambutol
Imipenem
Kanamycin
Methicillin, nafcillin
Penicillin G
Rifampin
Tetracycline
Trimethoprim
Vancomycin
Adequate with or without inflammation
Acyclovir
Chloramphenicol
Fluconazole
Foscarnet
Isoniazid
Metronidazole
Pyrazinamide
Sulfonamides
Vidarabine
Zidovudine

*Compiled with the assistance of R. Yogev, M.D.

TABLE A–16.
Aminoglycoside Serum Concentrations

	Therapeutic (μg/mL)		Toxic (μg/mL)	
	Trough	Peak	Trough	Peak
Amikacin	1–8	20–30	>10	>35
Gentamicin	0.5–2	6–10	>2	>12
Kanamycin	1–8	20–30	>10	>35
Netilmicin	0.5–2	6–10	>4	>16
Tobramycin	0.5–2	6–10	>2	>12

TABLE A–17.
Antibiotic Suspension Taste Ratings (From Best to Worst*

Trade Name	Generic Name
Suprax	(Cefixime)
Keflex	(Cephalexin)
Ceclor	(Cefaclor)
Ilosone	(Erythromycin estolate)
Gantrisin	(Sulfasoxazole)
Achromycin-V	(Tetracycline)
Augmentin	(Amoxicillin-clavulanate)
Grifulvin V	(Griseofulvin microsize)
Pediazole	(Erythromycin ES–sulfasoxazole)
Trimox	(Amoxicillin)
Erythromycin ES	(Erythromycin ethylsuccinate)
Sulfatrim	(Trimethoprim-sulfamethoxazole)
Vee Tids	(Penicillin VK)
Dynapen	(Dicloxacillin)

*Adapted from Ruff ME, et al: *Pediatr Infect Dis J* 10:30–33, 1991.

III. MISCELLANEOUS DRUGS

TABLE A–18.
Antifungal Agents

Drug	Indication	Route	Pediatric Dosage	Comment
Amphotericin B (Fungizone)	Invasive aspergillosis; candidemia or deep candidal infections; disseminated, meningeal, or severe pulmonary coccidiomycosis or cryptococcosis; disseminated, CNS, or chronic pulmonary histoplasmosis or blastomycosis mucormycosis; extracutaneous sporotrichosis	IV	0.25–1.0 mg/kg qd over 2–4 hr; may give 0.5–1.0 mg/kg qod after initial daily therapy	Test dose of 1 mg is given first; then gradually increase to 0.5–1.0 mg/kg daily; nephrotoxic
Clotrimazole	Oral or vaginal candidiasis; Esophageal candidiasis, Dermatoplytoses topical	PO	100 mg vaginal tabs or 10 mg tab 5 ×/day	
Econazole (Spectazole)	Cutaneous candidiasis, tinea cruris, or tinea pedis	Topical	bid	

Fluconazole (Diflucan); investigational in children	Systemic and mucosal candidal infections; Cryptococcosis (maintenance) Coccidiomycosis	PO IV	3–6 mg/kg/day 3–6 mg/kg/day	Precise role and pediatric dosing still being defined
Flucytosine (Ancobon)	Candidemia or deep candidal infection; disseminated or CNS cryptococcosis; frequently used for severe or chronic mucosal candidiasis; chromoblastomycosis	PO	50–150 mg/kg/day divided q6h	Generally used in conjunction with amphotericin
Griseofulvin (Grifulvin)	Dermatophyte infections (tinea capitis, onychomycosis)	PO	15 mg/kg/day	
Itraconazole Investigational	Aspergillosis	PO	Adult dose: 100–400 mg/day	Precise role and pediatric dosing being defined
Ketoconazole (Nizoral)	Blastomycosis; chronic mucocutaneous candidiasis; thrush; esophageal candidiasis; chromomycosis; pulmonary, extrapulmonary non-CNS coccidiomycosis; nonmeningeal cryptococcosis, dermatophytosis; disseminated or severe histoplasmosis in competent host	PO	5–10 mg/kg/day q12–24h	Potential hepatotoxicity

(Continued.)

TABLE A–18 (cont.).

Drug	Indication	Route	Pediatric Dosage	Comment
Miconazole (Monistat)	Severe *Pseudoallerscheria boydii* infection	IV	20–40 mg/kg/day q8h	Essentially replaced by ketoconazole
	Cutaneous or vaginal candidiasis; dermatophytoses	Topical	tid–qid	
Nystatin (Mycostatin)	Oral, cutaneous, or vaginal candidiasis	Topical, PO	200,000–600,000 U/dose qid	
Tolnaftate (Tinactin)	Tinea cruris, tinea pedis	Topical	bid	Nonprescription
Undecylenate (e.g., Desenex)	Tinea cruris, tinea pedis	Topical	bid	Nonprescription

TABLE A–19.
Antimalarial Agents

Drug	Pediatric Dosage	Indication	Comment
Chloroquine PO_4 (Aralen)	10 mg base/kg (max 600 mg base), then 1/2 dose at 6, 24, and 48 hr	Oral therapy for all but chloroquine-resistant *Plasmodium falciparum*	GI upset, pruritus, dizziness; may use hydroxychloroquine sulfate if chloroquine phosphate not available
	5 mg base/kg (max 300 mg base) once/wk	Prophylaxis	
Quinine dihydrochloride	25 mg/kg/day (max 1,800 mg/day) IV; give 1/3 over 2–4 hr; repeat q8h until oral drug is tolerated	Parenteral therapy for all including chloroquine-resistant *P. falciparum*	Available from CDC; cardiac monitoring required
Quinidine gluconate	10 mg/kg (max 600 mg) IV loading dose in normal saline solution over 1 hr; then continuous infusion of 0.02 mg/kg/min for 3 days max	Parenteral therapy for all including chloroquine-resistant *P. falciparum*	May be superior to quinine; may cause cardiac arrhythmia; monitoring required
Chloroquine HCl	0.83 mg base/kg/hr IV continuously over 30 hr, or 3.5 mg base/kg q6h IM or SC	Alternate parenteral therapy for all but chloroquine-resistant *P. falciparum*	
Quinine SO_4	25 mg/kg/day (max 650 mg/dose) in three doses for 3–7 days	Oral therapy for chloroquine-resistant *P. falciparum* (with Fansidar or tetracycline)	Investigational in U.S.

(Continued.)

TABLE A–19 (cont.).

Drug	Pediatric Dosage	Indication	Comment
Pyrimethamine-sulfadoxine (Fansidar)	Each tablet = 1,500/75 mg <1 yr: 1/4 tab × 1 1–3 yr: 1/2 tab × 1 4–8 yr: 1 tab × 1 9–14 yr: 2 tab × 1 >14 yr: 3 tabs × 1	Oral therapy for chloroquine-resistant *P. falciparum* (with quinine SO_4)	Can cause severe erythema multiforme bullosum or hepatic necrosis
Tetracycline	5 mg/kg (max 250 mg) qid for 7 days	Oral therapy for chloroquine-resistant *P. falciparum* (with quinine SO_4)	
Mefloquin (Lariam)	25 mg/kg (max 1,250 mg) × 1 Each tablet = 250 mg; 15–19 kg: 1/4 tab/wk 20–30 kg: 1/2 tab/wk 31–45 kg: 3/4 tab/wk >45 kg: 1 tab/wk Continue for 4 wk after leaving endemic area	Oral therapy for chloroquine-resistant *P. falciparum* Prophylaxis for chloroquine-resistant *P. falciparum*	Not approved for children; avoid with β-blockers, history of epilepsy, or psychiatric disorder; do not use with quinidine or quinine
Primaquine PO_4	0.3 mg base/kg/day for 14 days (max 15 mg base/day)	Oral therapy to prevent relapse of *Plasmodium ovale* and *Plasmodium vivax*	Hemolysis in glucose-6-phosphate dehydrogenase deficiency
Doxycycline	>8 yr: 2 mg/kg PO qd (max 100 mg/day)	Prophylaxis in areas with chloroquine-resistant *P. falciparum*	Can cause photosensitivity
Halofantrine	8 mg/kg (max 500 mg) Q6h × 3 doses	Oral therapy of chloroquine-resistant *P. falciparum*	

TABLE A–20.
Antiparasitic Agents

Drug	Indication	Route	Pediatric Dosage	Comment
Albendazole (Zentel)	Capillariasis	PO	200 mg bid for 20 days	Alternate therapy
	Echinococcus granulosus (hydatid cysts)		15 mg/kg/day for 28 days	Drug of choice
	Cysticercosis		15 mg/kg/day in three doses for 8 days; repeat prn	Alternative therapy
Amphotericin B (Fungizone)	Amoebic meningoencephalitis	IV	1 mg/kg/day	Investigational
	American leishmaniasis	IV	0.25–1 mg/kg/day qd or qod for up to 8 wk	Investigational; alternative therapy
Benznidazole (Rochagan)	*Trypanosoma cruzi* (Chaga's disease)	PO	6 mg/kg/day for 30–120 days	Not available in U.S.
Bithionol (Bitin)	*Fasciola hepatica* (liver fluke), *Paragonimus westermani* (lung fluke)	PO	30–50 mg/kg qod for 10–15 doses	Available from CDC
Chloroquine (Aralen)	Amebic liver abscess Malaria (see separate listing)	PO	10 mg base/kg/day (max 300 mg) for 2–3 wks	
Crotamiton (Eurax)	*Sarcoptes scabei* (scabies)	Topical, 10%		Apply; repeat at 24 hr; bathe at 48 hr
Dapsone	Prevention of pneumocystis	PO	1 mg/kg qd	

(Continued.)

TABLE A–20 (cont.).

Drug	Indication	Route	Pediatric Dosage	Comment
Dehydroemetine (Meban)	Intestinal or hepatic amebiasis	IM	1–1.5 mg/kg/day (max 90 mg/day) in two doses for up to 5 days	Less toxic than emetine
Diethylcarbamazine (Hetrazan)	Filariasis due to *Wucheria bancrofti, Brugia (W.) malayi,* loa loa	PO	Escalating doses up to 6–9 mg/kg/day in three divided doses, for 21 days	Lysis of filariae can produce severe allergic reaction
	Tropical eosinophilia, visceral larval migrans	PO	2 mg/kg tid for 7–10 days	
Diloxanide (Furamide)	Asymptomatic amebiasis	PO	20 mg/kg/day in three doses for 10 days	Available from CDC
Emetine	Intestinal or hepatic amebiasis	IM	1 mg/kg/day in two doses for 5 days (max 60 mg/day)	May cause arrhythmias
Furazolidone (Furoxone)	Giardiasis	PO	6–8 mg/kg/day in four doses for 7–10 days	
Iodoquinol (Yodoxin)	Amebiasis (all forms), *Balantidium coli, Dientamoeba fragilis*	PO	30–40 mg/kg/day in three doses for 20 days (max 2 gm)	
Ivermectin (Mectizan)	*Onchocerca volvulus*	PO	150 mg/kg × 1; repeat q6–12 mo	Investigational; available from CDC
Lindane (Kwell)	Lice, scabies	Topical		Two applications, 1 wk apart

Mebendazole (Vermox)	Angiostrongyliasis	PO	100 mg bid for 5 days	
	Ascariasis	PO	100 mg bid for 3 days	
	Capillariasis	PO	200 mg bid for 20 days	
	Enterobiasis (pinworm)	PO	100 mg × 1; repeat in 2 wk	
	Hookworm (*Ancylostoma, Necator*)	PO	100 mg bid for 3 days	Drug of choice for *A. duodenale*
	Trichinosis	PO	5 mg/kg tid for 14 days	Usually with steroids
	Trichuriasis (whipworm)	PO	100 mg bid for 3 days	
	Visceral larval migrans	PO	100–200 mg bid for 5 days	
Melarsoprol (Arsobal)	African trypanosomiasis with CNS involvement (sleeping sickness)	IV	18–25 mg/kg total over 1 mo; 0.36 mg/kg increasing to 3.6 mg/kg q1–5d for total 10 doses	Available from CDC
Metronidazole (Flagyl)	Intestinal or hepatic amebiasis	PO/IV	35–50 mg/kg/day in three doses for 10 days	
	Balantidium coli		35–50 mg/kg/day in three doses for 5 days	
	Dracunculosis (guinea worm)		25 mg/kg/day (max 750 days) in three doses for 10 days	
	Giarciasis		15 mg/kg/day in three doses for 5–7 days	
	Trichomoniasis		15 mg/kg/day in three doses for 7 days	

(Continued.)

TABLE A–20 (cont.).

Drug	Indication	Route	Pediatric Dosage	Comment
Niclosamide (Niclocide)	Intestinal flukes	PO	75 mg/kg/day in three doses for 1 day	
	Tapeworm *(Diphyllobothrium latum, Taenia saginata, Taenia solium, Dipylidium caninum, Hymenolepsis nana)*		11–34 kg: 1 g × 1; then 500 mg/day for 6 days >34 kg: 1.5 g × 1; then 1 g/d for 6 days	Follow-up doses needed only for *H. nana*
Nifurtimox (Lampit)	*Trypanosoma cruzi* (Chaga's disease)	PO	1–10 yr: 15–20 mg/kg/day in four doses for 90 days 11–16 yr: 12.5–15 mg/kg/day in four doses for 90 days	Available from CDC
Oxamniquine (Vansil)	*Schistosoma mansoni*	PO	20 mg/kg/day in two doses for 1 day	
Paromomycin (Humatin)	Asymptomatic or mild intestinal amebiasis; *Dientamoeba*	PO	25–30 mg/kg/day in three doses for 7 days	Alternative agent; available from CDC
Pentamidine (Pentam 300)	*Pneumocystis carinii* pneumonitis	IV/IM	4 mg/kg/day for 21 days	First alternative
	P. carinii prophylaxis	Aerosol	300 mg in 6 mL q4 wk	
	Leishmania donovani, kala azar	IM	4 mg/kg/day for 14 days	First alternative

Pentamidine	African trypanosomiasis (early)	IM or IV	4 mg/kg/day for 10 days	First alternative
Permethrin (Nix)	Lice, scabies	Topical, 5%		
Praziquantel (Biltricide)	Flukes:	PO		
	Clonorchis sinensis (Chinese liver flukes)		75 mg/kg/day in three doses for 2 days	
	Intestinal flukes; *Opisthorchis viverrini* (liver flukes)	PO	75 mg/kg/day in three doses for 1 day	
	Paragonimus westermani (lung fluke)	PO	75 mg/kg/day in three doses for 2 days	
	Schistosomiasis: *S. haematobium*, *S. mansoni*	PO	40 mg/kg/day in two doses for 1 day	
	S. japonicum, *S. mekongi*		60 mg/kg/day in three doses for 1 day	
	Tapeworms	PO	10–25/kg for one dose	
	Neurocysticercosis	PO	50 mg/kg/day in three doses for 14 days	Steroids used as adjunct
Pyrantel pamoate (Antiminth)	Ascariasis	PO	11 mg/kg once (max 1 g)	
	Enterobiasis (pinworm)	PO	11 mg/kg once; repeat in 2 wk	
	Hookworm (*Ancylostoma*, *Necator*)	PO	11 mg/kg (max 1 g) qd for 3 days	

(Continued.)

TABLE A–20 (cont.).

Drug	Indication	Route	Pediatric Dosage	Comment
	Moniliformis	PO	11 mg/kg once; repeat twice, 2 wk apart	
	Trichostrongylus	PO	11 mg/kg once (max 1 g)	
Pyrethrins (RID)	Lice	Topical	May repeat once, 1 wk later	
Pyrimethamine (Daraprim)	Toxoplasmosis (with sulfadiazine or trisulfapyrimidines)	PO	1 mg/kg bid for 3 days (max 100 mg/day), then 0.5 mg/kg bid for 4 wk (8–12 wk in immunocompromised patient)	Give 5–10 mg folinic acid qd
Quinacrine (Atabrine)	Giardiasis	PO	6 mg/kg/day (max 300 mg/day) in three doses for 5–7 days	
Spiramycin	Toxoplasmosis	PO	50–100 mg/kg/day for 3–4 wk	Alternative drug
	Cryptosporidium	PO	50–100 mg/kg/day for 3–4 wk	Unproved efficacy
Stibogluconate (Pentostam)	Leishmaniasis			Drug of choice
	American or visceral	IV/IM	20 mg/kg/day (max 800 mg/day) for 20–28 days	
	Cutaneous	IV/IM	10–20 mg/kg/day (max 600 mg/day) for 6–10 days	Available from CDC

Sulfadiazine	Toxoplasmosis (with pyrimethamine and folinic acid)	PO	25–50 mg/kg qid	
Suramin (Germanin)	Trypanosomiasis (African sleeping sickness), early	IV	20 mg/kg on day 1, 3, 7, 14, 21	Drug of choice; available from CDC
Thiabendazole (Mintezol)	Angiostrongyliasis	PO	75 mg/kg/day in three doses for 3 days (max 3 g/day)	
	Capillariasis	PO	25 kg/day in two doses for 30 days	
	Cutaneous larva migrans	Topical/PO	50 mg/kg/day in two doses for 2–5 days (max 3 g/day)	Drug of choice
	Dracunculus (guinea worm)	PO	50–75 mg/kg/day in two doses for 3 days	
	Strongyloidiasis	PO	50 mg/kg/day in two doses for 2–5 days	Drug of choice
	Visceral larva migrans	PO	50 mg/kg/day in two doses for 5 days	
Trimethoprim-sulfamethoxazole (Bactrim, Septra)	*Pneumocystis carinii* pneumonitis	PO/IV	20/100 mg/kg/day in four doses for 21 days	
	PCP prophylaxis	PO	5/25 mg/kg/day once 3×/wk	
	Isospora belli	PO	20/100 mg/kg/day in four doses for 10 days, then bid for 3 wk	
Trimetrexate	*P. carinii* pneumonitis (with leucovorin)	IV	45 mg/m^2 qd for 21 days	Use in TMP-SMX– and pentamidine-intolerant patients

TABLE A–21.
Antituberculous Antibiotics

Drug	Pediatric Dose (Maximum)	Adverse Reactions	Comment
First-line agents			
Isoniazid (INH)	10–15 mg/kg/day (300 mg/day) in 1–2 doses/day	Hepatotoxicity (rare in children); pyridoxine deficiency–related neuropathy (postpuberty)	Give pyridoxine, 15–50 mg/day if pubertal or older; IM available
Rifampin	10–15 mg/kg/day (600 mg/day) in 1 dose	Hepatotoxicity (unusual in children); orange urine, tears, sweat	IV available
Ethambutol (Myambutol)	15 mg/kg/day (2.5 g/day) in 1 dose	Optic neuritis	Monitor visual acuity and red/green vision
Pyrazinamide	25–30 mg/kg/day (2.0 g/day) in 1–3 doses	Hepatitis, gastritis	Can cause increase in uric acid

Streptomycin	20–30 mg/kg/day (1.0 g/day) in 1–2 doses **IM**	Ototoxic, nephrotoxic	Consider initially in meningitis, miliary, bone and joint infections
Second-line agents			
Ethionamide (Trecator)	10–20 mg/kg/day (1.0 g/day) in 2 doses	GI* intolerance, hepatotoxicity	Take with meals
Cycloserine (Seromycin)	7–10 mg/kg/day (1.0 g/day) in 2 doses	Psychosis, rash, seizures	Contraindicated in epilepsy
Kanamycin (Kantrex)	15–30 mg/kg/day (1.0 g/day) in 3 doses **IM**	Auditory, vestibular, nephrotoxicity	
Para-Aminosalicylic acid (PAS)	200 mg/kg/day (12 g/day) in 1–3 doses	GI distress, sodium load	Limited efficacy
Capreomycin	15 mg/kg/day (1 g/day) in 1 dose **IM**	Auditory, vestibular, nephrotoxicity	

TABLE A–22.
Antiviral Agents

Drug	Indication	Route	Pediatric Dosage	Comment
Acyclovir (Zovirax)	Primary genital HSV	200 mg cap or 200 mg/tsp syrup	200 mg 5×/day for 10 days	Response with recurrent episodes less dramatic
	Recurrent genital HSV		200 mg 5×/day for 5 days	
	Severe primary genital HSV, mucocutaneous HSV in compromised host	IV over 1–3 hr	250 mg/m^2 q8h; <1 yr: 15–30 mg/kg/day in three doses for 7–14 days	Renal dysfunction may occur, especially with rapid infusion
	HSV encephalitis; neonatal HSV, zoster or varicella in compromised host	IV over 1–3 hr	500 mg/m^2 q8h; <1 yr, including neonate: 30 mg/kg/day in three doses	
	Zoster in normal host	PO	20 mg/kg (800 mg max) 5×/day	
	Varicella in normal host	PO	20 mg/kg (800 mg max) 4×/day	
Amantadine (Symmetrel)	Prophylaxis and early treatment of influenza A	100 mg cap, 50 mg/tsp syrup	1–9 yr: 4.4 mg/kg/day in two doses (max 150 mg/day); >9 yr: 200 mg/days in two doses	Limited pediatric experience

Dideoxyinosine (Videx)	HIV infection	IV/PO	200 mg/m^2/day in two doses	Experimental agent, especially for AZT-intolerant patients
Foscarnet	CMV retinitis Acyclovir-resistant HSV and VZV	IV	60 mg/kg q8h 40 mg/kg q8h	Limited pediatric experience
Gancyclovir (Cytovene)	CMV infection, especially retinitis	IV	10 mg/kg/day in two doses or 7.5 mg/kg/day in three doses	Fairly toxic; chronic suppressive therapy recommended in immunocompromised patients
Ribavirin	Respiratory syncytial virus (RSV)	Aerosol	6 gm vial by aerosol generator q24h	Expensive; indicated in patients with underlying cardiac or pulmonary disease or with severe RSV infection
Trifluridine (Viroptic)	Primary HSV keratoconjunctivitis, recurrent keratitis	1% ophthalmic solution	1 drop q2h for up to 21 days	
Zidovudine (Retrovir, AZT)	Pediatric AIDS	100 mg cap, 50 mg/tsp syrup	720 mg/m^2/day divided q6h	Adverse effects have limited its use

CMV = cytomegalovirus, HSV = herpes simplex virus, VZV = varicella-zoster virus.

TABLE A–23.
Comparative Drug Costs for 10-Day Course of Oral Therapy for Urinary Tract Infection

Antibacterial Agent	Dosage	Average Wholesale Price
Ampicillin	250 mg q6h	$ 3.25
Carbenicillin	2 tab q6h:	111.75
Cephalexin	250 mg q6h	41.25 (generic $20.00)
Ciprofloxacin	750 mg q12h	91.15
Sulfamethoxazole	1 gm q12h	7.50 (generic $3.30)
Trimethoprim-sulfamethoxazole	1 DS tab q12h	17.10 (generic $3.00)
Tetracycline	250 mg q6h	1.05

TABLE A–24.
Alternatives to Penicillin for Penicillin-Allergic Patient

Bacteria	Antibacterial Agent
Streptococci, including *S. pneumoniae* but excluding enterococci	Erythromycin
Enterococci	Vancomycin
Staphylococcus aureus	Cephalosporin Clindamycin Vancomycin
Anaerobic bacteria	Clindamycin Metronidazole
Neisseria meningitidis	Chloramphenicol
Neisseria gonorrhoeae	Spectinomycin (genital disease) Tetracycline (systemic or articular disease)
Treponema pallidum	Erythromycin Tetracycline

INDEX

B

H

I

N

O

P

Q

R

T

W

X

Y

Z